Mobs and Microbes
Global Perspectives on Market Halls, Civic Order, and Public Health

MOBS AND MICROBES

Global Perspectives on Market Halls, Civic Order, and Public Health

Edited by

Leila Marie Farah & Samantha L. Martin

Leuven University Press

The publication of this work was supported by Toronto Metropolitan University's Faculty of Engineering and Architectural Science as well as the Department of Architectural Science, University College Dublin's Output-Based Research Support Scheme and the KU Leuven Fund for Fair Open Access.

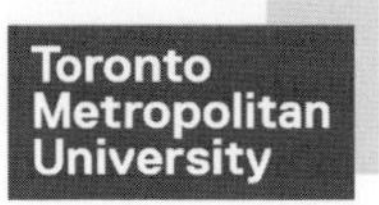

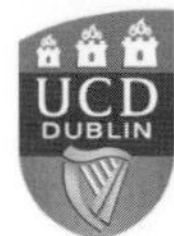

Published in 2023 by Leuven University Press/Presses Universitaires de Louvain/ Universitaire Pers Leuven. Minderbroedersstraat 4, B-3000 Leuven (Belgium).

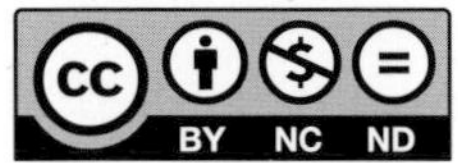

ISBN 978 94 6270 360 5 (Paperback)
ISBN 978 94 6166 495 2 (ePDF)
ISBN 978 94 6166 496 9 (ePUB)
https://doi.org/10.11116/9789461664952
D/2023/1869/3
NUR: 648
Cover design: Stephane De Schrevel
Cover illustration: Drawing of Borough Market by Lucinda Rogers
Layout: Crius Group

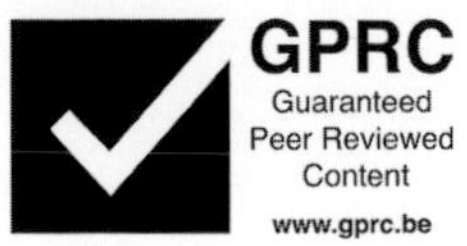

TABLE OF CONTENTS

Abbreviations 7

CHAPTER 1
Confluence 9
Samantha L. Martin & Leila Marie Farah

CHAPTER 2
Public Amenity or Public Threat? Epidemiology and Grassroots Activism in the Food Markets of New Orleans, 1900–1940 19
Ashley Rose Young

CHAPTER 3
The Crawford Market: Sanitary Problems, Engineered Solutions, and Symbolic Gestures in Late Nineteenth-Century Bombay 61
Daniel Williamson

CHAPTER 4
The Central Market in Hong Kong: Urban Amenities in a Speculative Field 99
Zhengfeng Wang

CHAPTER 5
Nairobi City Market: The Versatile Afterlife of a Colonial-Era Building in a Postcolonial World 129
Nkatha Gichuyia

CHAPTER 6
The St. Lawrence Market, Toronto: Changes and Continuity 157
Leila Marie Farah

CHAPTER 7
Between a Government Project and a Commercial Space for Ordinary Citizens: Dongan Market, 1903–1937 191
Xusheng Huang

CHAPTER 8
Hygiene, Urbanism, and Fascist Politics at Rome's Wholesale Market 227
Ruth W. Lo

CHAPTER 9
Modernization and Mobilization: Parisian Retail Market Halls, 1961–1982 245
Emeline Houssard

CHAPTER 10
Finding Food at Torvehallerne: Market Halls in Copenhagen between Gastrosexual Consumerism and the Coronavirus Pandemic 285
Henriette Steiner

CHAPTER 11
Pandemics and Marketplaces: A Coda from Viareggio, Italy 305
Andrea Borghini & Min Kyung Lee

About the Authors 313

Index 317

ABBREVIATIONS

APUR	Atelier parisien d'urbanisme
arr.	arrondissement
BHVP	Bibliothèque historique de la Ville de Paris
BMOVP	*Bulletin municipal officiel de la Ville de Paris*
CBD	Central Business District
CPP	Compagnie parisienne des parkings
ESA	École spéciale d'architecture
FFF	Foyer du Fonctionnaire et de la Famille
IPCC	Intergovernmental Panel on Climate Change
JO	*Journal officiel*
PC	Parti communiste
PHD	Public Health Department
PLU	Plan Local d'Urbanisme
PS	Parti socialiste
PSU	Parti socialiste unifié
PUD	Plan d'Urbanisme Directeur
RIBA	Royal Institute of British Architects
SPPEF	Société pour la Protection des Paysages et de l'Esthétique de la France
USDA	United States Department of Agriculture
WPA	Works Progress Administration

CHAPTER 1

CONFLUENCE

Samantha L. Martin & Leila Marie Farah

The idea for this volume first took root in 2018. The catalyst for the project was a desire to expand the breadth of research surrounding marketplaces in architectural history, in particular purpose-built food market halls. While there are standout monographs on individual markets, as well as pioneering studies of market complexes in specific countries, a wider, more global approach to this architectural type has eluded scholarly attention.[1] To address this lacuna, we organized a session at the annual meeting of the Society of Architectural Historians in 2019. As a way of highlighting how markets have been at the vanguard of urban development and renewal over the last century and a half, the session invited contributions that cross-examined these buildings through the dual focus of public health and civic order, two topics that are inextricably braided together in urban history.

Less than one year after this conference, the world ground to a standstill as the COVID-19 crisis unfolded. Given reports that a wet market was the likely origin of the virus outbreak, markets suddenly were front-page news. When the public turned its attention to the topic of food markets more generally, the academic community quickly followed suit. Historic market halls, long under the radar in research, were now in the limelight.

Markets have always been, on some level, anchors of community. Over the past several decades, these complexes have been cast as civic monuments and framed as centers of urban revitalization. Prior to 2020, whenever a newspaper or magazine featured a market hall, it was typically in the context of a heritage or conservation campaign.[2] But these places have always had a dark underbelly. The deep histories of marketplaces provide ample evidence of pestilence, violence, plots, and seedy intrigue.

In the post-Enlightenment period, the urban market was quite literally elevated to the position of institutional type; yet its Janus-faced character endured. As such, this groundbreaking book is ultimately an overdue reappraisal of the market hall, both as an architectural type and a handmaiden to politics. A timely aspect of the volume is the critical perspective it offers on how markets are used as instruments of soft power, especially within colonial and imperial contexts. We also consider whether governments and civic authorities will continue to use markets in this way in the future, in the course of post-pandemic urban planning.

By prioritizing the novel approach of combining civic order and public health, this book underscores the degree to which market buildings embodied transformations in architecture and urbanism from the mid-nineteenth century until the age of COVID-19. Crucial to this process are advancements in sanitation and hygiene and the inception of epidemiological and bacteriological research, all of which greatly influenced the spatial planning and physical design of markets. While regulations and inspections ordered these buildings, new scientific developments determined their location and connection to infrastructure, defined their layout, curbed pests, integrated natural light, ventilation, and mechanical systems, dictated materials, and regulated food stall design. Radical scientific interventions also mediated conflicting political and social interests. Through their rational designs, market halls intertwined with government policies and regulations that formalized, controlled, and literally imposed order on the market economy. In colonial contexts, these designs were often deployed at the expense of Indigenous and local knowledge. Furthermore, this was by no means a one-way process: while political powers sought to exert influence and project a particular image, citizens and market vendors mobilized opposition efforts to resist such pressures by displaying acts of resilience. Markets eventually also served as demonstration grounds for community-led mobilization efforts. Hence, besides architects, key protagonists involved in the development and transformation of markets have included public health officers, activists, politicians, and vendors.

At the same time, markets are always greater than the sum of their parts: while some have been integral to visions of urban sanitary reform, others were pivotal nodes in the long-standing food supply network of cities; and more recently, as mentioned above, markets have increasingly become essential components to the revitalization of urban public spaces. Like the foodstuffs they contain, the market halls in this collection evince the spread of ideas, the cross-pollination of methods, and the inflection of practices.

The Society of Architectural Historians conference session initially gathered papers that investigated markets in Beijing, Copenhagen, Mumbai, and Rome. This volume builds on this first public airing, substantially widening the geographical reach to include studies on markets in Hong Kong, Nairobi, New Orleans, Paris, Toronto, and Viareggio. By moving beyond purely descriptive, formal analyses to embrace top-down, bottom-up, and contextual perspectives, the contributions here clarify the market hall as an enduring phenomenon. These buildings are utterly typical and flicker with familiarity, and yet they are remarkable in their ability to leverage authority and negotiate order in the urban realm, often over an exceptionally long period of time.

This is the first book to consider the complex sociopolitical and public health roles of this kind of building type from a global perspective. Ultimately, this specific focus, in particular the relationship between marketplaces, disease, and sanitation, not only renders this volume especially relevant in the present day but also opens a window for reflecting on the lessons that historic markets may continue to offer us into the future.

The contributions presented here explore markets in ten cities across four continents. Although these studies follow a roughly chronological order, two contributions that directly foreground epidemics, one in the historical perspective and another in the present day, bookend the volume as a way of acknowledging the extraordinary period of time during which this project came to fruition. At the very start of her chapter, Ashley Rose Young points out that New Orleans, Louisiana, is a city known for extremes. "Public Amenity or Public Threat? Epidemiology and Grassroots Activism in the Food Markets of New Orleans, 1900–1940," dives into the public health crises that beset the city's market halls in the first half of the twentieth century. Salmonella, fly infestations, and cholera all galvanized competing stakeholders, from the government to vendors and customers. Young's chapter offers a valuable narrative that often goes overlooked: the struggles, resilience, and very public successes of women activists. New Orleans' many market buildings not only flourished as nexus points for the community but also gave rise to grassroots activism and advocacy, the effects of which can still be felt in the city today. Positioned at the other side of this narrative, both literally and figuratively, is a concluding essay by Andrea Borghini and Min Kyung Lee, "Pandemics and Marketplaces: A Coda from Viareggio, Italy." This contribution reflects on how the COVID-19 pandemic has impacted traditional food marketplaces. Based in Viareggio, Italy, during the first waves of the pandemic, the authors witnessed the tensions and conflicts facing civic market halls. Like Young's chapter, their argument highlights the intrinsic role these markets play in the communal, public life of towns and cities. Markets are often described as being consummate meeting places, but seldom have we considered what happens to these sites when people are forbidden to physically meet. Borghini and Lee revisit the uneasy relationship between traditional markets and supermarkets, asking how we might recuperate some of the civic values that are linked with food provisioning and that have been suppressed in the wake of COVID-19.

Covered market halls are one of the hallmarks of British colonial planning. They were not only integral to complex urban masterplans but also played a key role in engineering social and political order. Although these structures sprang up in vastly different geographical locations, they often harbored remarkable similarities in architectural design, technical innovation, and especially planning guidelines. Here, in this volume, we present a number of chapters that demonstrate how reforms in hygiene coalesced with developments in materials science and infrastructure under the British Empire. Daniel Williamson's contribution, "The Crawford Market: Sanitary Problems, Engineered Solutions, and Symbolic Gestures in Late Nineteenth-Century Bombay," exposes the way that the British regime utilized advancements in hygiene in tandem with building design to stage reform under the pretense of munificence. Williamson points out that contemporaneous commentators often overstate the dichotomies between East and West in market halls, casting them through an Orientalist lens. This contribution offers a different take on contradictions present in the Bombay market, in particular the incongruity between technological advancement, especially the use of iron, and a nostalgia for medieval architecture. This romanticized approach to building, seen also in Young's chapter on New Orleans, becomes part and parcel of market design more generally. In the interwar period, however, many markets in colonial cities became vessels for the spread of the modern movement in architecture. Two buildings featured in this volume, the Central Market in Hong Kong and Nairobi's City Market, both served as flashes of international modernism within rapidly developing colonial cities.

Zhengfeng Wang's chapter, "The Central Market in Hong Kong: Urban Amenities in a Speculative Field," examines how British authorities seized new developments in the use of iron, steel, and concrete to erect a monumental "clean machine" that would modernize the Crown colony in the 1930s. The Central Market thoroughly embodied ideas of sanitary bureaucracy that had become the norm in British planning: every eventuality and all possible circumstances in health and hygiene were considered in the market's design, from the most appropriate water storage tanks in the fish stalls to the best possible counters in the poultry section. Although the colonial administration encouraged segregation in many urban contexts, Central Market was an exception, one of the few places where Europeans, locals, and other foreigners commingled. The same could be said for another contemporaneous complex, the Nairobi City Market. Nkatha Gichuyia's contribution, "Nairobi City Market: The Versatile Afterlife of a Colonial-Era Building in a Postcolonial World," presents the first in-depth study of a landmark Art Deco building in East Africa. This chapter demonstrates how the development of Nairobi City Market paralleled large civic markets in other parts of the British Empire where government agendas sought to impose reforms, bureaucracy, and formal order on local cultures. Importantly, it also highlights colonial as well as postcolonial knowledge transfers, cultural exchanges, and public health concerns that contributed to shaping the urban order of Nairobi in the early part of the twentieth century. Ultimately, this chapter investigates how this market has evolved into a new role in the twenty-first century: a key protagonist in the endeavor to reimagine colonial legacies within the Global South.

Markets can be enduring places. Once they are established, they tend to grow roots and stay put in a given locale while co-developing with their surroundings, sometimes over hundreds of years. As such, while covered halls may be monumental and architecturally distinguished, they are very often later renditions of a long-standing tradition of buying and selling, converging and circulating. Leila M. Farah's chapter, "The St. Lawrence Market, Toronto: Changes and Continuity," explores the evolution of a market site since the early 1830s. This locale accommodated various markets central to the city's rich and vibrant history of industrialization, immigration, and modernization. The chapter examines rules and regulations pertaining to the order and sanitation of such infrastructures and visualizes both existing and disappeared market buildings in their urban context. This case can be useful for researchers dealing with changing urban and social landscapes and offers visualizations, methodological insights, and contributions to support their efforts to digitally model such developments through a variety of sources.

We tend to regard markets as repositories of sustenance, but they are equally political arenas, sites wherein governments test theories and experiment with new social policies. Xusheng Huang's chapter, "Between a Government Project and a Commercial Space for Ordinary Citizens: Dongan Market, 1903–1937," examines the ways that the Chinese government harnessed the paradigm of Western market hall architecture in its attempt to impose order on market sellers. At its core, this is a study of how a new market type emerged at the crossroad between traditional Chinese markets and Eurocentric retail spaces in the Republican period. Functionally, this large, covered street market in Beijing interweaved commercial areas and recreational activities; politically, it aimed to promote national identity and order, thereby catalyzing China's modernization.

The twin themes of modernity and political ideology coalesce as well in Ruth Lo's chapter, "Hygiene, Urbanism, and Fascist Politics at Rome's Wholesale Market." This contribution illuminates how market buildings in interwar Italy were at once harbingers of imperialist ambitions and facilities that underpinned biopolitics. Like other case studies in this volume, Rome's Wholesale Market was considered an engine for modernization. Yet under Mussolini food was not merely sustenance, but also a weapon. This chapter exposes the fascist party's ambitions to rethink the food supply of the city. Using sanitary reform as a justification, the party overhauled Rome's distribution systems, placing the Wholesale Market at the center of a vast infrastructure network. This contribution concludes with a coda that considers the decline and imminent redevelopment of the Wholesale Market, thus bringing the history of this site full circle.

The postwar era ushered in a period of decline for covered market halls. Supermarkets, car ownership, and the expansion of the suburbs brought a sea change in the ways that people shopped for and purchased food. Despite the fact that so many late nineteenth- and early twentieth-century halls were lauded at the time of their construction for technological advancements that foregrounded hygiene and sanitation, standards shifted in the second half of the century. These changes generated two different, often overlapping, trajectories: on the one hand, traditional markets were overhauled, sometimes from the ground up; on the other hand, market complexes became central to preservation efforts. Overall, these sites in many ways became literal and figurative scaffolds for urban regeneration. Emeline Houssard's contribution, "Modernization and Mobilization: Parisian Retail Market Halls, 1961-1982," casts light on an overlooked chapter of Paris's food history. While the rise and demise of Baltard's Les Halles is romanticized in literature and known even to undergraduate history students, few people are aware of the fate of other markets in the city, especially those built after World War II. Houssard's study combines architectural and planning history, showing how from the '60s onward French politics and bureaucracy reimagined the concept of a market hall, asking how it could respond to changing interpretations of public health needs. This paved the way for new multipurpose facilities while simultaneously mobilizing and undergirding calls for the preservation of historic market halls. The penultimate chapter in this volume, "Finding Food at Torvehallerne: Market Halls in Copenhagen between Gastrosexual Consumerism and the Coronavirus Pandemic," demonstrates the degree to which preservation efforts have successfully mainstreamed market halls in the late twentieth and early twenty-first centuries. In this contribution, Henriette Steiner speaks of the "market hall effect" in urban regeneration projects: urban centers harness the potential of new markets to promote a city as a brand, marketing it as a cultural destination that has food as a focus. Presenting a compelling case study of urban regeneration, this chapter offers a critical perspective on livability, particularly in the wake of the COVID-19 crisis.

While public markets are loci of contrasts, they can also be milieus of synthesis, a dialectical space where various perspectives meet and are creatively or antagonistically negotiated. Such have been the markets explored in this volume, across continents from the middle of the nineteenth century to the second decade of the twenty-first. The themes of antithesis and fusion permeate them.

Covered markets have always been places where the community gathers to safeguard its health through sustenance. Yet this objective has often faced competing theories of the spread of disease, ambiguous means of prevention, and dubious remedies. Put categorically, markets embody the inherently messy nature of human public interaction and congregation, often in tandem with the political imposition of order and discipline. They embrace tradition, while grappling with technological changes, and are sites where efforts to impose a particular vision have often clashed with a society in constant flux.

These polarities have resulted in the quest for and application of architectural solutions, processes, and mechanisms to negotiate them. Since the early waves of industrialization and globalization in the nineteenth century, the demands emanating from lateral demographic pressures necessitated the construction, expansion, and regeneration of markets. These structures made use of technological innovations and advances in public health to combat unhygienic practices, reduce direct or indirect pollution, and improve sanitation, turning them into models of scientific progress. In many ways, not only did they undergo transformation, but themselves also embodied change—in some cases serving as its drivers. At the same time, these buildings reflected the cultural and political realities of their times. While they were often used to project idealized and imagined visions of society itself, they exemplified power imbalances, became de facto vehicles of hegemonic discourse, and attracted activism. Numerous cases from this volume illustrate how citizens mobilized to have their voices heard about the fate of what they rightly considered their public realm.

Ultimately, as the contributions in this volume illustrate, markets have been serving both as mirrors that reflect a society's identity and sense of belonging, composition, output, and health, and as public laboratories that wrestle with modes and vectors of modernization, urbanity, and liberty. This characterization is also evident in the experiences of the recent COVID-19 pandemic, where the urban market has forced a renewed look at ventilation and other sanitation practices, as well as socialization and (re)connectivity with the community, its land, and its existing and evolving values.

All volumes of this nature rely on a diverse compendium of assistance, both tangible and intangible. We are grateful for the initial backing and support of the organizers of the 2019 Society of Architectural Historians conference, in particular Victoria Young. Our editor at Leuven University Press, Mirjam Truwant, has championed this project from its very beginning and has generously provided advice through the entire process. Thanks are also due to her colleagues at the press.

This publication received funding from KU Leuven Fair Fund for Open Access. We would like to express appreciation to Demmy Verbeke, head of KU Leuven Libraries Artes, research coordinator KU Leuven Libraries and his team for their support. We would also like to thank Toronto Metropolitan University's Faculty of Engineering and Architectural Science as well as the Department of Architectural Science for their financial support. Part of the publication expenses have also been underwritten by the Output-Based Research Support Scheme at University College Dublin.

In the process of compiling this book we received excellent support from four copyeditors, Irina du Quenoy, Lenore Hietkamp, Kathrine Morton, and Rebecca Bryan and from an indexer, Thomas Crombez. We are also grateful for the feedback from an external peer review by Victoria Kelley, at the

University for the Creative Arts, UK, and a second anonymous reviewer. It has been a pleasure working with all the authors in this volume and we are immensely grateful to them for sharing their research with us.

Notes

1. Here we use the term 'type' as it was construed by Post-Enlightenment architectural theorists; that is, as a classification system for buildings. See Jean-Nicolas-Louis Durand, *Précis of the Lectures of Architecture with Graphic Portion on the Lectures on Architecture*. Introduction by Antoine Picon, translation by David Britt (Los Angeles: Getty Research Institute, 2000). Architectural monographs on individual market halls are few and far between, but there is a growing body of existing literature on this topic more generally. A key resource is the volume by James Schmiechen and Kenneth Carls, *The British Market Hall: A Social and Architectural History* (New Haven: Yale University Press, 1999). Other important monographs include: Christopher Curtis Mead, *Making Modern Paris: Victor Baltard's Central Markets and the Urban Practice of Architecture*, Buildings, Landscapes, and Societies (Book 7) (University Park: Pennsylvania State University Press, 2012); Theodore C. Bestor, *Tsukiji: The Fish Market at the Center of the World* (Berkeley: University of California Press, 2004); and Yves Bergeron, *Les places et halles de marché au Québec. Collection patrimoines. Lieux et traditions* (Québec: Gouvernement du Québec, Ministère de la culture, 1993). Complementing these are standout projects that examine market culture in a broader sense, such as the work by Helen Tangires: *Public Markets* (New York: W. W. Norton, 2008); and *Movable Markets: Food Wholesaling in the 20th Century City* (Baltimore: John Hopkins University Press, 2019). For wide view on modern European market halls, see Manuel Guàrdia and José Luis Oyón (eds), *Making Cities through Market Halls: Europe, 19th and 20th centuries* (Barcelona: Ajutament de Barcelona, 2015). It is also worth highlighting sources that lie beyond architecture but that encompass market culture and the purveyance of food, particularly within cities. For example, Gergely Baics, *Feeding Gotham: The Political Economy and Geography of Food in New York, 1790–1860* (Princeton: Princeton University Press, 2017); Dorothée Imbert (ed), *Food and the City: Histories of Culture and Cultivation*, Dumbarton Oaks Colloquium on the History of Landscape Architecture 36 (Cambridge, MA: Harvard University Press, 2015); and Carolyn Steel, *Hungry City: How Food Shapes Our Lives* (London: Vintage, 2011).
2. Two of the most well-known public campaigns for the preservation of a market was Covent Garden in London and Les Halles in Paris, both of which galvanized activism globally for this type of edifice. See for example, Alvin Shuster, "Covent

Garden Plan Saves Some of Old," *New York Times*, January 16, 1973, 2; Pierre Schneider, "Paris: Timely Requiem for Les Halles," *New York Times*, May 25, 1970, 41. More recently, the Smithfield General Market in the City of London survived a substantial commercial redevelopment proposal and will now house the new Museum of London. Rob Winkley, "Crusaders Battle to Save Smithfield," *Planning* 1556 (2004): 5.

Bibliography

Baics, Gergely. *Feeding Gotham: The Political Economy and Geography of Food in New York, 1790–1860.* Princeton: Princeton University Press, 2017.

Bergeron, Yves. *Les places et halles de marché au Québec.* Collection patrimoines. Lieux et traditions. Québec: Gouvernement du Québec, Ministère de la culture, 1993.

Bestor, Theodore C. *Tsukiji: The Fish Market at the Center of the World.* Berkeley: University of California Press, 2004.

Durand, Jean-Nicolas-Louis. *Précis of the Lectures of Architecture with Graphic Portion on the Lectures on Architecture.* Introduction by Antoine Picon, translation by David Britt. Los Angeles: Getty Research Institute, 2000.

Guàrdia, Manuel, and José Luis Oyón (eds). *Making Cities through Market Halls: Europe, 19th and 20th Centuries.* Barcelona: Ajutament de Barcelona, 2015.

Imbert, Dorothée (ed). *Food and the City: Histories of Culture and Cultivation.* Dumbarton Oaks Colloquium on the History of Landscape Architecture 36. Cambridge, MA: Harvard University Press, 2015

Mead, Christopher Curtis. *Making Modern Paris: Victor Baltard's Central Markets and the Urban Practice of Architecture.* Buildings, Landscapes, and Societies (Book 7). University Park: Pennsylvania State University Press, 2012.

Schmiechen, James, and Kenneth Carls. *The British Market Hall: A Social and Architectural History.* New Haven: Yale University Press, 1999.

Schneider, Pierre. "Paris: Timely Requiem for Les Halles." *New York Times*, May 25, 1970.

Shuster, Alvin. "Covent Garden Plan Saves Some of Old." *New York Times*, January 16, 1973.

Steel, Carolyn. *Hungry City: How Food Shapes Our Lives.* London: Vintage, 2011.

Tangires, Helen. *Public Markets.* New York: W. W. Norton, 2008.

———. *Movable Markets: Food Wholesaling in the 20th Century City.* Baltimore: John Hopkins University Press, 2019.

Winkley, Rob. "Crusaders Battle to Save Smithfield." *Planning*, 1556 (2004): 5.

CHAPTER 2

PUBLIC AMENITY OR PUBLIC THREAT?

Epidemiology and Grassroots Activism in the Food Markets of New Orleans, 1900–1940

Ashley Rose Young

A Fundamental Dichotomy

Both historically and in the present day, in the United States and across the globe, a fundamental tension exists when it comes to marketplaces: they are simultaneously vital public amenities and a risk to public health.

Markets are much more than places of essential economic exchange. For vendors, they are a source of life-sustaining income; for customers, a source of life-sustaining goods, including food, clothing, and medicine. They are the stage upon which ordinary life plays out, sites for exchanging neighborhood gossip, training apprentices, throwing community socials, raising children, making art, hosting political rallies, collecting donations, staging protests, and more.

But the very coming together of people, information, and goods that makes public markets such rich cultural spaces is also the mechanism that causes the spread of deadly diseases. A byproduct of the economic, social, and cultural activities of the market is the refuse those interactions create, which over time threatens the cleanliness and sustainability of the marketplace. Concentrated interactions within heavily used marketplaces can turn them into breeding grounds and vectors of contagion.

New Orleans, a city already associated with extremes, is one such place where the dichotomy of markets has played out in everyday life. In this chapter, New Orleans serves as a case study through which to examine debates about public health and epidemiology, the role of government, and the local economy. This work offers a brief history of New Orleans's nineteenth-century public market system and then homes in on the role markets played in the opening decades of the twentieth century as salmonella and other diseases threatened the health and well-being of city residents.

Advocating for their personal and professional wellbeing, community members publicly complained about the conditions of the markets, which they argued led to disease outbreaks. Tensions came to a head in 1884, for instance, when conditions at the Dryades neighborhood market, a complex made up of two buildings, became unbearable for many food vendors. According to an article in the *Times-Picayune* titled "Inviting the Cholera," the floors of the Dryades Market were sticky and the thick air was ripe with the foul aroma of spoiled meat, fish, and produce. The wall paint had peeled, and the wooden eaves had rotted. The market, just like the fresh food it distributed, was slowly decomposing.[1] The author goes on to report:

> The condition of Dryades Market at present, from actual observation, is horrible. For the past 12 days the market has not been washed out, and the consequence is that a filthier place can souroely [*sic*] be imagined. The stench is intolerable, and numerous complaints are being made by the butchers, coffee and vegetable stand keepers. The facts have been reported but no attention is paid thereto.[2]

Despite the public outcry about these unsanitary conditions, the public markets went unchanged, and vendors and customers were forced to occupy these dilapidated buildings for several more decades.

In the opening years of the twentieth century, community members spoke out against the local government's apathetic approach to public health. Although people often think of such reforms as top-down, in the case of New Orleans's historic public markets, these improvements emerged from decades-long grassroots activism, highlighting the struggles and eventual success of community activist groups made up of both market vendors and marketgoers.

When city officials incorporated local activists' opinions and implemented large-scale renovations to the markets in the 1930s, they articulated a vision of a disease-free, modern society through market buildings that married emerging architectural styles with New Orleans's traditional market culture. In doing so, New Orleans maintained its commitment to local customs while at the same time embracing American progressivism and becoming a model for modern public markets across the country.

History of New Orleans's Public Markets

In the first half of the nineteenth century, New Orleans's local food distribution system reflected general public market culture in the Atlantic World, especially those areas that were or had been European colonies. Like most cities in the United States, New Orleans operated a central wholesale-retail market,

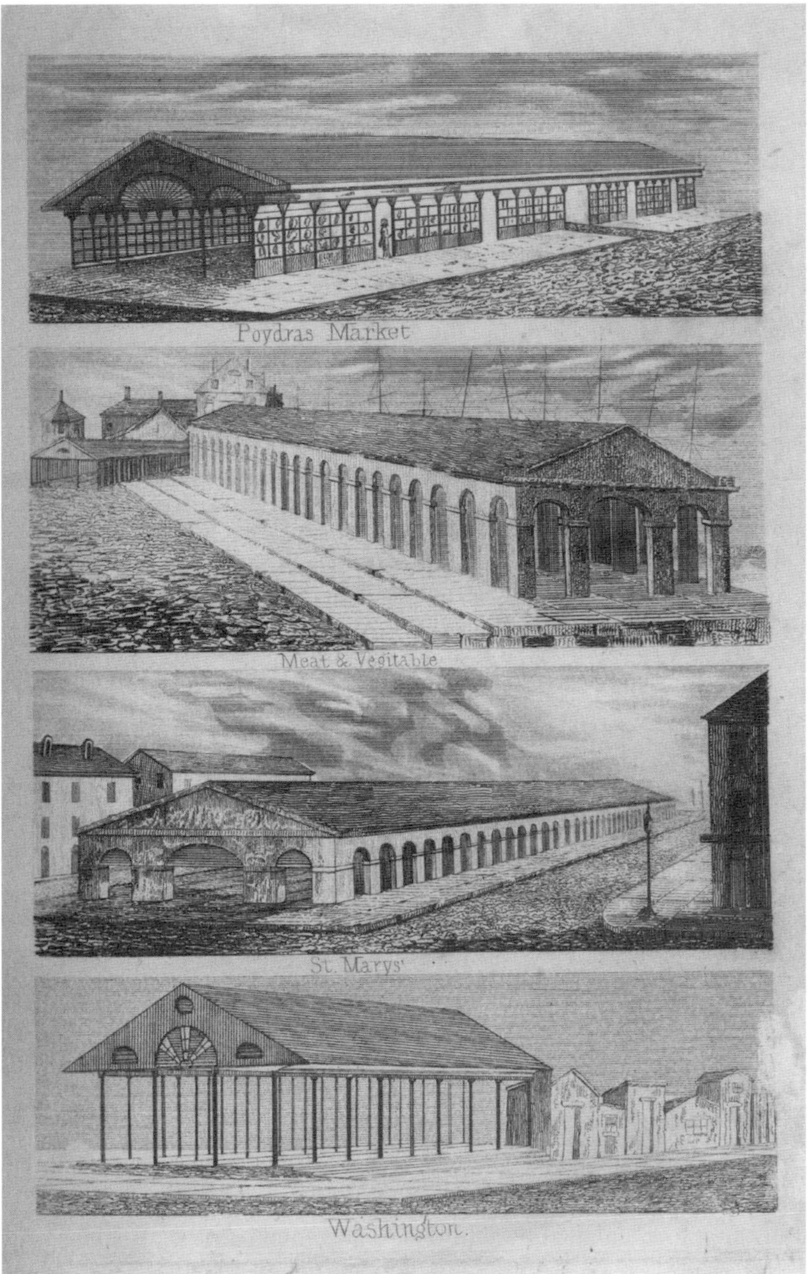

Figure 2.1. Engraving of Four Early Markets in Gibson's Guide and Directory of the State of Louisiana, and the Cities of New Orleans and LaFayette, 1838. Courtesy of the Historic New Orleans Collection, 87-085-RL.

the French Market, and, when needed, built auxiliary markets in growing neighborhoods. Several of New Orleans's early market structures as they appeared around 1838 are depicted in figure 2.1, including the Poydras Market, the Meat and Vegetable Market at the French Market complex, the St. Mary Market, and the Washington Market. These "pavilion markets" were essentially long colonnaded porticoes that provided vendors and marketgoers protection from the sun and rain. Because of New Orleans's role as a port city, the diversity of marketgoers reflected the diversity of the city's population, including Indigenous people, enslaved and free people of color, and migrants from throughout the Atlantic World. In the opening decades of the nineteenth century, a majority of vendors and customers at the French Market were enslaved and free Black women. Those demographics would shift over time as mass numbers of European migrants arrived throughout the first half of the nineteenth century.

People, animals, and goods easily moved through the markets, as did wind, dust, and other particles of urban life, some of them dirty and dangerous byproducts of industrialization. Exposure to the outdoors provided necessary natural ventilation, yet also invited unwelcome elements including pollution, vermin, and disease. Vendors and customers alike had contested relationships with open-air, pavilion markets and saw them as a public necessity that came with many dangers related to public health.

New Orleans' market culture dates back to the Spanish colonial period (1763–1802), during which time the local government first constructed a covered public market, primarily for the sale of meat, in 1780. The city replaced that structure in 1782 with a larger complex that burned down in 1788. Two years later, the city government began construction on the city's now iconic French Market, which opened to the public in 1791. As the population grew, the local government built more structures within the French Market complex to accommodate residents' needs. Eventually, the market consisted of five separate buildings: the meat market, vegetable market, fruit market, fish market, and bazaar. From 1791 to 1822, the French Market was the only municipally owned and operated market in the city. Urban and rural residents flocked to the market to trade and purchase fresh produce, meats, prepared foods, and other goods. As the population increased more rapidly in the 1820s, the French Market could no longer provision the entire city. The municipal government began building a series of smaller, neighborhood-based food markets to cater first to established neighborhoods surrounding its central core and then eventually to burgeoning communities beyond that.

The city government constructed the first neighborhood market, St. Mary Market, around 1822.[3] It was located upriver of the French Market, in a part of town known as "the American Sector" that had been steadily growing since

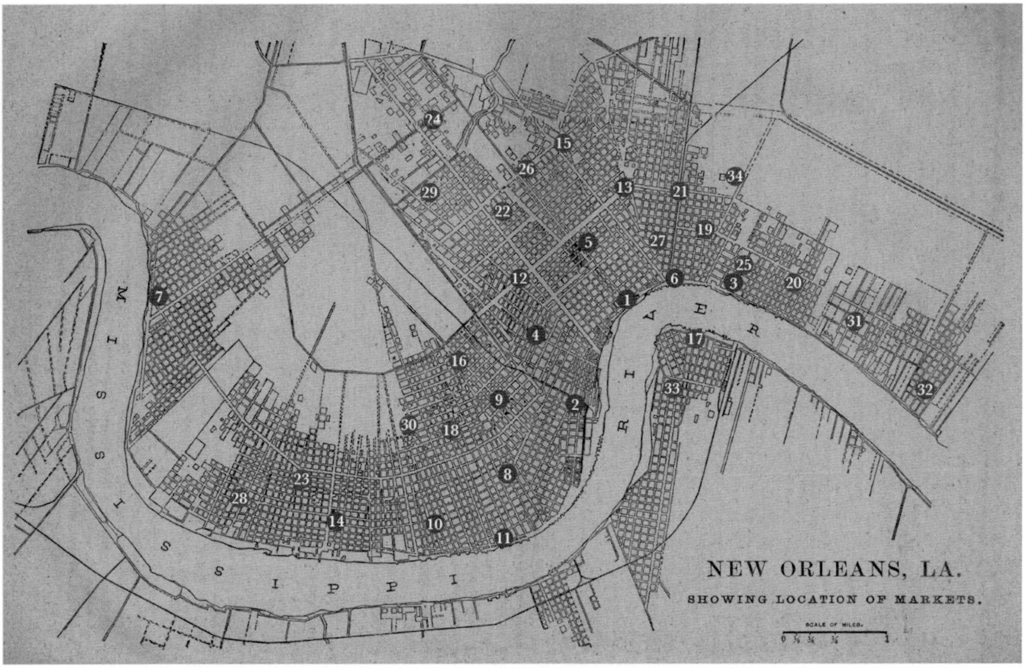

NEW ORLEANS, LA.
SHOWING LOCATION OF MARKETS.

pre-Civil War

1. French Market 1791
2. St Mary's Market 1822
3. Washington Market 1836
4. Poydras Market 1838
5. Treme Market 1840
6. Port Market 1840
7. Carrollton Market 1846
8. Magazine Market 1847
9. Dryades Market 1848
10. Ninth Street Market 1850
11. Soraparu Market 1852
12. Claiborne Market 1852
13. St. Bernard Market 1856
14. Jefferson Market 1860

☞ All market dates are approximate.

post-Civil War

15. Le Breton Market 1867
16. Keller Market 1867
17. St. John Market 1872
18. Second Street Market 1873
19. St Roch Market 1882
20. Guillotte Market 1882
21. Delamore Market 1882
22. Rocheblave Market 1882
23. Prytania Market 1890
24. Suburban Market 1896
25. Zengel Market 1900
26. Maestri Market 1900
27. Lautenschlaeger Market 1902
28. Ewing Market 1907
29. Memory Market 1907
30. Mehle Market 1907
31. Doullut Market 1907
32. Behram Market 1909
33. Foto Market 1910
34. McCue Market 1910

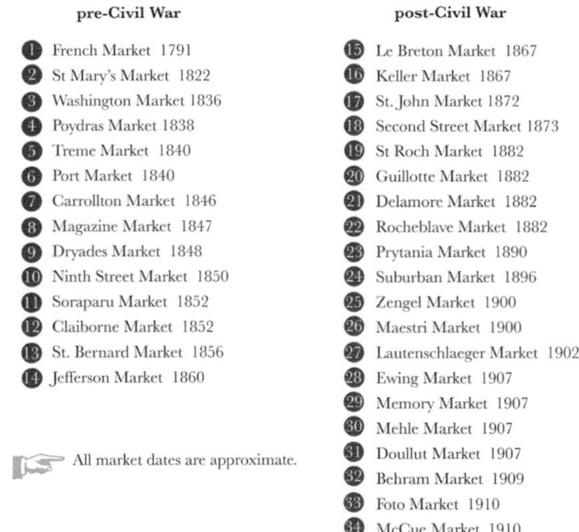

Figure 2.2. Public Markets Constructed in New Orleans pre- and post-Civil War. Market data compiled by Dr. Samantha Martin. Base map from Francis Joseph Reynolds, *The New Encyclopedic Atlas and Gazetteer of the World*. New York: Collier & Sons, 1917. Courtesy of the Perry-Castañeda Library Map Collection, University of Texas at Austin.

the US government acquired a large parcel of land from France through the Louisiana Purchase of 1803. Like in the French Market, "all kinds of meat, poultry, game, fish, vegetables and all other items destined for the daily supply of the city and its suburbs" could be bought and sold at St. Mary Market.[4] After St. Mary Market, the city built the Washington Market around 1836, located in what has become known as the Bywater, just two neighborhoods downriver of the French Quarter. Free people of color, French Creoles, and migrants from the Spanish colonial empire occupied the Bywater at that time.[5] Then followed the Poydras Market (around 1838), Treme Market (around 1840), and Port Market (around 1840). The first auxiliary markets were all constructed within a mile of the French Market complex. During this time, New Orleans became the third largest city in the United States, with a population in 1840 estimated at 102,193 (doubled since 1830).[6] From there, it continued to build markets for burgeoning neighborhoods, constructing a total of thirteen neighborhood markets between 1822 and 1860, as seen in figure 2.2. Indeed, New Orleans became a city of markets, with each market serving as the cultural and economic keystones of its neighborhood.

After the US Civil War (1861–1865), New Orleans's public market system deviated from that of other major American cities in both its architectural style and its geographic footprint. In the mid-nineteenth century, other major American centers adopted the model of the "modern" market hall, a larger and more ornate enclosed space for purveying foods. City officials saw them as civic symbols alongside libraries, museums, courthouses, etc. Philadelphia's Western Market, which opened its doors on April 20, 1859, was one of the first examples of the new market house model. A classically inspired pastiche, the market was "built of brick, ornamented with granite and brown stone, and externally presents a beautiful and tasteful appearance."[7] It had 280 stalls and boasted countertops hewn from Italian marble that had been polished until you could see your reflection in them. The market was also equipped with the latest ventilation technologies to promote airflow and reduce the smell of meat, seafood, and produce. In contrast, New Orleans's markets did not align with either the decorum of classically inspired brick and stone designs or the sheer size of the market buildings seen in cities like Philadelphia.

In New Orleans, city officials continued to build smaller, open-air, pavilion-style markets catering to growing neighborhoods.[8] The Magazine Market, depicted in figure 2.3, is a prime example of one of these post–Civil War pavilion-style markets. On average, New Orleans's public markets were about the size of a tennis court and continued to act as central commercial and cultural nodes for each neighborhood, attracting new brick-and-mortar businesses to open in the vicinity. In addition to those stores, peddlers clustered on street corners surrounding the market to hawk wares to customers en route to do

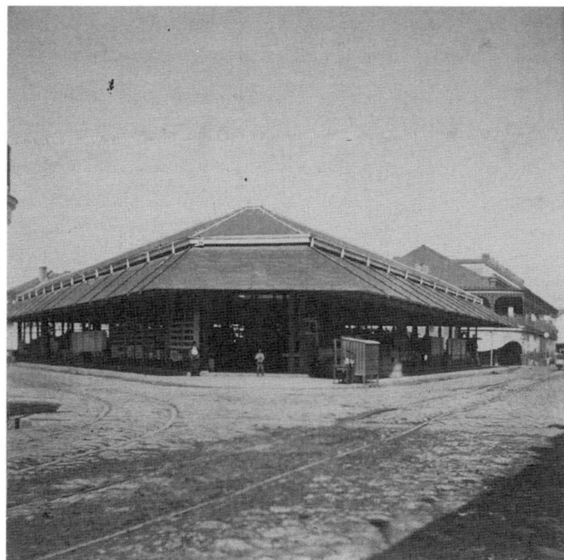

Figure 2.3. Pavilion Market. Magazine Market, New Orleans, around 1875. By S. T. Blessings. Courtesy of the Louisiana State Museum, 1979.126.84.

their daily shopping. The markets' simple, open architecture allowed for porosity—the easy flow of people and goods in and out of the market—that was lost in other US cities as they adopted the enclosed market house model. Throughout the second half of the nineteenth century, by contrast, New Orleans's focus remained on the hyperlocal rather than the fashion in other cities: a broader system of provisioning that relied on fewer, more ornate markets.

New Orleans's local laws played an important role in shaping the development of the city's unique local food economy. Whereas other cities had embraced a free market economy, enabling private markets to operate alongside public markets, local officials in New Orleans essentially made it illegal to do so. These privately owned markets most often took the form of a dry goods store, also known as a grocery store, that also sold fresh meat, seafood, and produce. They became known as a "green grocery." Fearful of competition, New Orleans officials instituted laws that prohibited private markets from selling fresh food (meat, seafood, and produce) within a range of six to twelve blocks of any public market.[9] In essence, they created a local food system in which the public markets had a monopoly over food distribution.

These laws helped city officials regulate the sale of fresh food by centralizing distribution, ensuring that what customers were buying was safe and fairly priced while the city's market system continued to grow. The government also did this to protect their investment in the public markets, which brought in money to New Orleans' general fund through rental fees and taxes. Throughout the second half of the nineteenth century, its officials used those funds to construct new markets (as seen in figure 2.2), while often neglecting repairs for existing ones. Additionally, they used market-raised money to fund other civic projects, leading to further disrepair of other markets already in existence.

By 1911 the city government of New Orleans had built thirty-three auxiliary neighborhood markets to supplement the French Market.[10] At its peak, New Orleans's public market system looked nothing like any other system in the country because of the sheer number of markets and individual communities to which they catered.[11] Additionally, the system appeared distinct within the United States because of the monopoly that the city government maintained over local food provisioning.

Although unusual in the US context, New Orleans's market system did mirror market systems in Europe and specifically that of Paris, which municipal governments throughout Europe and the United States saw as exemplary. Around 1910, Paris's market system consisted of one central market, Les Halles, and thirty-three auxiliary markets, the same number as in New Orleans by 1911. The parallels between New Orleans's and Paris's systems in the nineteenth and twentieth centuries suggests that the former likely drew inspiration from the latter. City residents openly acknowledged this transatlantic connection and Europe's longstanding influence on New Orleans. In a speech recounting the history of the city's market system, one citizen noted, "The French Market, if not physically as old as the city, was one of the European ideas brought over by the first settlers, and it has been along European lines of government that our market system has been run."[12]

Fly Infestation and Disease in New Orleans Public Markets

In 1911, just as the New Orleans's public market system swelled to its peak size, the city faced an alarming infestation of flies.[13] By early March, flies had found their way into every nook and cranny of public and private life. The markets' open-air designs exacerbated the issue. With no screens or walls, flies could easily swarm over the ornate and fragrant displays of fruits, vegetables, meat, and seafood. The small army of mule-drawn carts that clustered around the markets made conditions worse. Steaming piles of manure emitted noxious gases that also attracted flies, raising health concerns specifically tied to the spread of salmonella.[14]

During this crisis, the public markets were dramatically and directly tied to the spread of disease. In the twentieth century, salmonella was a major cause of food poisoning not only in the United States but worldwide. Scientists were all too aware that common flies, which hatched in manure, gravitated toward uncovered food on display in public markets. In the process, they flitted from a pile of dung to a barrel of apples, carrying bacteria on their bodies, and thus spreading disease. As scientists came to better understand the role of flies in the spread of salmonella, public health campaigns emerged to educate the public about how an everyday nuisance was also hazardous to one's health.[15]

New Orleans's public market history at the turn of the twentieth century shows that some of the hardest hit communities during a disease outbreak are those working in food industries. Vendors struggled to maintain customers' trust as conditions in the public markets worsened. Many did not have the economic means to leave the market to open up their own brick and mortar businesses where they could implement more stringent public health measures to prevent the spread of food-borne illnesses. Most of the city's food vendors were members of historically marginalized groups: recent migrants, women, and people of color. They worked in food provisioning because it was one of the only forms of entrepreneurship that did not require access to property. Vending in a market hall or selling at a street stand offered an economic toehold in a racist, classist, and sexist economic system that actively sought to keep them out of traditional businesses (i.e., brick and mortar). When fear of salmonella peaked at the turn of the century, threatening their very livelihoods, those vendors had few options. Not only that, their personal health was at stake. Market vendors, in particular, were incredibly vulnerable to the spread of the disease because their work necessitated daily engagement and close contact with the public, as they interacted with hundreds, if not thousands of marketgoers each day.

Market vendors in New Orleans, a majority of whom were white and many of whom were migrants from Europe, publicly expressed frustration over the terrible conditions of the public markets and criticized the laws that obligated them to sell fresh foods within them. Several of the vendors said they felt trapped by the system and argued that they could provide better services, higher quality products, and safer conditions in their own stores if municipal laws allowed private markets to sell meat, seafood, and fresh produce.[16] Paul Cendon, a butcher in one of the public markets, informed the City Council that while the fly problem was unbearable, flies were not the only creatures spreading food-borne illness. He noted that if the city officials visited the markets in the early morning, they would find dozens of feral cats and innumerable rats scampering over the meat that butchers were meant to sell to customers later that day. He criticized the City Board of Health for ignoring these conditions and for expressing little or no interest in the health of either vendors, customers, or the entire city. A fellow butcher added to the argument, stating that the City Board of Health's proposed solution to screen each individual stall was a terrible idea as it would further endanger the health of vendors and would, in fact, "make them sick."[17] Frustrated and seeking resolution, Cendon and his fellow vendors argued that the markets were "unfit to be used and that they ought to be torn down and remodeled."[18]

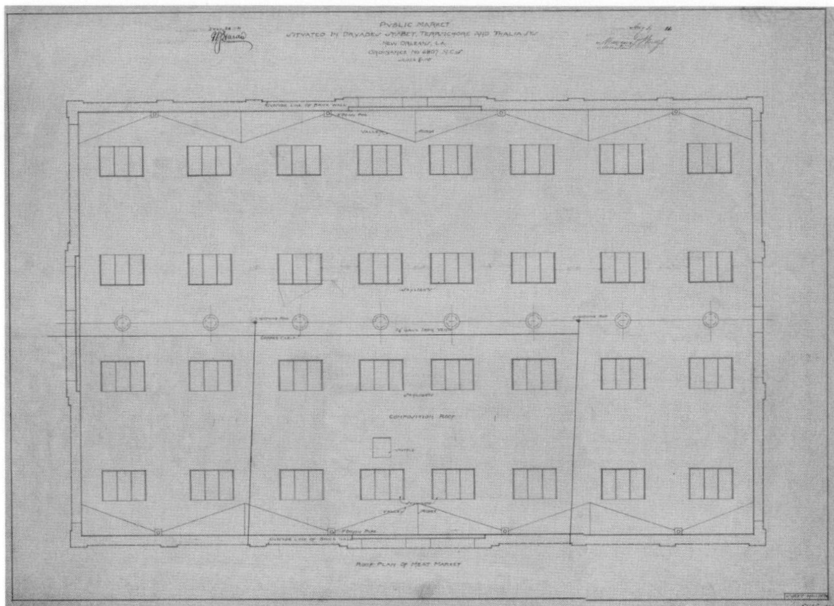

Figure 2.4. Roof Plan of Dryades Market Building A, New Orleans, 1911. Courtesy of the Louisiana Division/City Archives of the New Orleans Public Library.

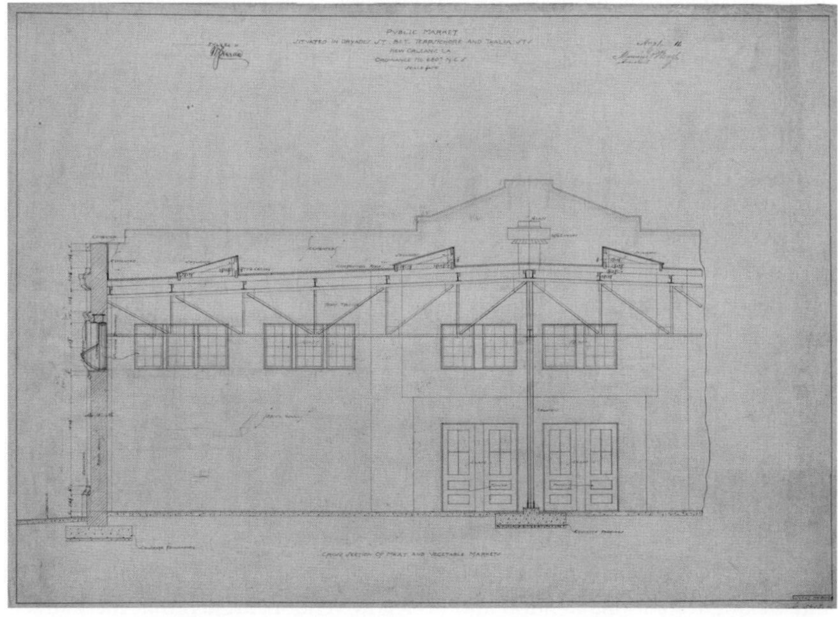

Figure 2.5. Cross Section of Dryades Market Building A, New Orleans, 1911. Courtesy of the Louisiana Division/City Archives of the New Orleans Public Library.

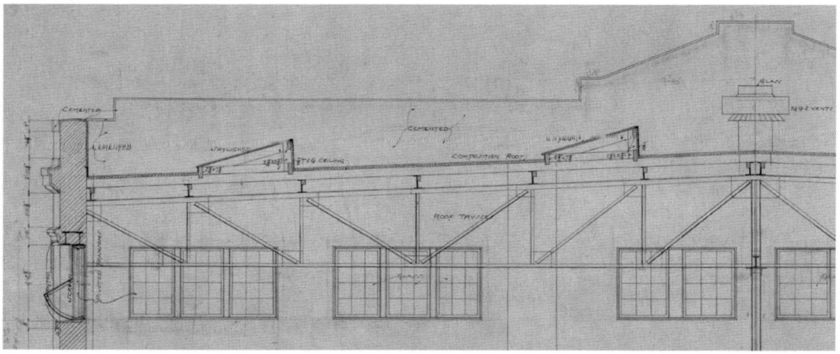

Figure 2.6. Detail of the Cross Section of Dryades Market Building A, New Orleans, 1911. Courtesy of the Louisiana Division/City Archives of the New Orleans Public Library.

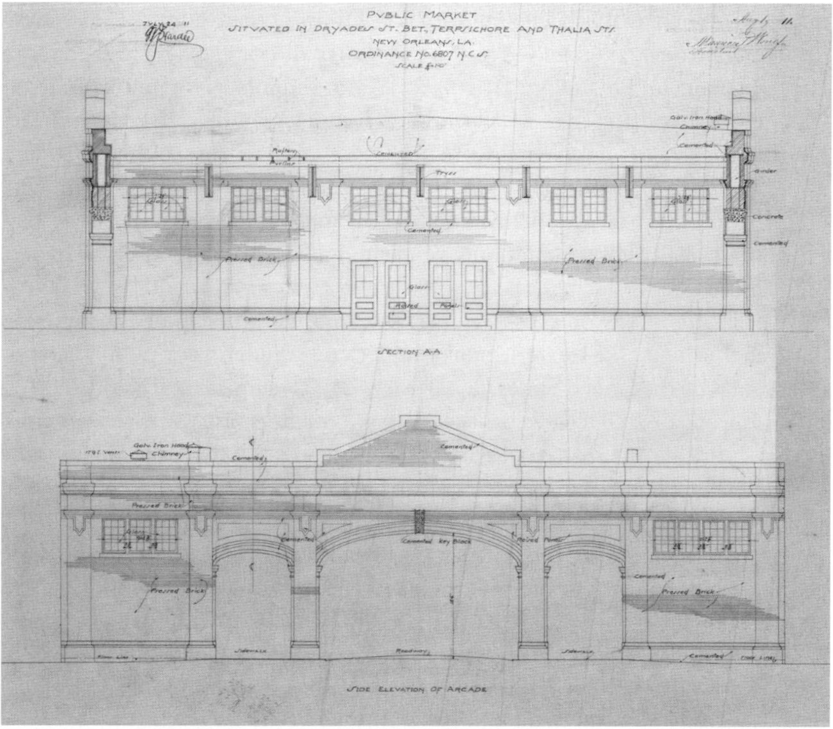

Figure 2.7. Front Elevation of Dryades Market Building A (top) and Side Elevation of Arcade Between Building A and B (bottom), New Orleans, 1911. Courtesy of the Louisiana Division/City Archives of the New Orleans Public Library.

City councilmen took the concerns of these vocal vendors into consideration. According to the *Times-Picayune*, at a public forum held in March of 1911, city councilmen had

> been considerably moved by the argument of the market people that the city forces them into the markets at a high rental when they might, if left to themselves, get fine shops with modern improvements outside, and as it is they are obliged to charge the public high and give inefficient service because they are up against high rents and poor facilities.[19]

Privately owned markets (i.e., green grocers) seemed like an increasingly better option than the public markets, but at this point in New Orleans's history, they were still largely illegal because of the ordinance banning their operation within nine blocks of any public market. The private markets afforded entrepreneurs greater control over the sanitary conditions of their businesses (whereas in the public ones, vendors were at the mercy of the city government to make improvements and maintain structures). Some vendors in the public markets wanted that freedom. To combat growing clamoring for private groceries, city officials rushed to make patchwork improvements to ease public concern, afraid that if they lost vendors' support, the entire system would collapse. City officials approved measures to screen some markets to keep insects at bay. However, the city government only renovated a few, leaving most unscreened and exposed.

For example, city officials began renovations with the Dryades Market, as illustrated in figures 2.4 to 2.7, marrying federal standards for public markets established by the United States Department of Agriculture (USDA) with traditional European architecture. In the early twentieth century, the USDA envisioned the ideal American city as one that operated modern market halls for the benefit of the people. This vision was tied into the City Beautiful Movement, which when it came to the architecture of public markets, embodied the federal government's epidemiology efforts. As a result, New Orleans became a melting pot for American progressivism that drew upon European traditions. New Orleans officials assessed the current conditions of the two-building Dryades Market structure, which had served as the keystone of its neighborhood since 1849. Each building carried different products. Vendors sold butchered meat, game, and seafood in the first building, known by locals as the Meat Market and hereto referred to as "Building A." Meanwhile, vendors sold fruits and vegetables in the second building, known as the Vegetable Market and hereto referred to as "Building B." The two buildings were connected by a covered walkway. Ultimately, city officials decided to demolish and completely rebuild the Dryades Market because the condition of the existing structures was so poor.

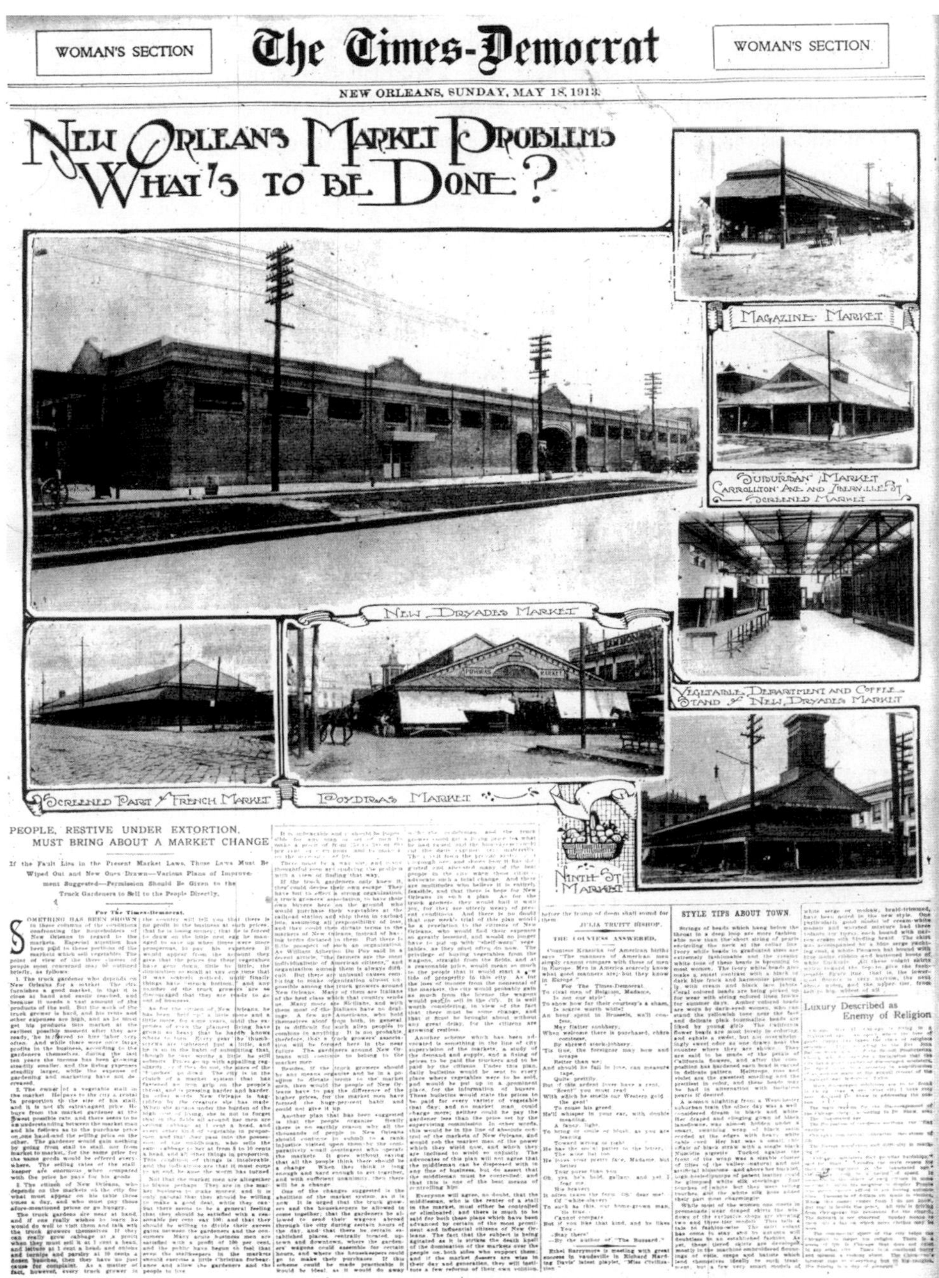

WOMAN'S SECTION | The Times-Democrat | WOMAN'S SECTION

NEW ORLEANS, SUNDAY, MAY 18, 1913.

NEW ORLEANS MARKET PROBLEMS
WHAT'S TO BE DONE?

SUBURBAN MARKET CARROLLTON AVE. AND ZINARY... ST

MAGAZINE MARKET

SCREENED MARKET

NEW DRYADES MARKET

VEGETABLE DEPARTMENT AND COFFEE STAND OF NEW DRYADES MARKET

SCREENED PART OF FRENCH MARKET

POYDRAS MARKET

NINTH ST. MARKET

PEOPLE, RESTIVE UNDER EXTORTION, MUST BRING ABOUT A MARKET CHANGE

STYLE TIPS ABOUT TOWN.

Luxury Described as Enemy of Religion

Figure 2.8. New Dryades Market alongside Pavilion Markets, New Orleans, 1913. In "New Orleans Market Problems: What's to Be Done?" *Times Democrat*, May 18, 1913.

As much as Dryades neighborhood residents derided the unsanitary conditions of the old market structures and were thrilled that new, more sanitary structures were to be built, they were saddened by the loss of such an important and historic community center. Upon hearing the news that the market buildings would be razed to make way for the modern market, they proposed that "a tablet [be] placed to commemorate them."[20] Their sense of loss and compulsion to memorialize the old, dilapidated structures speaks to the fundamental dichotomy that lies at the heart of many historic urban markets: that they are simultaneously a center of culture and a vector of disease.

City officials wanted "to make the new market one of the finest in the country" and a symbol of New Orleans's commitment to national standards of public health and public provisioning.[21] In order to fulfill those commitments, they planned to furnish the new Dryades Market with the latest technologies, including modern lighting, ventilation, and refrigeration systems.[22] City architects, for example, planned for thirty-two skylights (as shown in figure 2.4) and numerous windows (as shown in figures 2.5 and 2.6) to enable natural light to illuminate the retail space. They also planned to have 8 twenty-four-inch galvanized iron vents along the center line of the roof (as depicted in figure 2.4) to allow rising air perfumed with the smell of the marketplace to escape. Further, they included pivoting screens (as depicted in figures 2.5 and 2.6) to encourage airflow through side windows. Screened windows were not the only way to keep insects and vermin at bay. As seen in figures 2.5 to 2.7, city architects planned to enclose the market, constructing brick walls where once wooden columns had existed—a departure from the colonnaded portico style of the pavilion market predominant throughout the city. This transition away from New Orleans's traditional market architecture is perhaps best captured in an article published in the city's newspaper, which juxtaposes the enclosed Dryades Market with other neighborhood markets around the city (as seen in figure 2.8).

The New Orleans commitment to technologies and architectural elements that improved public health mirrored the commitments of city officials in other US cities. For example, when the West Side Market opened in Cleveland, Ohio, in November 1912, newspapers focused on narratives of improved public health. One article starts off with, "Sanitation. That is going to be the watchword at the new West Side market house."[23] According to the article, the aesthetic design of the West Side Market was reminiscent of hospital white: "The building is lined with white tile from the gleaming white counters to the lofty roof."[24] Architects chose these elements to distinguish the new market from the old and to reaffirm the cleanliness of the new facility: "Everything has been eliminated which would tend to breed noxious germs."[25] Like the West Side Market, the new Dryades Market buildings also had white interiors that reflected the city's commitment to the new aesthetic of cleanliness and sanitation. The city's newspaper captured the luminescent interior in a photograph labeled "Vegetable Department and Coffee Stand of New Dryades Market" (as seen in figure 2.8). The modern amenities and aesthetic designs of the West Side Market and the new Dryades Market not only strove for national standards of public health through architectural design but also came to exemplify them.

Although the New Orleans government was willing to make strategic renovations as a symbolic gesture toward its commitment to improving public health, it did not have and did not allot funds to overhaul the entire market system—a widespread renovation that residents desperately needed. Behind the celebrations of the new Dryades Market, pervasive public health issues continued to threaten the sustainability of the public markets and made private markets, which were typically more sanitary and modern, an increasingly appealing option for residents.

Women Consumer-Activists and the Policing of New Orleans Public Markets

In the following year, unrest continued to brew among the city's populace, much of it a carryover from the debates over the fly infestation and market screening debacle of 1911. Although generally supportive of the initial renovation efforts, customers wanted to see a renovation of the *entire* system, not just one or two select markets. They wanted one that, across the board, eliminated the threat of food-borne illnesses. When the Louisiana State Board of Health stepped in to assess the public markets, the results were abysmal.[26] The Poydras and Prytania Markets had dirty refrigerators, the Ninth Street Market had a rat infestation, and the Treme Market had dysfunctional iceboxes. These public health infractions exemplified the terrible condition of the whole market system. State Board of Health officials were finally catching on to what angry and concerned citizens had been expressing for decades. At a meeting with the State Board of Health in September 1912, New Orleans resident Raymond de Lord argued that a city that could not take care of its markets should not have them.[27] De Lord's opinion reflected an increasingly popular sentiment in the city: the public markets should be shut down or privatized.

Concerned citizens realized that shutting down the public market system in the 1910s was a long shot. The markets were too entrenched in the politics of the city, and too critical to the city government's general fund. Citizens, though, had other strategies in mind to ameliorate issues in the local food system. For inspiration, they looked to other American cities like New York, where modern market halls and grocery stores coexisted in a free market economy. In these cities, both public and private markets were fitted with electricity and refrigeration—necessary amenities for safe provisioning. In the eyes of New Orleanians, people in those other cities had choices of where to shop whereas New Orleanian customers did not. They felt forced to shop in the subpar public markets. So, they began organizing to petition the local government to give them more options.

Women consumer-activists formed organizations that were key players in market reform in the 1910s, creating leverage and shaping narratives about the markets that influenced policy about public health. Their voices rang out alongside the voices of city officials, public market vendors, and private market operators and vendors—almost all men—whose involvement in the public markets had been reported in the newspapers. Given the racial prejudices entrenched in New Orleans's segregated society at the time, the city's main newspaper, the *Time-Picayune*, privileged white women's voices over Black women's. Women activists' efforts demonstrate how important grassroots organizations remained in shaping public health at a time when the federal government was becoming increasingly involved in the regulation of food in America.[28]

One such group of women activists belonged to the Era Club, which worked with the State Board of Health to create "model markets." Members suggested ways to improve both sanitation and efficiency in New Orleans's market system. For example, Mrs. Gordon Sargent visited the Dryades Market in September 1912 and "tried to get them to place refrigerator [*sic*] down middle aisle, so that same ice would serve for butchers in both aisles, and for greater convenience in serving public and less handling of meat."[29] Her grassroots activism, alongside that of her peers, shaped the very physicality of the markets and behavior of the people who worked and shopped within them.

Another group of women activists involved in the creation of model markets was the Market Committee formed by the Housewives' League Division of the City Federation Clubs.[30] The Market Committee members' ideal vision of New Orleans's local food economy was one based on an American model of a free-market economy that would give shoppers a choice about where they acquired their food. They believed that such an arrangement would enable more sanitary and modern private markets to open in the city. These markets, direct competitors of the public ones, would encourage the city government to renovate the city's public markets to stay competitive, thus improving overall public health within the local food economy. In order to make their vision a reality, they needed to convince public officials that private markets were essential to the city's success and that they were in fact necessary to the survival of New Orleans. One of the ways the committee members sought to gain officials' favor was to demonstrate the poor conditions of the public markets by conducting inspections that listed public health infractions, which they reported to the city government. They also collected data from heating, lighting, ventilation, and refrigeration experts about best practices in market facilities across America, comparing and contrasting the conditions in New Orleans with those in other US cities.[31]

Members of the Housewives' League Division of the City Federation Clubs were particularly keen on providing greater opportunity for private markets to operate within the city and often lobbied on behalf of private retailers. For example, at a Housewives' League Division board meeting, Miss Hudson objected to a drafted market ordinance that required private markets to have "holes in the roofs" to provide ventilation.[32] Said ordinance would make it impossible for retailers to live above their stores. Members of the division proposed a slightly modified architectural approach with "transoms or opening in the walls, up close to the roof" that would ensure airflow while also allotting for living space. They strengthened their argument by citing examples of other markets whose upper floors served as community spaces. Harriet Barton, for example, noted a structure in Dayton, Ohio, "where above [the market] were the clubrooms of one of the prominent men's clubs of the day."[33] Helen McCants drew upon another example in Houston, "which is climatically not unlike New Orleans," where the "city administration offices were erected over the public market."[34] Such efforts demonstrate that the Housewives' League Division's activism included direct engagement with and suggestions about the architectural design of marketplaces, both private and public. Their focus on market architecture was just one angle in their efforts to transform the local food economy of New Orleans by shaping local law.

In the spring of 1914, the efforts of the Housewives' League Division paid off when the city government passed three new ordinances pertaining to the public markets.[35] The first governed the construction of private and public markets, and the second repealed a prior ordinance barring private markets from operating within nine blocks of the St. Mary, Delamore, Soraparu, Guillotte, St. John, and Carrolton Markets.[36] Commissioner E. E. Lafaye of the Department of Public Property would propose the third ordinance, which expanded private markets' operating hours throughout the day, to the City Council in December.[37] These laws were a major victory for the women-operated committee, bringing it one step closer to its vision of a modern New Orleans free of the public markets' monopoly over local provisioning. A report drafted by the committee drew attention to particular aspects of the laws that its members identified as "important points." One of the ordinances, for example, focused on improving public health through the built environment of the public markets and the amenities installed within.[38] Creating space for the movement of fresh air was key. Market structures were required to stand alone, separate from any other structures, and had to be constructed of iron-concrete or brick-concrete. Alleys between buildings had to be at least five feet wide to allow for ventilation. The ordinance also required metal ventilators to provide adequate airflow in any attic space of the market, despite the Housewives' League Division's previous objections, and mandated that each market have at least one electric fan over each entrance. To maximize airflow while keeping flies and other creatures at bay, any openings in the market walls had to be screened with eighteen-inch mesh bronze wire. The interior designs of the markets were made to resemble sterile, cleanly places akin more to a hospital than the city's markets of old. The ordinance required laid stone or tile flooring graded to drain into city sewers. The interior surfaces of all foundation walls had to be full-glazed white enamel brick or tile.[39] All other interior walls as well as the ceiling had to be plastered "perfectly smooth" and given three coats of white paint.[40] These interiors would plainly show any speck or splatter, making the market's cleanliness readily apparent to vendors and customers.

Guidelines for the construction of markets were just one piece of the legal reform that drew the attention of the Market Committee. Another element of special importance to them was the lifting of the nine-block radius rule in some sections of the city, mainly where the most recent public markets had been constructed and in the largest commercial district in New Orleans (the historic neighborhood markets nearer to the city center were still protected by the nine-block radius rule). According to the ordinance, as long as those private markets "comply with the sanitary provisions" outlined in the other market ordinance, they were clear to operate.[41] This new law would allow "the modern sanitary grocery, restaurant, fruit-store, or department store to sell fresh meat[,] fish, or game, as in other cities."[42] Celebrating their contributions to these major changes, the committee noted that "in framing the three ordinances, the suggestions made by our committee members were freely used [...] and in almost every case the specifications suggested were inserted."[43] The efforts of concerned citizens led to one of the most significant changes in the city's food economy in decades. The women on this committee knew, however, that these ordinances would only create real change if the city enforced them.[44]

Soon after these new ordinances passed, the Market Committee met with Commissioner Lafaye to make a strategic plan for the future. During this meeting, he noted that these ordinances were the first step in completely revolutionizing New Orleans's local food economy. Lafaye stated, "I confidently hope that these changes will bring new blood into our market business, and that both local and Northern capital will open retail green groceries [i.e., ones that sell fresh food] here similar to those in other cities."[45] Later that year, after the market ordinances had been in place for several months, Lafaye once again publicly acknowledged the critical role that the Housewives' League Division played in "bringing about better market conditions in New Orleans" and pledged to continue his support of the division's policies.[46]

The 1914 ordinances made inroads for modern private markets, enabling them to embed themselves into the changing food culture of the city, one that was beginning to look more like other American cities. New Orleans's suburbs were growing, stretching out toward Lake Pontchartrain, and these new residential communities provided opportunities for private markets to legally operate outside of the nine-block radius concentrated in the historic heart of the city. Able to tailor their business practices to the needs and the desires of their customers, private retailers invested in refrigeration technologies, allowing them to keep longer operating hours and improve the quality and shelf life of their products. This was the beginning of the transformation of small-scale private markets into supermarkets, ones that would develop on the outskirts of New Orleans proper as suburban populations grew.

At the city center, the public markets continued to face public health problems throughout the 1920s and into the early 1930s because of the city government's decision, once again, to place market profits into its general fund rather than into market upkeep.[47] The issues, laid bare by the local newspapers, were eerily similar to those of the preceding decades due in large part to the municipal government's refusal to invest in overhauling the entire market system to improve public health. In 1920, for example, the State Board of Health issued an injunction against several of New Orleans's public markets, most of which remained unscreened and therefore open to insects, vermin, and dangerous forms of nature that spread disease.[48] They were also condemned for their poor sanitary conditions because refuse and food debris were not washed out of the markets.[49] In 1930, Dr. Dowling, the former president of the State Board of Health, described the conditions of the market as "unspeakably filthy."[50] He noted that he had condemned the public markets in 1911 and that conditions had improved, "but not much," over the last twenty years.[51] The threat of disease was still very much a reality for vendors and customers alike. New Orleans's public provisioning was stuck, unchanging for the most part, as new technologies and improvements thrived in supermarkets on the city's periphery.

Planning for More Sanitary Public Markets

In a similar condition and state of financial distress as the public markets in 1911, city officials again decided to invest in the public markets in the early 1930s.[52] This time, though, they were willing to overhaul the entire system, providing citizens with the amenities they had so desperately needed for generations. They believed that with the market overhaul, they had the potential to see threefold profits, thereby justifying their investment in the markets' renovations.[53]

Yet conditions were slightly different in the 1930s from what they had been nearly twenty years earlier. Stronger external pressures from the federal government likely weighed on city officials in New Orleans who had shown a commitment (albeit a wavering one) to meeting national standards. In 1913, when the municipal government had invested in the construction of a new Dryades Market, the first "modern" market in the city, the US Department of Agriculture had just established the Bureau of Markets, whose purpose was to identify model market systems and create standards for their construction and management. The bureau's creation testified to the federal government's belief that modern cities needed modern market halls. Across the country, city governments heeded the call and reinvested in their historic market halls, many of which had been originally constructed in the nineteenth century. The New Orleans local government took note of other municipal governments' renewed interest in their markets and the reasons why those cities invested in their renewal: for the economic and commercial advantage of both city government and local entrepreneurs.[54] New Orleans officials wanted to do the same. Confident in its plan to reboot the city's market system, the local government assessed "The Markets of the Past" to determine the best path forward for the markets of the future.[55]

The municipal government tasked Theodore Grunewald with updating the city's public market system. In order to do so, he visited Washington, DC, Detroit, Baltimore, Philadelphia, New York, and Chicago to observe their systems and devise a plan to bring New Orleans's system up to date.[56] After conducting his fieldwork, Grunewald created a plan that would consolidate the city's public market system. In December 1930, at a community meeting at the Orleans Club, he recommended that instead of operating its remaining twenty-three markets, the city government should focus on operating just three major facilities: a central wholesale-retail market and two retail markets.[57] Essentially, he suggested that the city government completely abandon its traditional market system.[58]

Furthermore, Grunewald also plainly pointed out the city government's detrimental financial interests in the markets. As reported in the *Times-Picayune*, he stated, "The public markets have been political stepchildren. The revenue collected by the city government from the public markets does not go for the rehabilitation or upkeep of the markets. It goes into the general fund and is diverted to other uses."[59] Grunewald wanted to depoliticize the markets. His report, as one might imagine, incited major outcries not only from city residents, but from government officials as well. The next morning, the *Times-Picayune* reported that city officials opposed many of his recommendations, saying they "would not be taken seriously."[60]

Grunewald's proposed plan involved implementing the best national standards in New Orleans. Those standards, however, conflicted with New Orleanians' commitment to local economic culture. That dispute demonstrated the staying power of local custom in a period marked by the popularization of national standards and mass consumer culture. Outspoken New Orleanians, many of them food entrepreneurs, were not willing to give up the culturally significant neighborhood markets that were pivotal to their livelihoods and sense of community. In a public letter published in the *Times-Picayune*, city resident Sam Blum argued that the public markets "are essential in the neighborhood which they are located" and should not be converted into private markets.[61] Common public sentiment was that all of the public markets should be renovated, as previously agreed to by the City Council when it formed the Municipal Markets Commission in the spring of 1930. Otherwise, too many citizens would lose jobs, city residents argued.[62] Secretary of the New Orleans Live Stock Exchange, Major John S. South, pointed out that Grunewald's plan did not take into account the unique cultural makeup of the city: "The people of New Orleans are different from people of the cities Mr. Grunewald visited in making his market study."[63] Acknowledging those sentiments, and agreeing with citizens who spoke out against Grunewald's plan, City Councilman Miles A. Pratt, head of the Municipal Markets Commission, noted that "the council's intention [is] to preserve the public markets system for the public."[64]

Largely ignoring Grunewald's recommendations, the City Council adopted a hybrid plan, one that preserved elements from New Orleans's historic market system while adopting modern amenities and architectural design from national standards of excellence that addressed public health concerns. The council wanted to keep open as many public markets as possible. An initial bond of $1 million from the city government helped initiate the market renovations. The US government's Works Progress Administration (WPA) further funded the completion of the public market renewal project in the late 1930s, illustrating the ever-increasing involvement of the federal government in local affairs.[65] Through projects like the revitalization of the markets, the federal government played a key role in unifying Americans around a common culture and shared sense of American citizenship, while still allowing for sustained local traditions. At the same time, the federal government educated local governing officials about the best public health practices within food distribution to protect American consumers.

A New Modern Market System

After decades of failed promises, the New Orleans city government finally rebuilt or renovated the public markets throughout the 1930s, transforming them into the impressive, cleanly, modern structures that city residents had wanted for generations. The markets were aesthetically stunning, with terrazzo tile, wrought iron detailing, flowerbeds, flag stone patios, fireplaces, etc. They were smaller than the market houses in most other American cities, but that reflected the architectural norms within New Orleans's historic market culture. The first markets opened to the public in 1931, and the last were finished in the late 1930s with the help of the WPA. City officials consolidated the markets' management and regulation under one department, the Department of Public Markets, with Theodore Grunewald as director.[66] With these amenities in place and a centralized department to regulate the markets, the city managed the maintenance and cleanliness of the markets. The department employed a team of janitors who were hired to prevent the markets from transforming back into marginalized spaces.[67] Janitors cleaned a number of market amenities, including stalls, refrigerators, toilets, ceilings, walls, sidewalks, window, doors, and light fixtures. They were in charge of garbage and repair issues related to plumbing, electricity, furniture, and hardware. These maintenance efforts proved crucial in upholding the city's promise to keep disease out of the public markets.

The rebuilt or renovated New Orleans markets became some of the finest examples of public markets in the country and sported functional designs that enabled vendors to safely handle and prepare food for sale. Detailed architectural plans remain for at least seven of the nineteen renovated markets.[68] They were fitted with hot- and cold-water lines and electricity and furnished with the latest refrigeration and ventilation technologies. Stalls were equipped with expansive counters for food preparation as well as large display cases to showcase vendors' wares. Plans for the Dryades Market Building A, for example, indicate that there were twenty-three vendor stalls in total (depicted in figure 2.9).[69] Twenty were designated for the sale of meat and game and three were designated for the sale of fish. Of the twenty-three stalls, eight were equipped with walk-in coolers (6 ft. x 8 ft.) for easy access to refrigerated items. Display cases were twelve feet long in the meat department and six feet long in the fish department. The fish department also had a separate shared preparation area for fishmongers behind the display cases. In a plan for a smaller market, the Suburban Market, there were eleven vendor spaces to vend meat, fish, and vegetables. Six of the stalls, presumably for meat, had refrigerators. The one fish stall had two fish boxes to keep seafood cold. The vegetable stalls, however, did not seem to require refrigeration. The architects also took into consideration the needs of vendors by equipping them not only with refrigeration and display cases but also flexible work environments that could be changed to suit the individual needs of each vendor. Another proposed architectural plan, for example, grouped together layouts of vegetable vendors' stalls in six different markets; a moveable counter at each workstation allowed spatial flexibility.

For New Orleanians, the markets represented the city's advent into the modern age of America and its renewed commitment to public health. City officials promoted the new markets with great gusto, claiming that they "rival[ed] in complete detail and efficiency as well as artistic design any public market in the country."[70] They were the opposite of the unsanitary pavilion markets that had faced a constant encroachment from Louisiana's natural environment and the byproducts of New Orleans's industrial sector. The designs of Sam Stone Jr. & Co., the firm hired by the city government to design the new markets, eradicated all evidence of debris, dust, dank, and disease that had plagued the markets for generations. People who frequented these once-marginalized spaces had to interact with these newly renovated spaces and with each other in different ways. The *feel* of the market was different in that it moved from dilapidated to sterling, from dark to light, from dirt floors to tiled ones as captured in photographs of the interior of St. Roch Market before and after its renovation (figures 2.10 and 2.11).

Aesthetically, the new markets' architecture reflected styles that were not necessarily historically representative of New Orleans but popular throughout the United States at that time, inspired by a variety of distinctive architectural movements in the United States, including Art Deco and Mission Revival. The entrances to the Dryades, Zengel, Ewing, and Suburban Markets, for example, show influence from Art Deco, especially in the handles of their brass doors, which were framed by polished marble (figures 2.12–2.16). The Zengel, Ewing, and Suburban Markets also have an ornate aluminum grille, influenced by the same style, located above the main entrance of the market. By drawing upon the Art Deco aesthetic for the entrances, the architects were also drawing upon the style's underlying themes of opulence and faith in social progress. However, they did so in a way that was not *too* radical. The market designs found a middle path between high modern and traditional architectural design, reflecting the tensions reverberating in New Orleans between its past and future, between antiquation and modernization, and between local and national.[71] The city was not inclined to hover toward one pole, but rather occupied an interstitial space that accommodated that balance.

The Magazine Market, in contrast to the Dryades Market, was modeled heavily after Mission Revival architecture, with its terracotta tiled roof, arched porticos, flagstone porch, and stucco exterior walls (as shown in figures 2.17

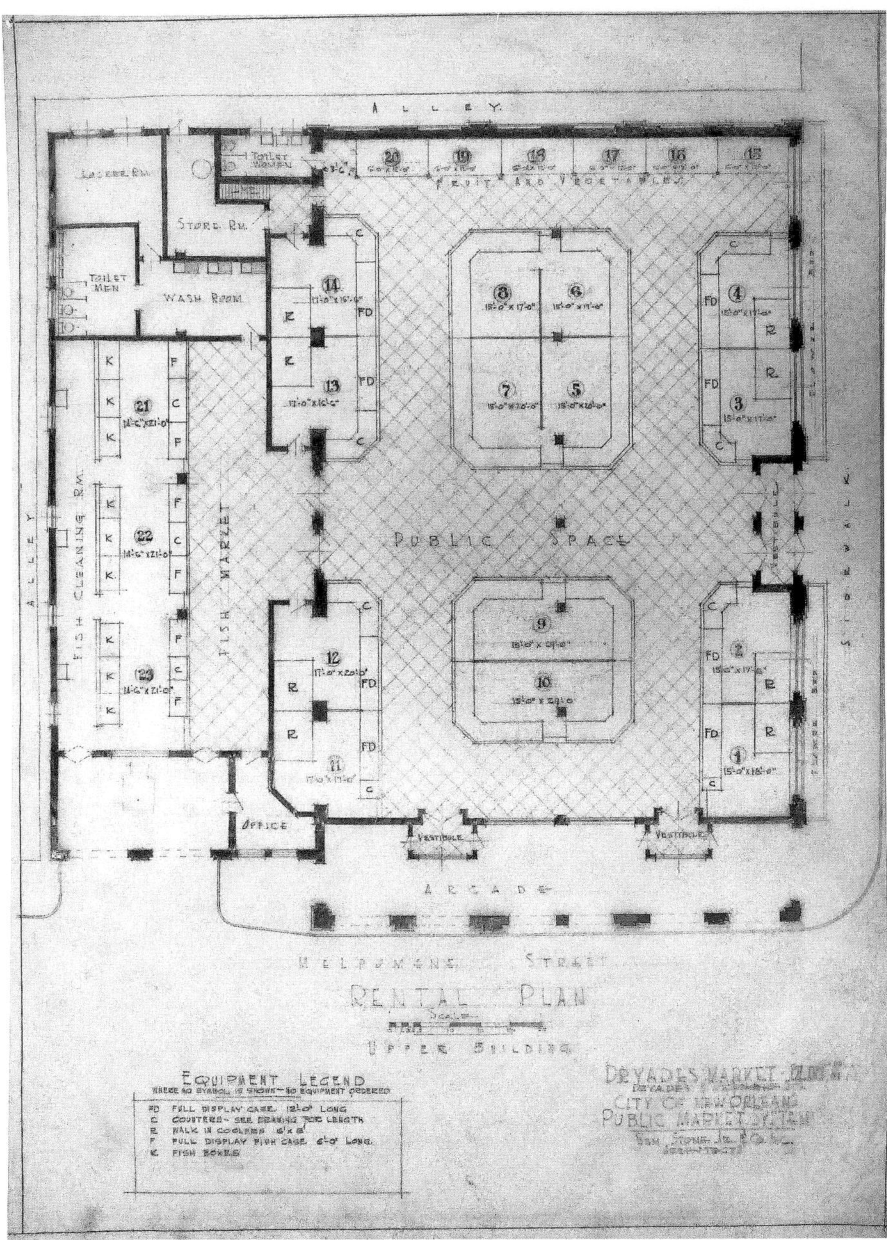

Figure 2.9. Rental Plan of Dryades Market Building A, New Orleans, around 1931. Drawing by Sam Stone Jr. & Co., Inc., Architects. Courtesy of the Southeastern Architectural Archive, Tulane University.

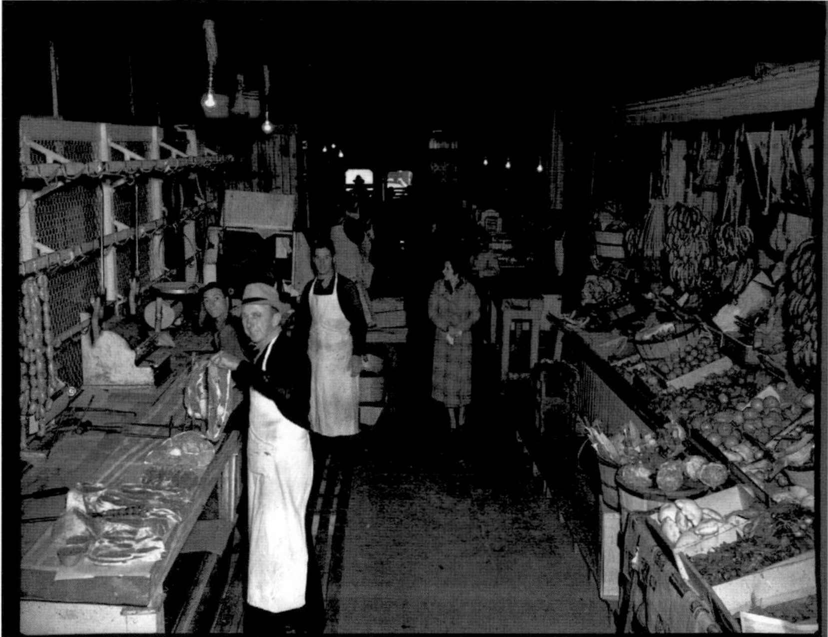

Figure 2.10. Interior of St. Roch Market before WPA renovation, New Orleans, October 1, 1937. Courtesy of the Louisiana Division/City Archives of the New Orleans Public Library.

and 2.18). Whereas Art Deco suggested civic progress through luxuriant metal ornamentation, the humbler Mission Revival design of this building gestured toward nostalgia for the American Southwest, where Mission architecture had historic roots. Similarly, Sam Stone Jr. & Co. architects designed the St. Bernard Market in the Mission Revival style, complete with a copper-embellished copula and wood rosettes on the arcade ceiling of the tower (as shown in figures 2.19 and 2.20). By adopting Mission-style markets, New Orleans embraced an architectural style that romanticized the American Southwest. The city, therefore, contributed to the popularization of an aesthetic form that othered an American region. New Orleans, which had historically been othered by Americans as an "exotic" and "antiquated" city, was now itself participating in that process of othering.

There was also another dynamic at play that merits discussion here. White citizens' views of modernization and their visions of ordered society reflected prevalent notions of racial segregation, during a time period when public spaces like streetcars, schools, pools, parks, and restaurants were thus segregated.[72] For segregationists, the act of consumption, the ritual of the communal

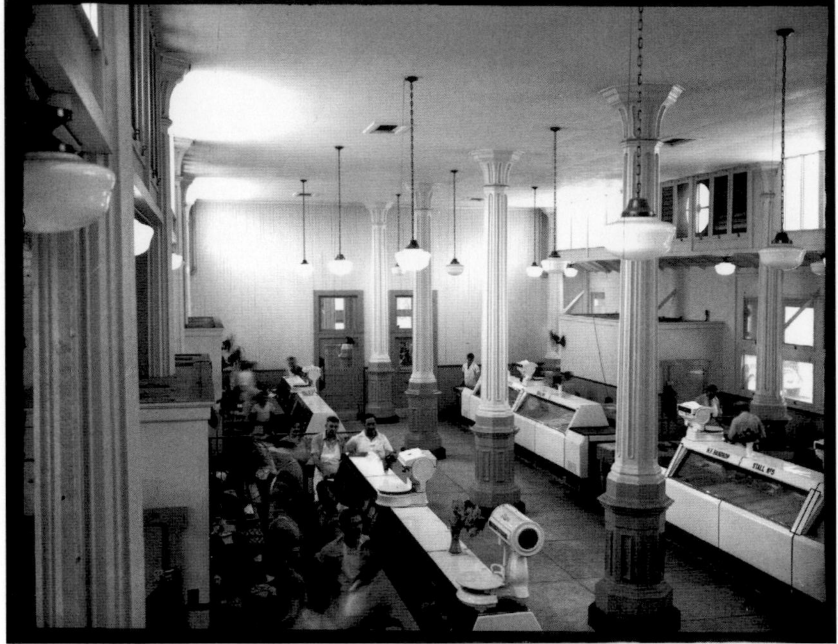

Figure 2.11. Interior of St. Roch Market after WPA renovation, New Orleans, June 31, 1938. Courtesy of the Louisiana Division/City Archives of the New Orleans Public Library.

meal, and the bonds formed over a single table were too intimate and sensual for white and Black diners to share. Still, of the neighborhood markets that we have detailed architectural plans for, the Dryades Market is the only one that shows evidence of spaces designed for racial segregation, specifically in Building B, which had a lunch counter (i.e., a public eatery).[73] The early plans for Building B had four bathrooms that were segregated by race. In the original plans, the white women's and Black women's restrooms were similar sizes and were right next to each other (the same for white and Black men's restrooms). Later, however, the Black men's and Black women's restrooms were placed next to each other, and those two restroom designs were much smaller than those designed for white customers and staff. The lunch counter in the early plans was not specified as a racially segregated space. Over the course of implementing changes into the architectural plans, however, the space became a segregated one.[74]

The final layouts of the Dryades Market drawn up by the Sam Stone Jr. & Co. architects segregated both the lunch counter and the bathrooms in Building B. Because dining was associated with a certain physicality—consumption being considered an intimate bodily activity—the segregationist

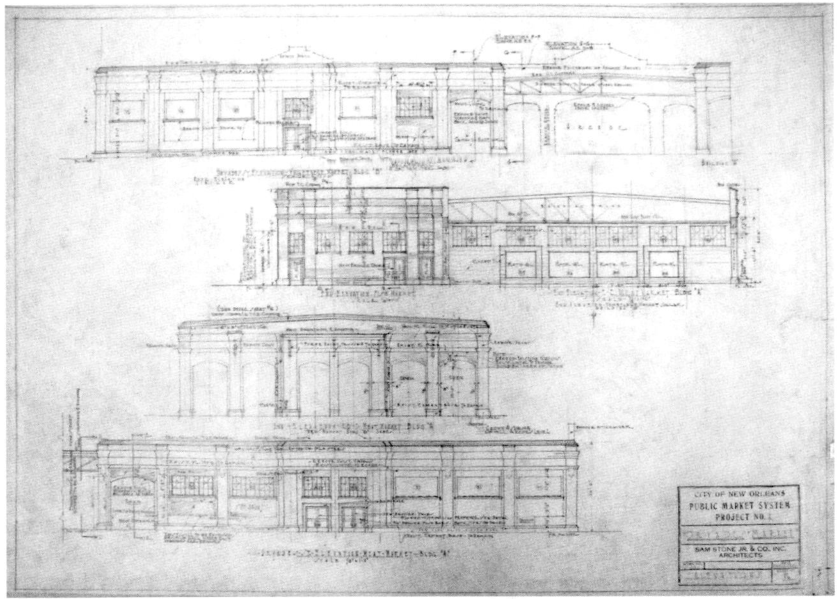

Figure 2.12. Elevations of Dryades Market Building B (top elevation) and Building A (bottom three elevations), New Orleans, May 6, 1931. Drawing by Sam Stone Jr. & Co., Inc., Architects. Courtesy of the Southeastern Architectural Archive, Tulane University.

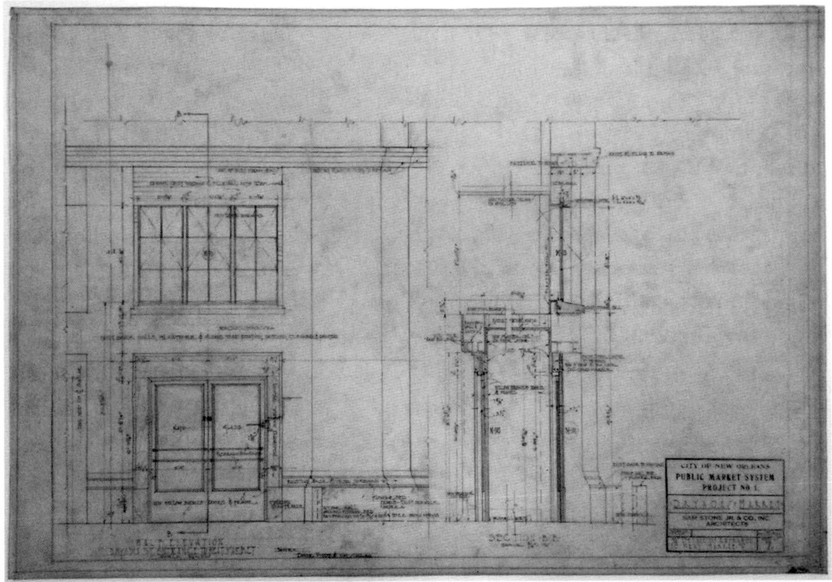

Figure 2.13. Details of Entrance of Dryades Market Building A, New Orleans, around 1931. Drawing by Sam Stone Jr. & Co., Inc., Architects. Courtesy of the Southeastern Architectural Archive, Tulane University.

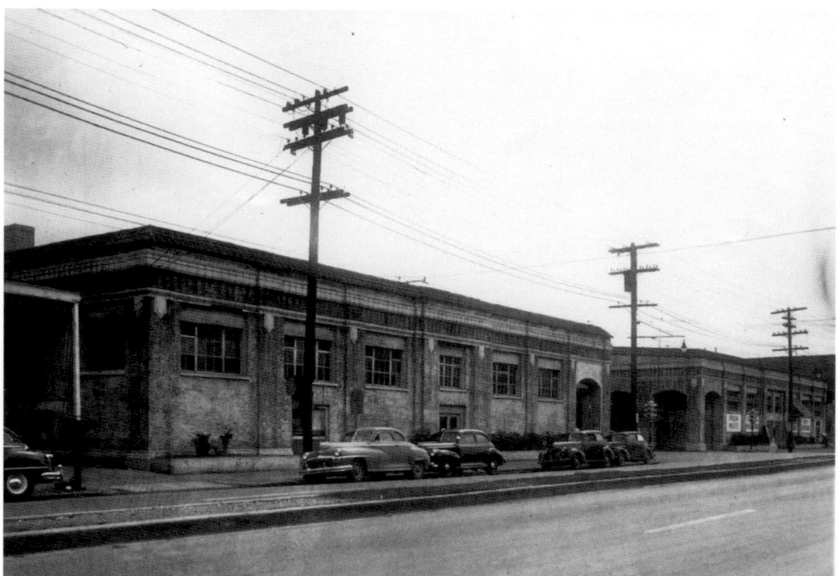

Figure 2.14. Market House. Dryades Market Building A (foreground) and Building B (background), New Orleans, around 1940. Courtesy of the Charles L. Franck Studio Collection at the Historic New Orleans Collection, 1979.325.3960.

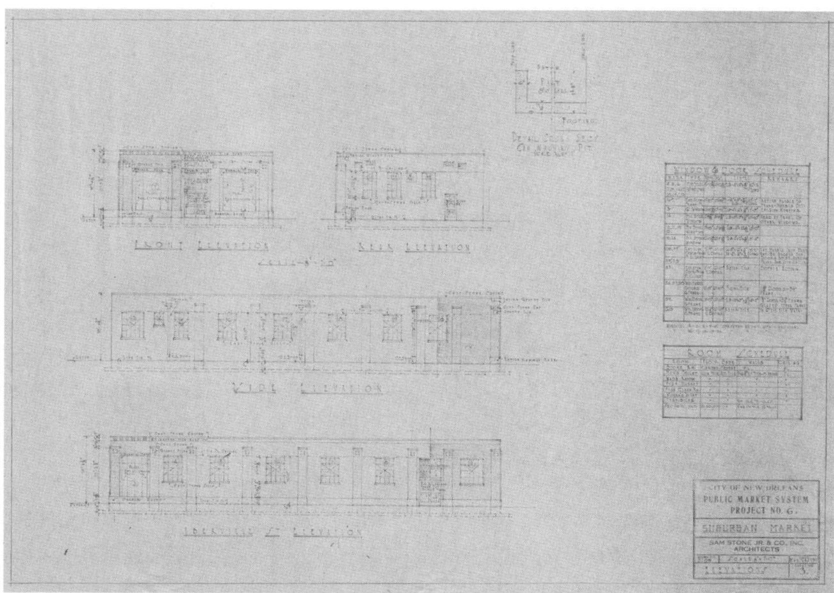

Figure 2.15. Elevations of Ewing Market, New Orleans, 1931. Drawing by Sam Stone Jr. & Co., Inc., Architects. Courtesy of the Louisiana Division/City Archives of the New Orleans Public Library.

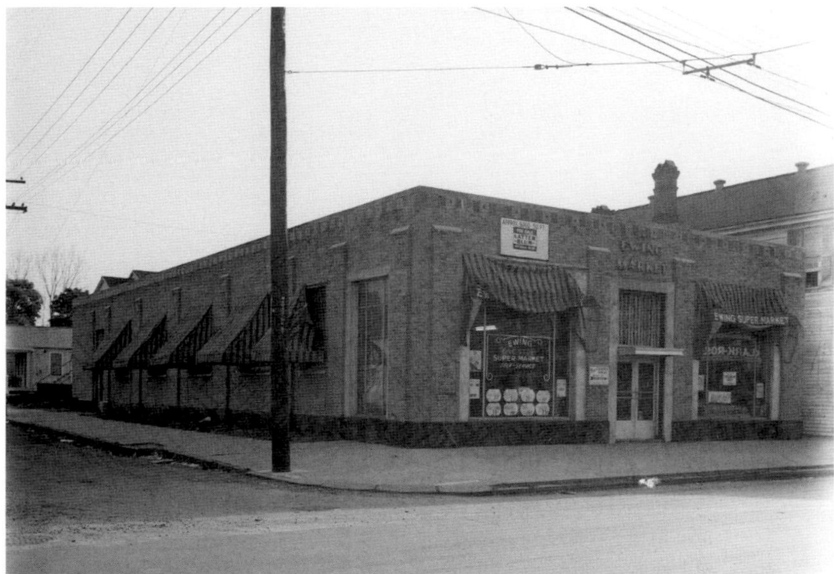

Figure 2.16. Market House. Ewing Market, New Orleans, around 1940. Courtesy of the Charles L. Franck Studio Collection at the Historic New Orleans Collection, 1979.325.3962.

instinct was to racially segregate eateries. The building was also constructed at a time when race relations in the city were increasingly marked with violence and local officials sought to control people's movement and behavior through a seemingly benign medium: architecture. The design of Building B and its impacts on social interactions and cultural formation, however, were anything but benign. Renovations of the markets were also an attempt to control Black and white bodies, limiting their mobility and barring Black people from fully accessing the market's facilities.

The segregationist instinct, however, did not extend to the market stalls themselves, indicating that the purveying and purchasing of foods was not viewed as an intimate bodily act in the same way as eating, digesting, and defecating. Furthermore, segregating the markets would not have been feasible because the city depended too heavily upon the exchange of food between the city's diverse populations. Feeding the city remained a priority even as segregation laws clenched tighter around other food spaces such as restaurants. Consequently, markets—particularly the French Market—remained meeting grounds for the entire city, an occasion to interact with people outside of one's immediate community. Historically, the French Market drew more diverse customers, whereas each neighborhood market was tied more closely to the ethnic, racial, and socioeconomic identity of its particular locality and drew a

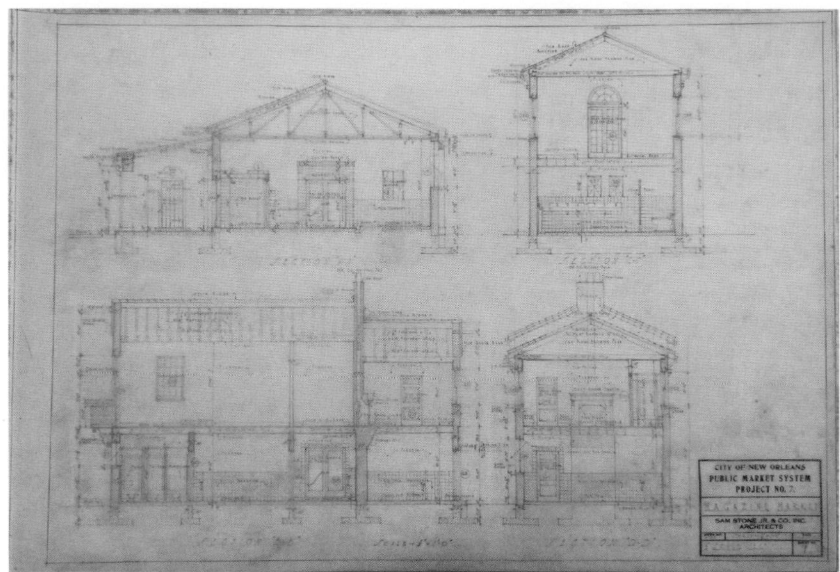

Figure 2.17. Scale Section of Magazine Market, New Orleans, 1931. Drawing by Sam Stone Jr. & Co., Inc., Architects. Courtesy of the Louisiana Division/City Archives of the New Orleans Public Library.

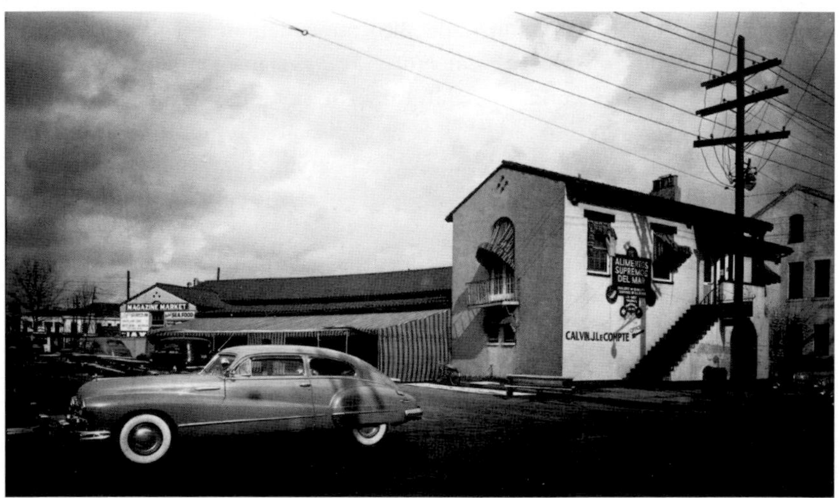

Figure 2.18. Market House. Magazine Market, New Orleans, around 1940. Courtesy of the Charles L. Franck Studio Collection at the Historic New Orleans Collection, 1979.325.3978.

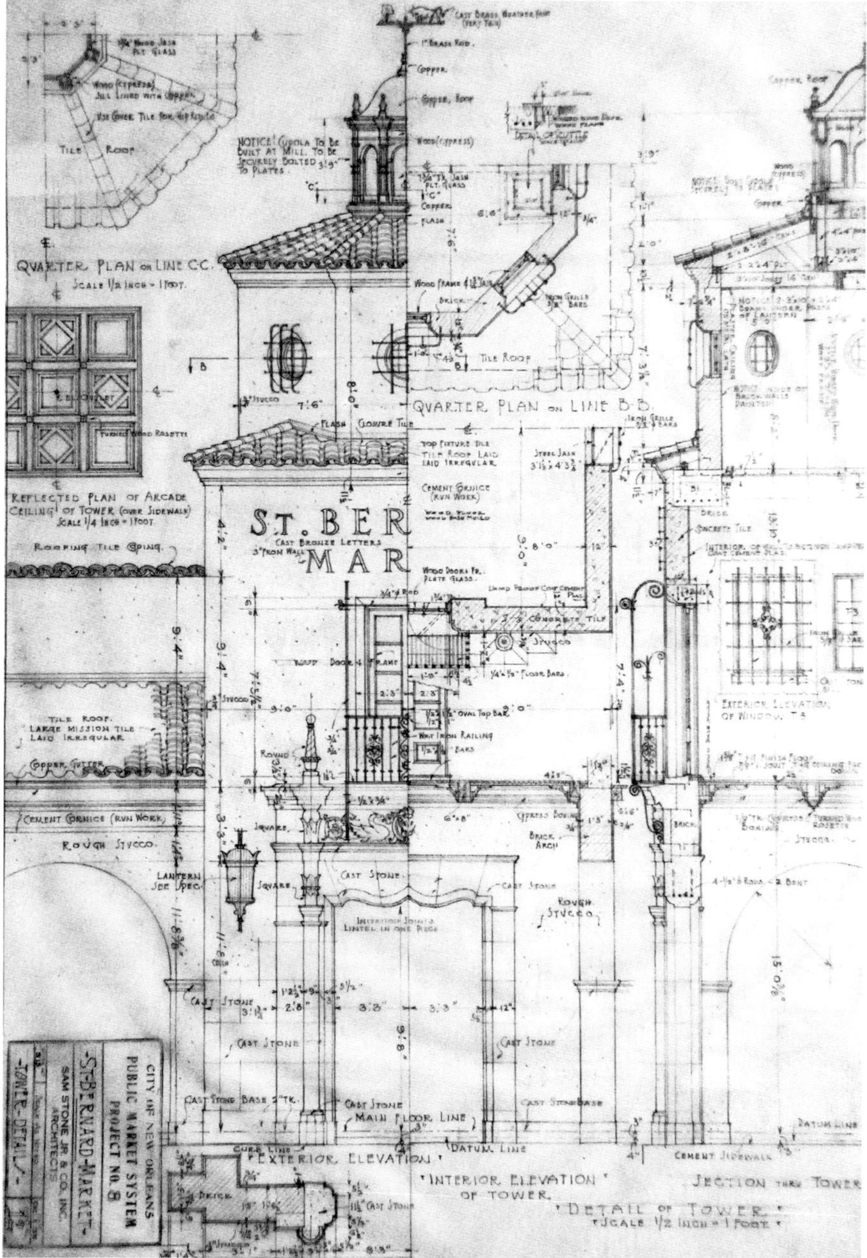

Figure 2.19. Elevation and details of St. Bernard Market, New Orleans, around 1931–1932. Drawing by Sam Stone Jr. & Co., Inc., Architects. Courtesy of the Southeastern Architectural Archive, Tulane University.

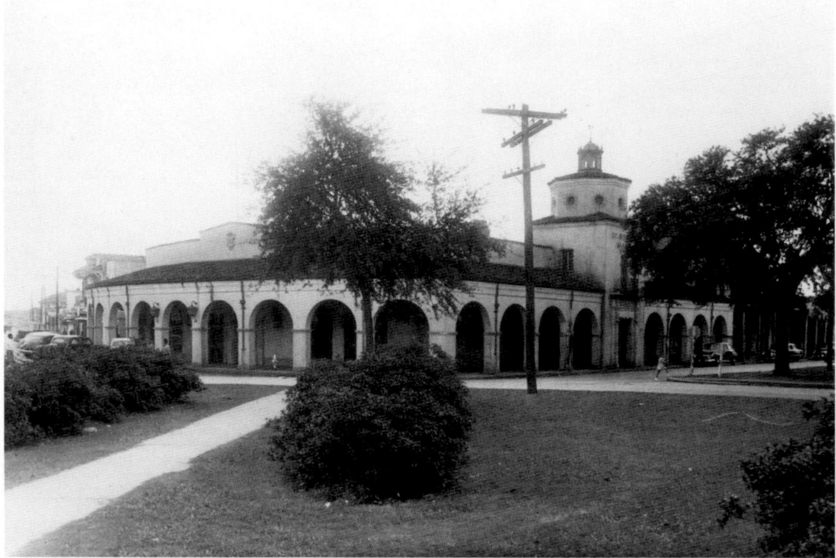

Figure 2.20. Market House. St. Bernard Market, New Orleans, around 1940. Courtesy of the Charles L. Franck Studio Collection at the Historic New Orleans Collection, 1979.325.3987.

more homogenous customer base. New Orleanians tended to live intimate lives, ones that functioned within the bounds of their immediate communities. Shopping at the public markets disrupted that tendency. For example, Millie McClellan Charles, a Black New Orleanian who lived uptown, recalls how she rarely came downtown, "except for with my grandmother who went to the French Market every Saturday."[75] The market broke the cycle of isolation and the instinct to stay within one's neighborhood, introducing Charles to the city's multiethnic, multiracial populace that frequented the market.

Although the interiors of the public markets were not racially segregated, the enclosure of the public markets had unintended consequences that disproportionately affected itinerant vendors and the working poor, many of whom were African American. The markets were enclosed for many reasons, one of the largest being public health—to shut out dangerous insects and vermin and provide electricity, refrigeration, and other amenities to ensure the sale of quality products and to prevent the outbreak of disease. At the same time, the market enclosures also shut out roving vendors and limited the fluid interactions throughout the market that contributed to the city's fusion food culture. Public health concerns about the spread of disease, therefore, were laid on top of structural inequalities that forced many Black people into peddling rather than into the public markets. Unlike the public market vendors working in brand new facilities, street peddlers worked in crowded, muddy streets littered with the refuse of city life. They hawked foods that were exposed to the smoke, dust, and gas emitted from neighboring factories. They had little to no protection from insects, vermin, and disease that ignited so many fears among public market customers. Peddlers did not benefit from the amenities of the public markets. If anything, those renovations damaged their livelihoods in that peddlers often set up near the public markets hoping to catch passersby en route to the market. By erecting walls that impeded the movement of people and goods in and out of the markets, the city government was blocking a crucial, historic connection between street food vendors and public markets. As the municipal government finally modernized the New Orleans's local food economy, the city's street food vendors were getting swept away by that wave of "progress."

A Way Forward

Years of grassroots activism on the part of market vendors and customers brought about drastic changes within New Orleans's local economy. Due in large part to their efforts, the renovated public markets of New Orleans proved to be fitting food distribution centers. Vendors no longer had to fear for their own health as essential workers. They had workspaces fitted with technologies that enabled them to vend food safely while ensuring their own health and safety and that of their customers. Under the improved conditions of the markets, they could rebuild trust with customers who, like the vendors themselves, had endured unsanitary conditions for generations. That trust was crucial to the viability and sustainability of the municipal markets in the years to come. The success of New Orleans's public markets, therefore, relied on incredibly intimate interactions between market vendors, customers, and the local government. Although the federal government played an increasingly important role in communities across the United States, smaller networks of influence remained at the heart of food provisioning in New Orleans, particularly those of women consumer-activists and the vendors themselves.

These vocal citizens along with city officials transformed New Orleans's market system by merging ideologies from the City Beautiful Movement and the Works Progress Administration with new practices in public health and epidemiology. The City Beautiful Movement represented New Orleans's long-standing connections to European culture that are rooted in the city's French and Spanish colonial histories. The Works Progress Administration's involvement reflected the country's understanding and belief that New Orleans's unique culture should be documented, preserved, and celebrated in public architecture. Their convergence in 1930s New Orleans—made possible by the grassroots activism of community members—created a distinct brand of American progressivism articulated in the very structures of urban provisioning: the public markets.

The aesthetic design of the new markets was diverse, ranging from Art Deco to Mission Revival, and signaled city officials' and residents' embrace of an eclectic Americana. These structures nodded to the country's past, while also gesturing to a progressive future. By steering away from traditional architectural styles in New Orleans, and instead embracing ones increasingly popular throughout the United States, the city boldly articulated its overlapping identity as American and Creole. City officials and residents alike understood that the two seemingly incongruent cultures could coexist within the new market houses.

Many of these structures still stand today. Although the buildings no longer function as public markets—and are instead the sites of retail shops, private housing, offices, and even a school gymnasium—their walls stand testament to and memorialize the collective effort of New Orleanians to transform markets that were once a threat to public health into a public amenity that embodied community safety and fit their vision of a better, disease-free future for their city.

Notes

1. "Inviting the Cholera," *Times-Picayune*, July 13, 1884, 11; "The Dryades Market," *Times-Picayune*, July 16, 1884, 2.
2. "Inviting the Cholera," 11.
3. The exact date ranges of a market's construction are difficult to determine because most of the municipal records of the public markets were destroyed. Regularly, the city would approve the construction of a public market, making a public announcement in the local newspapers. The city engineer or private contractors would not break ground until several months later, thus the date of the city government's approval of a market does not necessarily correspond with the date of the market's construction.
4. Donatien Augustin, *A General Digest of the Ordinances and Resolutions of the Corporation of New-Orleans* (New Orleans: J. Bayon, 1831), 2011.
5. Richard Campanella, *Bienville's Dilemma: A Historical Geography of New Orleans* (Lafayette: Center for Louisiana Studies, University of Louisiana at Lafayette, 2008), 174.
6. The city's population consisted of 59,519 white residents, 23,448 enslaved Black residents, and 19,226 free Black residents. Campanella, *Bienville's Dilemma*, 32–33.

7. The remainder of the paragraph draws upon evidence presented in Helen Tangires, *Public Markets and Civic Culture in Nineteenth-Century America* (Baltimore: Johns Hopkins University Press, 2002), 112–14; "Local Intelligence: Open for Inspection," *Philadelphia Inquirer*, April 12, 1859, 1; "The Western Market House," *Press*, April 20, 1859, 2; Agricultural Department of the United States, *Report of the Commissioner of Agriculture for the Year 1870* (Washington, DC: Government Printing Office, 1871), 245.
8. After the Civil War, the city government lost control of its public markets. During Reconstruction, the state legislature of Louisiana took control of them and decided to privatize the markets, which was not uncommon in US cities at the time. The city council of New Orleans regained jurisdiction over the markets in 1878. At that time, the city government continued to lease them out for contracts to private market managers ranging from one month to twenty years. "Sale of the Revenues of the Public Markets for the Year 1879," *Times-Picayune*, December 19, 1878, 6; "City Hall Affairs: Cost of Recorder's Courts—The Market War," *Times-Picayune*, April 28, 1879, 1; "Public and Private Markets," *Times-Picayune*, June 4, 1900, 4; "The Market Question Plainly Set Forth," *Times-Picayune*, January 8, 1901, 9; Beth A. Jacob, "New Orleans' Historic Public Markets: Reviving Neighborhood Landmarks through Adaptive Reuse" (master's thesis, Tulane University, 2012), 63.
9. For examples of said laws restricting the sale of meat, seafood, game, and fresh produce, see: Ordinance 7607, C.S., published May 25, 1893, and Ordinance 312, N.C.S., published October 23, 1900.
10. This number includes quasi-public markets. Quasi-public markets were erected by private entrepreneurs with the permission of the city government. This agreement was memorialized in a contract between the municipal government and a private entrepreneur. The entrepreneur then agreed to pay the city a monthly fee to lease the building and maintain its use as a fresh food market. They did so for a specific period of time, typically twenty to thirty years. Then, the market would become city property. I treat quasi-public markets as public markets because they were still subject to the regulations of the municipal government and operated in a similar way to public ones. As noted in the *Times-Picayune*, "The only difference between [quasi-public markets] and the public markets is that the dues are collected by the contractors, and not by the city." "The 'Quasi' Market Facts and Figures," *Times-Picayune*, January 24, 1901, 7; Robert A. Sauder, "The Origin and Spread of the Public Market System in New Orleans," *Louisiana History* 122, no. 3 (Summer 1981): 288. "Committee of Streets and Landings," *New Orleans Times*, June 14, 1866, 3; "Extension of Poydras Market," *Times-Picayune*, December 14, 1866, 9; "The Pilie Market," *New Orleans Times*, February 1, 1867, 2; "Sale of Revenues of the Public Markets," *Times-Picayune*, May 20, 1876, 1.

11. In fact, New Orleans's system paralleled those of several major European cities that had a central wholesale-retail market and a series of auxiliary markets. Antwerp, for example, had a robust system consisting of twenty-one markets in the early twentieth century. Clyde Lyndon King, "Municipal Markets," *Annals of the American Academy of Political and Social Science* 50 (November 1913): 11.
12. Speech made at Round Table Club, around 1915, Box 1, Folder 985-1-5, 985 City Federation of Clubs Records, Louisiana Research Collection, Howard-Tilton Memorial Library, Tulane University, New Orleans, Louisiana.
13. "Fly Ordinance Again," *Times-Picayune*, March 21, 1911, 10; "Crescent City Notes," *New Advocate*, March 21, 1911, 1; "Fly Ordinance Finds No Favor," *Times-Picayune*, March 24, 1911, 4.
14. "Modern Model Public Markets: Dryades to Be First Rebuilt," *Times-Picayune*, July 31, 1910, 4.
15. See Hardy's work on Great Britain as a case study for the scientific and cultural awareness of germ theory and specifically how it impacted cultures of consumption at the turn of the twentieth century. Anne Hardy, *Salmonella Infections, Networks of Knowledge, and Public Health in Britain, 1880–1975* (Oxford: Oxford University Press, 2015), 69–71.
16. "Fly Ordinance Finds No Favor," 4.
17. "Fly Ordinance Finds No Favor," 4.
18. "Fly Ordinance Finds No Favor," 4.
19. "Fly Ordinance Again," 10.
20. "Fly Ordinance Again," 10.
21. "Modern Model Public Markets," 4.
22. "Modern Model Public Markets," 4; "Budget Committee Matters," *Times-Picayune*, November 12, 1910, 5; "New Dryades Market," *Times-Picayune*, September 8, 1911, 4; "Mayor Behrman Urges Acceptance of Delgado Trade School Bequest. Dryades Market Refrigerator," *Times-Picayune*, March 27, 1912, 5; Notes from State Board of Health 1912, Box 1, Folder 985-1-1, 985 City Federation of Clubs Records, Louisiana Research Collection, Howard-Tilton Memorial Library, Tulane University; Beth A. Jacob, "Seated at the Table: The Southern Food and Beverage Museum's New Home on Oretha Castle Haley Boulevard," *Preservation in Print* 41, no. 8 (November 2014): 22–23.
23. "Views of New Market House That Was Opened Yesterday," *Plain Dealer*, November 5, 1912, 5.
24. "Views of New Market House," 5. For works analyzing the evolution and significance of hospital architecture as it relates to increased understandings of sanitation, cleanliness, and germ theory, see: Jeanne Kisacky, "Germs Are in the Details: Aseptic Design and General Constructors at the Lying-In Hospital of the City of New York, 1897–1901," *Construction History* 28, no. 1 (2013): 83–106; Jeanne Kisacky, *Rise of the Modern Hospital: An Architectural History of Health and*

Healing, 1870–1940 (Pittsburgh: University of Pittsburgh Press, 2017), 56–57; Christine Stevenson, *Medicine and Magnificence: British Hospital and Asylum Architecture, 1660–1815* (New Haven: Yale University Press, 2000); Leslie Topp, *Freedom and the Cage: Modern Architecture and Psychiatry in Central Europe, 1890–1914* (University Park: Penn State University Press, 2017).

25. "Views of New Market House," 5.
26. Notes from State Board of Health 1912, 985 City Federation of Clubs Records.
27. Notes from State Board of Health 1912, 985 City Federation of Clubs Records.
28. The Pure Food and Drug Act of 1906, which prevented the distribution and sale of adulterated or harmful foods as well as drugs, medicine, and liquor in the United States, was a major example of the growing federal presence in communities across the country.
29. Notes from State Board of Health 1912, 985 City Federation of Clubs Records.
30. Report of the Market Committee, Housewives' League Division, City Federation of Clubs, March 24, 1914, Box 1, Folder 985-1-2, 985 City Federation of Clubs Records, Louisiana Research Collection, Howard-Tilton Memorial Library, Tulane University, New Orleans, Louisiana.
31. "Women's Work to Cheapen Living," *Times-Picayune*, January 21, 1914, 13; Report of the Market Committee, 985 City Federation of Clubs Records.
32. "Women's Work to Cheapen Living," *Times-Picayune*, January 21, 1914, 13.
33. "Women's Work," 13.
34. "Women's Work," 13.
35. Report of the Market Committee, 985 City Federation of Clubs Records.
36. Ordinances 1231 CCS and 1232 CCS, respectively.
37. "Markets to be Open at All Hours of Day," *Times-Picayune*, December 16, 1914, 6.
38. Ordinance 1231 CCS.
39. For works that interpret the significance of the color white in architecture, see: Suellen Hoy, "Whiter Than White—and a Glimmer of Green," in *Chasing Dirt: the American Pursuit of Cleanliness* (New York: Oxford University Press, 1995) and Mark Wigley, *White Walls, Designer Dresses: The Fashioning of Modern Architecture* (Cambridge, MA: MIT Press, 1995).
40. Ordinance 1231 CCS
41. Report of the Market Committee, 985 City Federation of Clubs Records.
42. Report of the Market Committee, 985 City Federation of Clubs Records.
43. Report of the Market Committee, 985 City Federation of Clubs Records.
44. Report of the Market Committee, 985 City Federation of Clubs Records.
45. My emphasis added. Report of the Market Committee, 985 City Federation of Clubs Records.
46. "Housewives' League of City Federation of Women' Clubs," *Times-Picayune*, December 27, 1914, 25.
47. Sauder, "The Origin and Spread," 288.

48. "Improving Markets," *Times-Picayune*, January 17, 1914, 5; "Ninth Street Market," *Times-Picayune*, February 5, 1914, 4; United States Bureau of the Census, *Municipal Markets in Cities Having Populations of over 30,000: 1918* (Washington: Government Printing Office, 1919), 29; Sauder, "The Origin and Spread," 288; Jacob, "New Orleans' Historic Public Markets," 68, 139.
49. "Board Now after Keller Market," *Times-Picayune*, January 11, 1920; Sauder, "The Origin and Spread," 289.
50. "Public Market Reorganization Plans Outlined," *Times-Picayune*, December 17, 1930, 14.
51. "Public Market Reorganization," 14.
52. "Grunewald Mart Report Will Be Studies [*sic*] Today," *Times-Picayune*, January 21, 1931, 3.
53. "Grunewald Mart," 3; "Entire Markets Committee Will Conducting Hearing," *Times-Picayune*, January 22, 1931, 1.
54. "Markets Bureau Is Recommended for City System," *Times-Picayune*, December 7, 1930, 20.
55. "Commissioner Pratt, Civic Head and Theodore Grunewald to Talk at Orleans Club," *Times-Picayune*, December 14, 1930, 8.
56. "Grunewald Back from Market Tour," *Times-Picayune*, June 22, 1930, 13.
57. "Public Market Reorganization," 1.
58. "Public Market Reorganization," 1.
59. "Public Market Reorganization," 14.
60. "Plan for Private Markets Lease Denied by Pratt," *Times-Picayune*, December 18, 1930, 3.
61. "Letters from Readers: Public Market Problem," *Times-Picayune*, December 21, 1930, 30.
62. "Public Markets Rehabilitation Plans Opposed," *Times-Picayune*, December 31, 1930, 1.
63. "Grunewald Market Plan Denounced as Menace to Independent Business," *Times-Picayune*, January 6, 1931, 1.
64. "Grunewald Again Urged to Speed Markets Report," *Times-Picayune*, January 7, 1931, 10.
65. "Market Repairs to Be Discussed: Proposal to Seek WPA Funds Will Feature Conference," *Times-Picayune*, October 24, 1935, 4; "Market Repairs Planned by City: Skelly Says Work Depends on Assistance of WPA," *Times-Picayune*, October 26, 1935, 16. For key works on the role of the WPA in funding civic projects in American cities see: United States Work Projects Administration, *Jobs: The WPA Way* (Washington, DC: Works Progress Administration, 1936); David A. Horowitz, "The New Deal and People's Art: Market Planners and Radical Artists," *Oregon Historical Quarterly* 109, no. 2 (Summer 2008): 318–28; Nick

Taylor, *American-Made: The Enduring Legacy of the WPA: When FDR Put the Nation to Work* (New York: Bantam Books, 2008).

66. "Business Starts Today at City's Six New Markets," *Times-Picayune*, June 27, 1932, 13.
67. Department of Public Markets City of New Orleans, Reports of Custodial Worker (St. Bernard Market) around 1948. Box 1, Folder City Board of Health Reports – Private Markets, Department of Public Markets Old Records, Department of Public Markets Miscellaneous Files ca. 1923–1949. The Louisiana Division/City Archives of New Orleans.
68. At the Louisiana Division/City Archives at the New Orleans Public Library and the Southeastern Architectural Archive at Tulane University, I examined the detailed architectural plans created by the Sam Stone Jr. & Co. for the following seven markets: Dryades, Magazine, Suburban, Zengel, Ewing, Jefferson, and Ninth Street Markets.
69. Rental Plan, "Dryades Market – Bldg. A," Sam Stone Jr. & Co., Inc. Architects, Southeastern Architectural Archive, Tulane University, New Orleans, Louisiana; Rental Plan, "Suburban," Sam Stone Jr. & Co., Inc. Architects, Southeastern Architectural Archive, Tulane University, New Orleans, Louisiana.
70. "Business Starts Today," 13.
71. Richard Striner, "Art Deco: Polemics and Synthesis," *Winterthur Portfolio* 25, no. 1 (1990): 21.
72. In the early twentieth century, the patronage of restaurants in the American South was dictated more by class than by race. However, the major customer base were white residents, and mainly men. At that time, it was not customary for women to eat with men, although some establishments were defying those social conventions. Typically, though, public eateries were seen as places where white women could be exposed to what were thought to be inappropriate behaviors, "race mixing," among them. As restaurant culture changed approaching midcentury and women dined with men on a regular basis, the popular belief that public dining should remain segregated stayed in place. Angela Jill Cooley, *To Live and Dine in Dixie* (Athens: University of Georgia Press, 2015), 47.
73. The remainder of the paragraph draws upon the following sources created by Sam Stone Jr. & Co., housed in the Southeastern Architectural Archive: Floor Plan, "Additions to Bldg. 'B' Dryades Market," November 19, 1931, revised December 30, 1931; Floor Plan, "Additions to Bldg. 'B' Dryades Market," January 21, 1932, revised January 21, 1932, revised February 5, 1932; Features, "Showing Addition to & Changes in Floor Layout-Bldg. – 'B,'" June 20, 1931; Floor Plan, "Additions to Bldg. 'B' Dryades Market," January 21, 1932. Revised March 2, 1932 and March 9, 1932, Sam Stone Jr. & Co., Inc. Architects, Southeastern Architectural Archive, Tulane University, New Orleans, Louisiana.

74. It is possible that the early plan for the lunch counter was also one that had a segregated lunch counter. The early plan is minimal; there are no markings designating spaces by race. However, judging upon changes made to the public restrooms based on race, I determined that a similar attempt to keep white and Black people separate in public spaces is reflected in the lunch counter.
75. Quoted in Lakisha Michelle Simmons, *Crescent City Girls: The Lives of Young Black Women in Segregated New Orleans* (Chapel Hill: University of North Carolina Press, 2015), 31.

Archival sources

New Orleans, Louisiana
- Louisiana Division/City Archives & Special Collections, New Orleans Public Library
  - New Orleans (La.) Dept. of Public Markets Records
  - Building Plans Records
- Louisiana Research Collection, Tulane University
  - Market Committee Records, 1913–1916 (Manuscript Collection 985)
- Southeastern Architectural Archive, Tulane University
  - Sam Stone Jr. Office Records (Collection 85)

Newspapers

New Orleans, Louisiana, USA
- *Times-Picayune*
- *New Orleans Times*
- *New Advocate*
- *Plain Dealer*

Philadelphia, Pennsylvania, USA
- *Philadelphia Inquirer*
- *Press*

Bibliography

Agriculture Department of the United States. *Report of the Commissioner of Agriculture for the Year 1870.* Washington, DC: Government Printing Office, 1871.

Augustin, Donatien. *A General Digest of the Ordinances and Resolutions of the Corporation of New-Orleans.* New Orleans: Printed by J. Bayon, 1831.

Campanella, Richard. *Bienville's Dilemma: A Historical Geography of New Orleans.* Lafayette: University of Louisiana at Lafayette, 2008.

Cooley, Angela Jill. *To Live and Dine in Dixie: The Evolution of Urban Food Culture in the Jim Crow South.* Athens: The University of Georgia Press, 2015.

Hardy, Anne. *Salmonella Infections, Networks of Knowledge, and Public Health in Britain, 1880–1975.* Oxford: Oxford University Press, 2015.

Horowitz, David A. "The New Deal and People's Art: Market Planners and Radical Artists." *Oregon Historical Quarterly* 109, no. 2 (2008): 318–28.

Hoy, Suellen. "Whiter Than White—and a Glimmer of Green," in *Chasing Dirt: The American Pursuit of Cleanliness*, 151–78. New York: Oxford University Press, 1995.

Jacob, Beth A. "New Orleans' Historic Public Markets: Reviving Neighborhood Landmarks through Adaptive Reuse." Master's thesis, Tulane University, 2012.

Jacob, Beth A. "Seated at the Table: The Southern Food and Beverage Museum's New Home on Oretha Castle Haley Boulevard." *Preservation in Print* 41, no. 8 (November 2014): 22–23.

King, Clyde Lyndon. "Municipal Markets." *Annals of the American Academy of Political and Social Science* 50, no. 1 (1913): 102–17.

Kisacky, Jeanne. "Germs Are in the Details: Aseptic Design and General Constructors at the Lying-In Hospital of the City of New York, 1897–1901." *Construction History* 28, no. 1 (2013): 83–106.

———. *Rise of the Modern Hospital: An Architectural History of Health and Healing, 1870–1940.* Pittsburgh: University of Pittsburgh Press, 2017.

Sauder, Robert A. "The Origin and Spread of the Public Market System in New Orleans." *Journal of the Louisiana History* 22, no. 3 (1981): 281–97.

Simmons, LaKisha Michelle. *Crescent City Girls: The Lives of Young Black Women in Segregated New Orleans.* Chapel Hill: University of North Carolina, 2015.

Stevenson, Christine. *Medicine and Magnificence: British Hospital and Asylum Architecture, 1660–1815.* New Haven: Yale University Press, 2000.

Tangires, Helen. *Public Markets and Civic Culture in Nineteenth-Century America.* Baltimore: Johns Hopkins University Press, 2003.

Taylor, Nick. *American-Made: The Enduring Legacy of the WPA: When FDR Put the Nation to Work.* New York: Bantam, 2008.

Topp, Leslie. *Freedom and the Cage: Modern Architecture and Psychiatry in Central Europe, 1890–1914.* University Park: Penn State University Press, 2017.

United States Bureau of the Census. *Municipal Markets in Cities Having a Population of over 30,000: 1918.* Washington, DC: Government Printing Office, 1918.

United States Works Progress Administration. *Jobs: The WPA Way.* Washington, DC: Works Progress Administration, 1936.

Wigley, Mark, *White Walls, Designer Dresses: The Fashioning of Modern Architecture* Cambridge, MA: MIT Press, 1995.

CHAPTER 3

THE CRAWFORD MARKET

Sanitary Problems, Engineered Solutions, and Symbolic Gestures in Late Nineteenth-Century Bombay

Daniel Williamson

The Crawford Market is one of the sights of Bombay. Outside, with its steep roofs, belfry and projecting eaves, it has a rather English Gothic look, but inside the scene is entirely oriental, crowded with natives in all sorts of colours, moving among fish, fruit, grain, and provisions of all kinds, buying and selling amid a clamour of tongues—a busy scene of colour and variety, in a symphony of smells, dominated by that of the smoke of joss-sticks kept burning at some of the stalls as well as a suspicion of opium, which pervades all the native quarters in Indian cities.

—Walter Crane, *Indian Impressions*, 1907

[The Crawford Market] stands on a corner site, and like some English country market buildings it has a prominent clock tower crowned by a cupola, with a gable to each frontage and open timber galleries beneath ... A visit to the markets is one of the most compelling experiences in India. The noise is deadening, the crowd suffocating and the senses are assaulted by such an array of sights and smells that the unprepared visitor fresh from the order and calm of a European city emerges reeling.

—Philip Davies, *Splendours of the Raj*, 1985[1]

Introduction

Nearly eighty years separate the two commentators above, yet the treatment of their subject, the Arthur Crawford Market in Bombay (renamed the Mahatma Jyotiba Phule Market and Mumbai respectively), is nearly identical (figures 3.1 and 3.2).[2] Both Walter Crane and Philip Davies present the Crawford Market, designed and built between 1866 and 1869, as a contradictory building. They do so by contrasting the staid, English Gothic appearance of the exterior, expressed through the building's style, with the "oriental" activity of the people

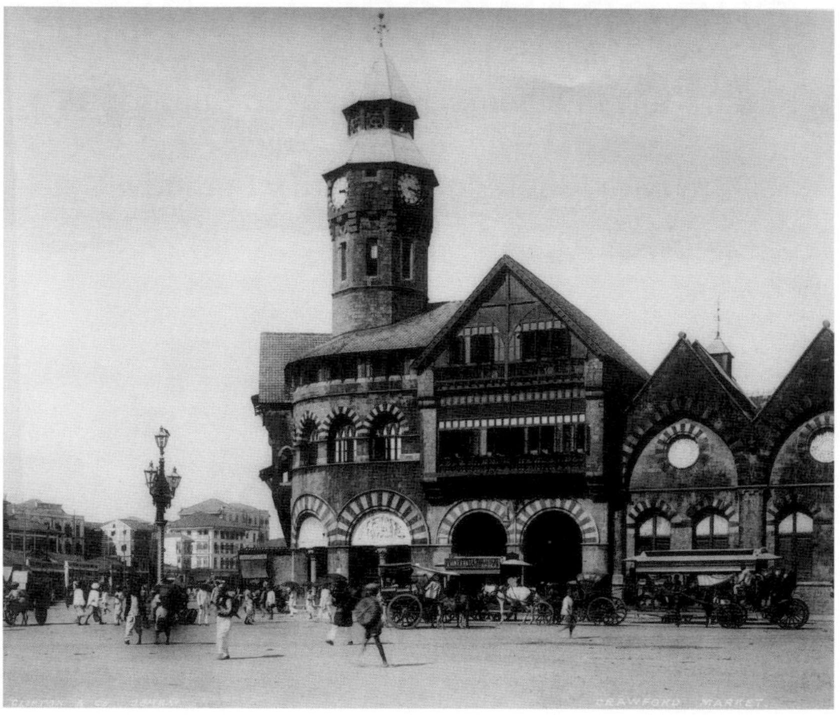

Figure 3.1. Crawford Market, Mumbai, India, ca. 1880. Photograph by Clifton & Company. 28 x 23.5 cm. Private collection.

in the interior, which they characterize as an energetic sea of life that "assaults" the senses. In the commentators' eyes, the building becomes a symbol of the contradictions of British colonial rule: a genteel, taming structure constraining an interior whose chaotic bustle is emblematic of what Anand Yang has called the "'Oriental Market,' that exoticized Other place of Western imagination."[3] The authors' delight in the thrill of spectacle and their reliance on a readymade binary epistemic framework of East and West prevents them from interrogating this contradiction any further. Moreover, their focus on reading the crowd through an Orientalist lens obscured the fact that their observations were built on a common, long pedigreed trope in travelogues that paint markets as scenes of great diversity, spectacle, and cacophony.[4] Nevertheless, their observations raise important questions about the purpose of the market hall and its role in Colonial Bombay's urban development. To move beyond this framework requires placing the building in its historical context, both in terms of evolving urban policies in British colonial cities and the broader history of the market hall as a building type.

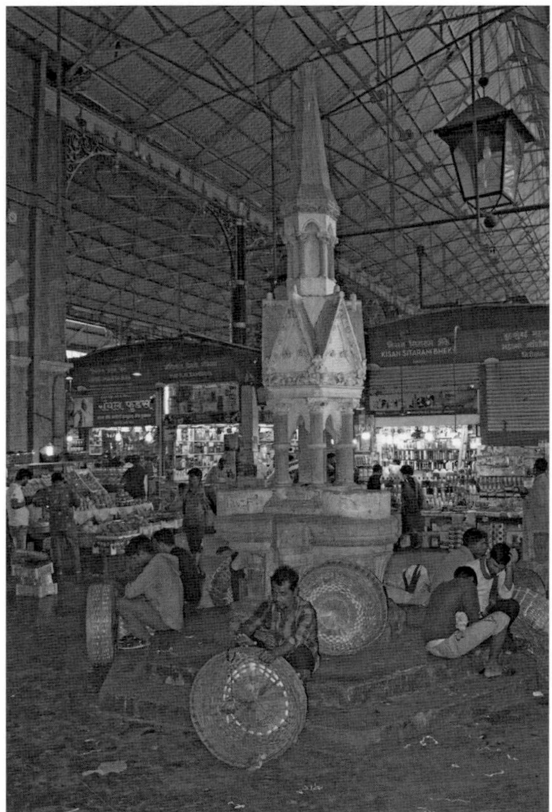

Figure 3.2. Crawford Market interior with fountain donated by Cowasji Jehangir Readymoney in foreground and ironwork and shed roof in background. Photograph by author, 2019.

A distinction between the inside and outside of the market hall was acknowledged by the three figures primarily responsible for the building, the Bombay municipal commissioner Arthur Crawford, municipal engineer Russell Aitken, and architect William Emerson. For them, however, this distinction centered on aesthetics and engineering, the picturesque stone façade and decorative Gothic ironwork of the street-facing markets giving way to rationally organized interiors pragmatically shaded by iron sheds.[5] Indeed, later descriptions focused on a chaotic and disorienting interior would have disappointed them, as their purpose had been to subject shoppers and vendors to a moral and sanitary order. As Russell Aitken claimed about market reforms in Bombay in 1867, "the order and cleanliness which … prevails when compared with the former inconvenient markets must exercise a powerful moral effect for good on the minds of the native community frequenting them."[6]

In the late nineteenth century, English reformers conflated good sanitary habits with moral virtues. English market halls were presented by city administrators not just as a mechanism to improve hygiene but as a means to reform the behavior of the working class.[7] In the colonial context, blurring the distinction between sanitary and moral reform became a justification for Britain's authoritarian hegemony. In the name of addressing serious sanitary issues in the city, the proposed reforms expanded British surveillance and regulation of Indigenous shoppers and shopkeepers. Moreover, the markets were designed to present the solutions to the moral and sanitary degradation of the city's populace as uniquely arising from an assumed British technological and cultural superiority. Yet British morality was not the only kind accommodated in the markets' designs. Hindu and Muslim moral attitudes toward food and pollution required Crawford, Russell, and Emerson to consult a variety of different religious and community leaders of various factions in Bombay as they planned their designs.

The supposed contradiction between European building and Indian user that many European observers noted when visiting the markets concealed more fundamental ones in the project that threatened to undermine the clear connection between sanitary improvement and British rule. These included the contradiction between British technophilia and medieval nostalgia, which further manifested in the debates about the proper role of architect and engineer in the design process. Another contradiction emerged between the market hall as a device to reform the moral character of Indian subjects, and colonial buildings as a staging of the character of Indian subjects as unchanging and therefore subject to perpetual British administration.[8]

These contradictions resulted in part from the inability of Crawford, Aitken, and Emerson to distinguish clearly between practical solutions to specific sanitary problems in their design and theatrical and symbolic gestures toward sanitary practices, regardless of their actual effectiveness. This blurring mirrored the blurring between sanitary and moral reform, because if sanitation was a moral problem, then solutions required an architecture of persuasion as much as an architecture of hygiene. Further, the moral message that the market projected could not be controlled by the authorities responsible for the reforms. Instead, they became diffuse as different stakeholders in Bombay's food supply read different meanings into the building. While wealthy Indian businessmen, particularly those among the Parsi community, lent their support to the project as a means of civic boosterism, others questioned whether the building's extravagant gestures were the most efficient means to address sanitary concerns. These included British and Indian taxpayers who balked at the market's costs and butchers and shopkeepers who saw the encroaching economic and social control exerted by the British primarily in terms of power and resistance.

Urban and Sanitary Reform in Bombay after 1857

The Crawford Market was the visually prominent architectural synecdoche of a broader project of sanitary reform in Bombay initiated by the city's newly established municipal corporation in 1865.[9] Named for the municipal commissioner who planned the project, placed in a prominent new location adjacent to other new administrative buildings, and dressed in lavish Gothic architectural ornament, the market would serve as the visual representation of a series of reforms that were less visible and humbler in their architectural pretension. These sanitary reform projects ranged from large-scale drainage projects to the building of new latrines. They also included less lavishly designed, pragmatic market reforms in less prominent parts of the city, and the criminalization of unsanitary practices, with harsh punishments including incarceration for the sale of spoiled meats.[10]

Sanitary reform itself was part of a larger transformation of Bombay in the 1860s that was spurred by two intertwined events: the establishment of Crown rule and the cotton boom. The 1857 Sepoy Rebellion and its suppression led the British to transfer the management of its Indian colonies from the British East India Company to the British Crown. Along with this change came a much more expansive bureaucracy that increased the data collection and surveillance of the local populace.

While the goal of all this data was more efficient management of the colonial subjects, the Sepoy Rebellion also led many colonial policy makers to conclude that Indians were culturally and racially opposed to British culture in a timeless and unchanging way.[11] Arthur Crawford, Bombay's municipal commissioner, wrote a memoir of his time as an Indian police official in which he referred ominously to the "darker side of Indian character," which was offset by "good traits; such as unbounded hospitality, kindliness of disposition, the rugged fidelity of the servant to his master."[12] For Crawford, this supposed essential character served as justification for the British administration of India. At the same time, without noticing any contradiction, Crawford posited that "I trust I may have sown the need for incessant watchfulness in the administration of a conglomeration of nationalities, creeds and castes such as exist in India."[13] Thus, for him, Indian subjects could be reduced to an essential character, whose qualities (like fidelity) implicitly justified British rule. Yet simultaneously, India contained such an admixture of distinctive communities that British rule was necessary to maintain peace and order. Such a paternalistic attitude undergirded Crawford's projects as municipal commissioner, particularly the Crawford Market.

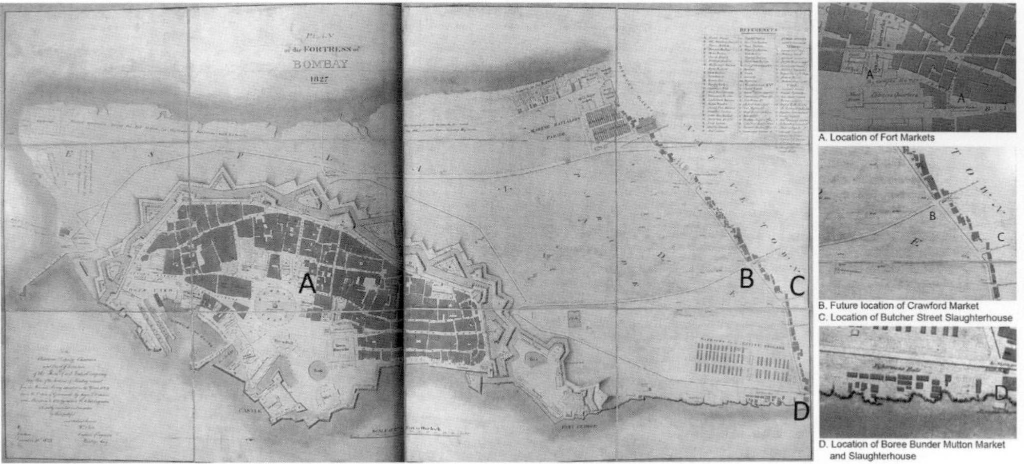

Figure 3.3. Plan of the Fortress of Bombay, 1827. William A. Tate. 73.7 x 132.1 cm. © The British Library Board, IOR/X/2642.

In Bombay, the need to house Britain's expanding administrative bureaucracy and to exert more symbolic authority over the Indian populace led Bartle Frere, the governor of the Bombay Presidency, to call for a major building campaign and reordering of the city. Prior to the 1860s, the British conceived of central Bombay as divided into the original British settlement in the Fort and a densely packed "Native Town," with the walls of the Fort and a green esplanade acting as a buffer between them (figure 3.3).[14] Frere removed the walls of the Fort and erected the new administrative core on the Esplanade, which was housed in buildings designed in the Gothic Revival style. These projects and others were largely funded through the taxes and charitable donations of the city's wealthiest businessmen, English and Indian alike, who were experiencing unprecedented profits due to a cotton boom in Bombay, spurred by the US Civil War.[15]

As the British expanded the administrative state, sanitation became a category for controlling bodies and justifying rule. Concern about sanitation in English cities had grown steadily since the 1840s, when Edwin Chadwick called attention to the unhygienic condition of much of Britain's working population. His assessment relied on a theory of disease that focused on miasmas or the stench emitted by stagnant waters and rotting meats.[16] Sanitary zeal initially arrived in India through concern about British troops but soon spread to urban environments.[17] In Bombay, an initial, blistering sanitary report was prepared in 1855 by Henry Conybeare, who explicitly referenced the work of Chadwick in London.[18] Conybeare's report dealt primarily with the water

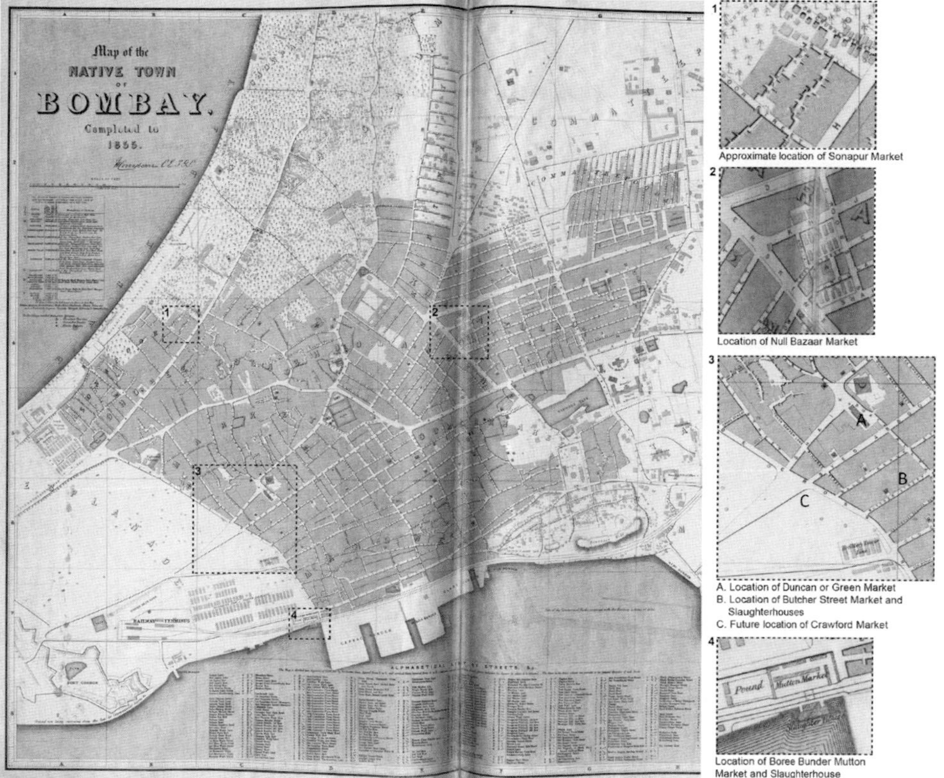

Figure 3.4. *Map of the Native Town of Bombay Completed to 1855.* Henry Conybeare. 84 x 102 cm. Library of Congress. https://lccn.loc.gov/2015588078.

supply, but it was expanded on by Andrew Leith, a local doctor, in his 1864 *Report on the Sanitary State of the Island of Bombay*. Leith's forty-six-page report detailed sanitary problems that ranged from increased disease due to overcrowding, inadequate drainage in most of the city, dangerously unstable houses, and inadequate infrastructure to handle human waste. Leith too owed a debt to Chadwick's theories of miasmas, citing "aqueous vapour" as contributing to disease and focusing his ire at unsanitary conditions on their stench.[19]

Leith found one source of disease in Bombay's markets, particularly those attached to slaughterhouses.[20] The latter were primarily divided between those for oxen on Butcher Street and one for sheep and goats on the Esplanade (figure 3.4). The Esplanade slaughterhouse particularly met Leith's ire, as it was "[A] shed built on stakes just below the highwater-mark on the foreshore of the harbor, and the blood and offal fall upon the mud. … The operations of the butcher are imperfectly screened from public view, and the offensive putrid mud around cannot but be very unwholesome."[21] Sir Dinshaw E. Wacha, a wealthy Parsi citizen of Bombay who was educated in England and became an early member of the Indian National Congress, recalled in his memoirs that the slaughterhouses and their adjacent markets were "bloody, reeking, stinking, abominable … the very sight of [them] used to give us a shock."[22] For both Leith and Wacha, stench was the primary denotation of unsanitary conditions. At the same time, in their focus on the unsightliness of animal slaughter, they blurred the distinction between sanitary concerns and concerns about propriety. Their attitudes reflected an emerging consensus about urban organization that certain necessary but disturbing activities should be pushed to more marginal parts of the city, out of the sight of middle and upper classes.

The immediate result of Leith's report was the establishment of the Municipal Corporation of Bombay, a body with the power to levy taxes, borrow money, and enact the sweeping measures thought necessary for sanitary reform.[23] One of the corporation's first acts was to appoint Arthur Crawford, then a thirty-year-old police officer, as the city's first commissioner. Dinshaw Wacha saw him as "our local Haussmann" to whom "Bombay owes a deep debt of gratitude … for all he accomplished," but whose "finances were in a condition of chronic embarrassment."[24] Crawford's tenure as commissioner would end in scandal in 1871, when his excessive taxation and expenditures led to a revolt by the city's taxpayers, spearheaded by James A. Forbes and prominent businessmen like Sorabji Shahpurji Bengalee and backed by the editorial page of the *Times of India*. The Crawford Market became emblematic of Crawford's excesses. As an anonymous petitioner who supported Crawford complained in 1871, "It is not more than a year or two ago since the Bench requested Mr. Crawford to allow his name to be applied to the new markets … and yet you now say, 'We cannot afford to have this man any longer. We do not want either Mr. Crawford or his markets any longer' we will have a new regime."[25]

Market Reform under Crawford

From Crawford's perspective, the sanitary improvement of Bombay's markets focused on several intertwined reforms: reduction of overcrowding through larger allocations of land for markets, the decoupling of meat markets from the slaughterhouses, the use of iron sheds to better protect from weather and to increase ventilation, the use of stone paving to reduce muck and mud, and greater observational control by market authorities.[26] As Crawford explained, he "found on taking charge in July 1865" that "the so-called public markets of Bombay [were] places the very sight of which was loathsome and disgusting and to which no one would resort if he could help it. It seemed to me that reform of the Markets and Slaughterhouses was the most pressing duty to be undertaken."[27] At the same time, secondary concerns become clear in his municipal reports. One was the desire to generate more revenue by taxing the shopkeepers and butchers for use of the new facilities. The other was the need to remove certain slaughterhouses and markets that were in the way of the improvements being undertaken by the Bombay Presidency as part of its rampart removal plans.[28]

Andrew Leith had identified ten public markets in the city.[29] In addition to those attached to the city's main slaughterhouses, four others were distributed throughout "Native Town" and four served the wealthy Indian merchants and British residents of the Fort area. Each market's operations and goods on sale were adapted to cater to the particular community it served. The two major meat markets and slaughterhouses were adjacent to predominantly Muslim neighborhoods. A small market in Sorunpur, a neighborhood of Christians and Chinese immigrants, was the only market in the city that sold pork (figure 3.4).[30] The main market in the Fort was located near the Bombay Mint adjacent to an open public square (figure 3.3). Compared to the other markets in the city, it was "clean and well kept," at least according to the wealthy merchants who lived nearby, and it was one of the few that had a market officer maintaining order.[31] For Dinshaw Wacha, who found the sights and smells of the slaughterhouses so disturbing, this was "the only market approaching to the rudimentary conception of a market of the mid-Victorian age."[32]

The most popular market, meant to cater to the largest cross-section of the city's population, was the Duncan, or Green, market located near the Jama Masjid on Sheikh Memon Street in "Native Town" (figure 3.3). Sheikh Memon Street was the city's major shopping district, lined with cloth markets and the houses of prominent cloth and jewelry merchants. While it was established in the 1770s as a private market known as Mahomed's market, Jonathan Duncan, governor of Bombay, took over its rebuilding after it burned down in the early nineteenth century. Afterwards, Duncan set limits on the goods sold to vegetables, fruits, and flowers and decreed that the government would collect no revenue from the vendors.[33] Given its location in the central shopping district of "Native Town," the limit to fruits and vegetables ensured that it would be frequented by all communities. This placed a tremendous strain on the market, as it served one of the densest sections of the city on a relatively small lot. Crawford described the market as "a few ranges of low-tiled open sheds, indifferently paved and drained, very crowded and hot, and dirty to a degree, containing about 1300 square yards."[34]

Crawford's original plan was to close the Duncan market, slaughterhouse markets, and the markets in the Fort area and combine all of them into a new, fifty-five-thousand-square-foot site on the Esplanade at the entrance to Sheikh

Memon Street (figure 3.4). The site was two hundred meters from the Jama Masjid and the Duncan market in "Native Town" and adjacent to "Frere Town," the emerging administrative center on the former esplanade. In petitioning the Bombay Presidency for the land, Crawford used the pretext that the Fort markets were in the way of a new boulevard constructed as part of Frere's rampart removal scheme. Thus, the elites in the Fort, or at the very least their servants, would now more freely mix with other communities in a single central market. The combination of several community markets into a central hall was often justified in market halls back in England precisely as a means to "morally improve" the working classes by having them mix with middle and upper classes.[35] However, on finding that markets would be moved outside of their neighborhood, the citizens of the Fort protested, led by the Parsi newspaper publisher K. N. Kabraji, forcing Crawford to rebuild the Fort markets a stone's throw from their old site with simple improvements, including iron sheds and new stone flagging, all imported from England.[36]

Having failed to bring the Fort markets into the central one, Crawford nevertheless persevered in closing the slaughterhouse markets and Duncan market in order to bring them into his new central market hall. Symbolically and practically, then, removing them from their locations in "Native Town," where the massive flow of people and the less-ordered urban fabric denied control and oversight, and relocating them onto the Esplanade, where government administrative buildings were being planned, allowed a mostly British government to claim tighter control of the markets. In placing the central market hall near the new government buildings Crawford was, as he put it, "bound, as well for the appearance of the town as by the government grant, to erect a building with some architectural pretensions."[37] Given the less-visible nature of most of the city's other sanitary reforms, the market hall would now serve as the most prominent expression of sanitary reform in the city.

In casting sanitary reform as culturally British, Crawford came to believe that the solution to market reform in Bombay could be found in the city market halls emerging as a new building type in England. Thus, in the spring of 1866, he advertised a competition for the design of the Bombay market in London, with notices appearing in the *Builder* and the *Building News*.[38] The winner was a London-based architect named John Norton, who had not yet designed any market halls but had rather built a career designing churches and country houses, including one for a maharajah in Suffolk.[39] In August 1866 the top three designs were sent to Bombay with William Emerson, an architect from the High Victorian Gothic architect William Burges's office, who would take over the design of the markets after the proposals from England were rejected. Emerson was traveling to Bombay to act as supervising architect for the Sir Jamsetjee Jeejeebhoy School of Art, designed by Burges as one of the new projects in "Frere Town" funded by its namesake, the most prominent Parsi businessmen in Bombay.[40] Emerson would go on to design several buildings in India, including the Victoria Memorial in Calcutta, and would eventually serve as president of the Royal Institute of British Architects.[41]

The idea that an English architect who had never been to India would be unsuited to understanding the climatic and cultural realities of Bombay was picked up on almost immediately by both the architectural press in London and by Bombay's municipal corporation. The *Builder* ran an anonymous article warning that the "peculiar and exceptional conditions that attend the climate and the population of Bombay" would flummox "professional men in no way specially qualified by their local knowledge to meet the difficulties of the case."[42] For the author, the building's role as a mechanism of imperial order and moral reform was self-evident, but so was the necessity of local knowledge in its design. As he explained, "in the face of a population of other blood and other manners than our own … and over whom our hold is rather a moral than a physical one, we cannot afford to blunder."[43] In Bombay, the municipal engineer, Russell Aitken, found that "the arrangements of the Markets, however suitable they may have been for European requirements, were not adapted for India, where caste prejudices and other circumstances necessitate peculiar arrangements to meet them."[44]

Aitken did not elaborate on what precisely he meant by "caste prejudices and other circumstances," but one concern was certainly the variety of food prohibitions that served as a means of achieving moral purity and a marker of identity for Jains, upper Hindu castes, and Muslims. Meat had to be placed under separate roofs from vegetables and grains, because Jains and high caste Hindus found the mere presence of meat in the same interior with other food stuffs to be polluting. In addition, prohibition on beef was quickly becoming a central plank in the Hindu revivalist movement that would coalesce in the 1870s around *gauraksha sabhas* (cow protection societies).[45] These societies used abstention from beef as a way of fostering a nationalist identity that excluded both the British and Muslim populations and cast them as morally inferior. For Muslims, it was essential that pork be kept separate from other meats and that slaughterhouses follow the halal rules.

Crawford and Aitken were largely dismissive of the motivations for these concerns, even as they recognized the necessity of addressing them. While Crawford consulted with Brahmin priests and Muslim leaders in the design of new slaughterhouses to go along with the markets, he too complained about their beliefs as "prejudices" that "showed themselves at every step and in the most trivial detail."[46] In this, Crawford cast his project in the voice of the paternalistic colonial government official tasked with placating unreasonable native demands, without losing sight of his own goals.

As evolutionary psychologists have argued, however, the purity/pollution dyad is a largely universal "moral module" driven primarily by the emotion of disgust.[47] As we have seen, the supposedly objective sanitary reports of Leith and the municipal reports of Crawford are full of these emotive outbursts. In this, British administrators' own claims for reform often rested on the same underlying emotive "moral module" as Hindu and Muslim prohibitions. Moreover, evolutionary psychologists argue that as purity/pollution prohibitions evolve in cultures, disgust often moves from a focus on food and the body to moral judgments.[48] This helps explain the conflation of sanitation and moral virtue in the design of market halls. Only as germ theory came to the fore in the late nineteenth century did moral intuitions derived from disgust give way to more rationally based sanitary prescriptions.[49] Given the early stages of this theory and the continuing belief in miasmas of the sanitary authorities in Bombay, it is no surprise that the line between rational sanitary reform and moral posturing became blurred in the design of the Crawford Market.

The Slaughterhouses

The need to balance Muslim and Hindu moral codes with British sanitary reform also drove the decoupling of the slaughterhouses from the markets. For Crawford, the redesigned slaughterhouses were an opportunity to demonstrate British technology and supervision as a means of achieving new sanitary conditions (figure 3.5). Hence, they were removed to a location eight miles outside of the city along the emerging railway networks so that fresh meat could be efficiently shipped daily by railway to the market. Russell Aitken, the municipal engineer, designed the complex with an emphasis on efficient organization and visual control. The slaughterhouses were fanned out along the railway with separate facilities for mutton and beef, and one for the military to maintain separation of meats. A tall wall strictly separated beef slaughterhouses from the rest, which was paralleled on the meat trains by the separation of cars for beef and mutton. A sentry box for the inspector was placed between cattle holding pens and the slaughterhouses to streamline the process of inspection.

Overall, they were relatively simple structures that emphasized ventilation and light. Double tiered iron roofs provided ventilation over rubble walls touched up with simple Classical details, including arches with accentuated voussoirs and quoins. These ornamental details, along with the iron roof, were meant to explicitly tie the sanitary reform of the slaughterhouses with British values. Iron's status as a modern, Western technology automatically infused it with a superiority in the minds of many of the engineers who employed it, even if this superiority was exaggerated. T. Roger Smith, an architect who

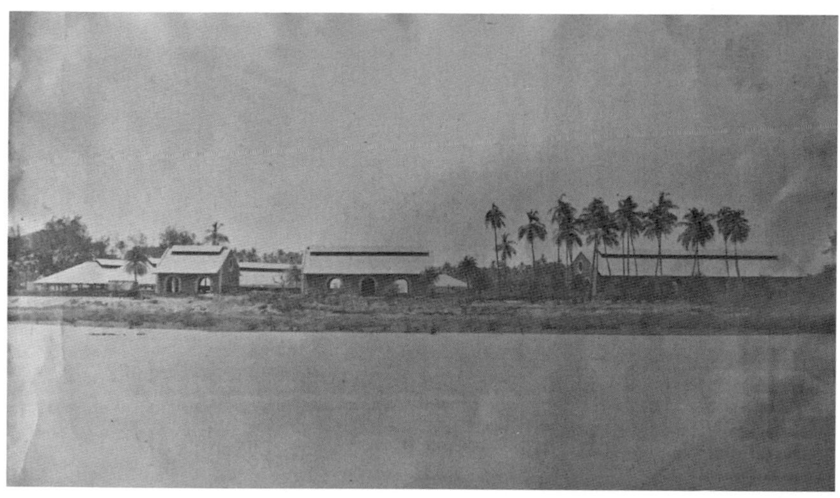

Figure 3.5. View of the Bandora Slaughterhouses, 1867. In Arthur Crawford, *Annual Report of the Municipal Engineer of Bombay for the Year 1867*. © The British Library Board, IOR/V/24/2722.

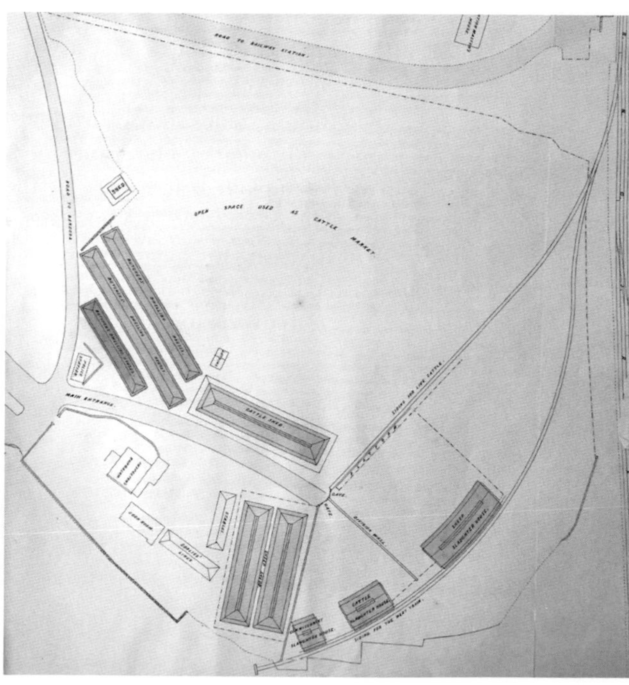

Figure 3.6. Plan of Bandora Slaughterhouses, 1867. Russell Aitken. In Arthur Crawford, *Annual Report of the Municipal Engineer of Bombay for the Year 1867*. © The British Library Board, IOR/X/2642.

worked in Bombay in the early 1860s and consulted with Bartle Frere on his grand architectural vision, contrasted iron favorably with tile roofs, which he considered "an extremely bad roof covering."[50] Even as Smith admitted that iron conducted heat easily, making it "not altogether well suited to the climate … it is still an improvement on the tiles."[51]

The layout of the slaughterhouses was accompanied by other buildings that demonstrated the exertion of colonial control (figure 3.6). The main entrance to the complex from the road was flanked on the south by the inspector's bungalow and to the north by the police station, two buildings dedicated to order, control, and authority. Immediately behind the police station, the houses for the butchers and their workers stretched in three long, narrow buildings. The contrast between the bungalow, a free-standing building whose name had become synonymous with the quarters of the civil servant class in India, and the chawls for the butchers, a catch-all term for single room workers' housing projects in Bombay, clearly reflects the subordinate status of the latter. In addition, the butchers had to pay a five-rupee license fee to use the government slaughterhouses, as well as rail fares for themselves, their workers, cattle, and meat.[52]

The end result satisfied Crawford, who boasted, "I doubt if many towns in Europe possess better abattoirs than these."[53] The butchers, however, were not pleased, and in March of 1866 they went on strike to protest the removal of the slaughterhouses from their neighborhoods. When their strike failed, rumors began to spread through the Hindu community that the mutton was slaughtered in the same houses as beef and transported in the same railway cars. Crawford suspected that the butchers were behind the gossip, though he could not prove it. In the meantime, they attempted to supersede Crawford and appealed directly to the government of the Bombay Presidency. The government replied that "the measure against which they complain is necessary to the Health and Comfort of the Inhabitants of the City of Bombay."[54] A final failed strike on January 1, 1867, ended with Crawford forcing the butchers to sign a "substantial guarantee for their future good behavior," in which they promised not to strike and to abide by the fee structure set up by the municipality.[55]

Sanitation and the Crawford Market Layout

As meat was now meant to travel by railway from the new slaughterhouses to the new market hall in central Bombay, it was essential that the latter be integrated with rail lines from the nearby terminus, which were partially rerouted to the rear of the market's triangular site. After abandoning the designs from England, Russell Aitken organized the new markets to meet local moral requirements and create this efficient relationship with the rail lines (figure 3.7). Fruit,

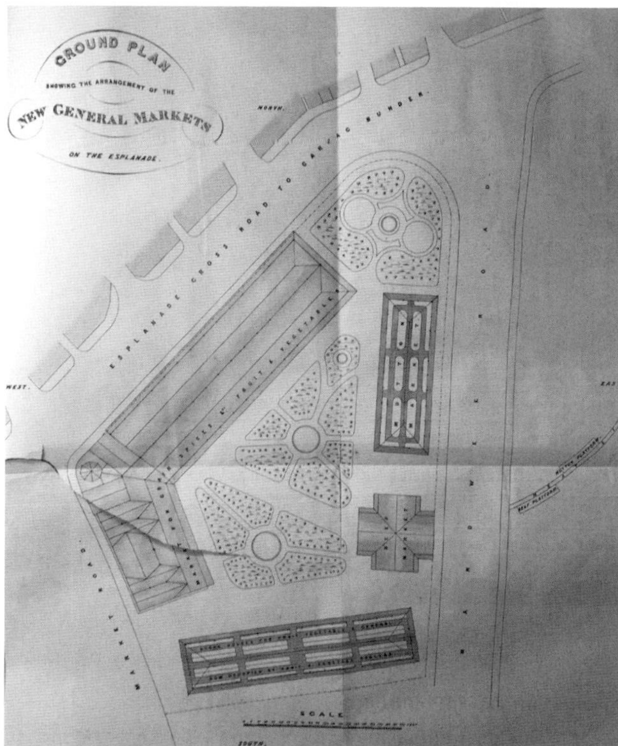

Figure 3.7. *Ground Plan Showing the Arrangement of the New General Markets on the Esplanade*. Russell Aitken and William Emerson. In Arthur Crawford, *Annual Report of the Municipal Engineer of Bombay for the Year 1867*. © The British Library Board, IOR/V/24/2722.

grain, and vegetables were gathered in the largest, most prominent market building at the corner of the site, in front of the entrance to Sheikh Memon Street. Mutton and fish were placed in one market shed at the rear of the site. Beef was placed in its own shed, designed in a cruciform shape with metalwork that had to be specially ordered from England to completely block views into the interior that might offend high-caste Hindu visitors to the market (figure 3.8). The rear placement of the meat halls not only hid them from the view of the city's vegetarians but also provided easy access to the rail lines so that meat could be efficiently unloaded into the markets directly from the meat train.

A central triangular garden with an ornamental fountain at the center served as a buffer between the vegetable, fruit, and grain market and the meat markets (figure 3.7). This helped reinforce the spatial separation of meat and vegetable markets, but it also was designed to reduce overcrowding, one of Crawford's major sanitary concerns. The creation of a calming garden in the heart of the market was also supposed to play a moralizing role, promoting the virtues of orderliness, calmness, and introspection.

While the meat and wholesale markets were simple utilitarian sheds, the vegetable and fruit market was the public face of the building and required

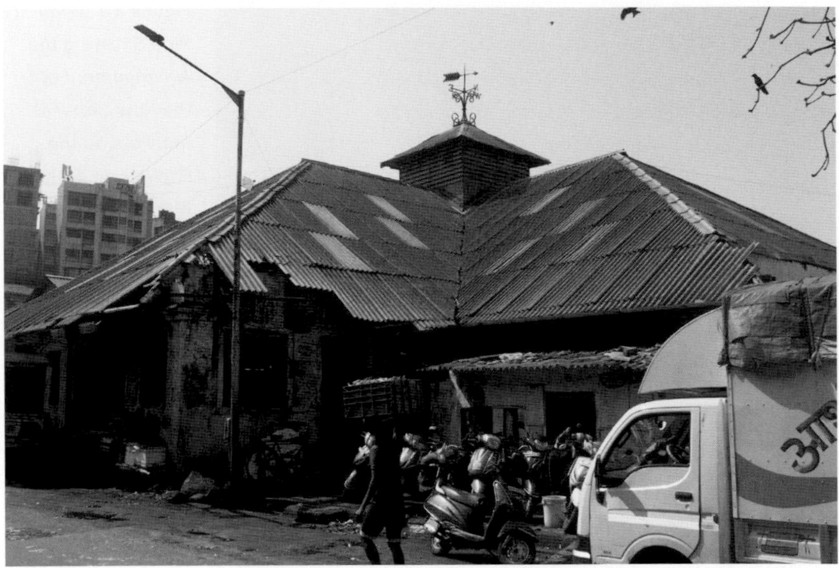

Figure 3.8. Crawford Market, Beef Market Shed. Photograph by author, 2019.

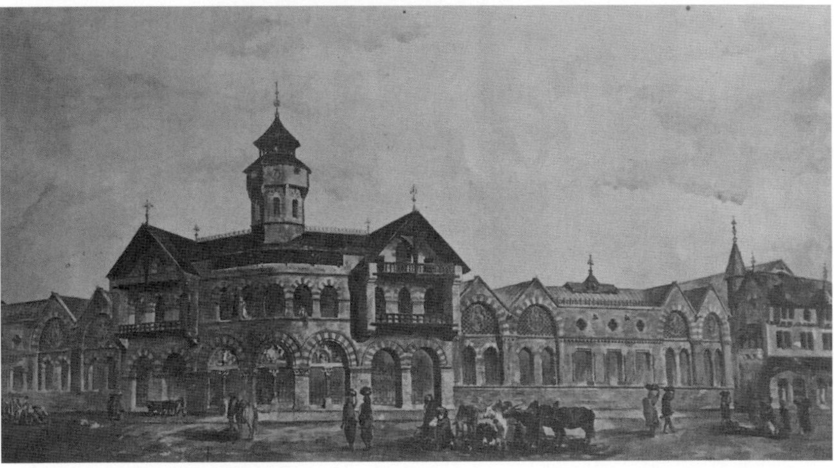

Figure 3.9. *The New General Markets in Course of Erection on the Esplanade*, 1866. Watercolor by William Emerson. Reprinted (from the original, now lost) in Arthur Crawford, *Annual Report of the Municipal Engineer of Bombay for the Year 1867*. © The British Library Board, IOR/V/24/2722.

architectural elaboration. Aitken prepared a design, but he later admitted that "I found that architecture is not a science which comes kindly to an engineer, as he is usually brought up to consider questions of utility only."[56] Crawford turned to William Emerson, the assistant from Burges's office who had brought the competition designs and had arrived to oversee Burges's design of the Sir Jamsetjee Jeejeebhoy School of Art.[57] Emerson was given the task of designing the building's stone street elevation and the ornamental work for the interiors, which included griffin-shaped gas jets, foliate brackets, and Gothic detailing (like quatrefoils on iron cross beams and railings). Aitken, meanwhile, designed the roof structure, using a lightweight, structurally advanced set of bolted trusses to support the same corrugated iron, double-tiered shed roof that he had employed at the slaughterhouses.

Emerson's earliest design for the façade was exhibited in Bombay in October of 1866 along with the rejected designs from England.[58] A watercolor from that exhibit shows that while there were a few significant modifications made in the construction process, Emerson's initial design is remarkably similar to the finished building (figure 3.9). He anchored the building to its corner site with a tall clock tower wrapped by a curving, arched façade and flanked by two porches projected on solid stone corbels with expressed wooden trusses. This central block was flanked by two symmetrical wings that served as the grain and vegetable markets respectively. Each wing consisted of two pairs of gables connected by a horizontal block from which projected the double shed roof capped by a lantern and vane. Attached to the vegetable market, a house that emulates the English medieval vernacular—complete with turret and projected upper story—was meant to serve as the house of the market inspector.[59]

In the final design, the eastern wing along what is now Lokmanya Tilak Road was replaced by an open iron shed to provide increased ventilation, open the market to street traffic, and save costs. The market inspector's house was similarly eliminated for reasons of cost. Nevertheless, the inspector's presence was expressed architecturally in other ways. The inspector's offices and residence were placed on the second floor of the central block behind one of the corbelled porches, with additional windows facing the garden, reinforcing the idea of perpetual surveillance.[60] Stalls in the market were organized in gridded rows for easier monitoring. This heightened surveillance of market activity was highlighted by statistical records in the municipal reports that show a marked increase in the confiscation of spoiled foods and meats and the levying of fines.[61]

Moral Order and the Façade Features

Both the market's porches and the clock tower played a significant role in presenting the buildings as a project of moral reform. Porches were rarely found on the market halls of England. Instead, Emerson seems to have been inspired by the ornate, projecting balconies supported by intricately carved brackets that were a common feature of the houses of the Fort Area and "Native Town" of Bombay (figure 3.10). The delicate woodwork was inspired by haveli architecture in Gujarat, and a taste for these porches was likely brought to the city by Gujarati merchants.[62]

For the British, these were the most striking features of the domestic architecture of Bombay. Louis Rouslett, for example, described houses with "fronts adorned with verandas the pillars of which are delicately carved and painted in lively colours, afford[ing] a peculiarity of appearance altogether unknown

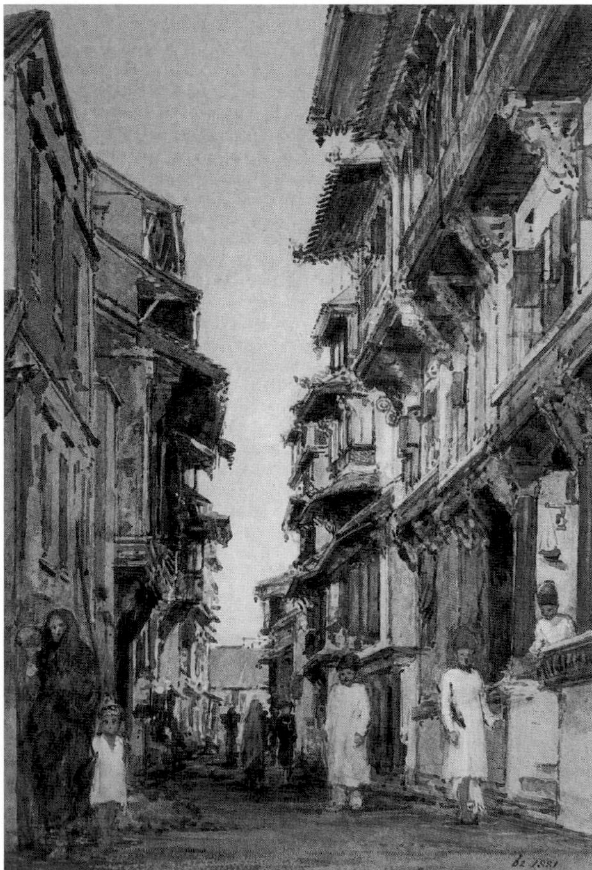

Figure 3.10. *A Street in the Native Town, Bombay*. Watercolor by William Carpenter, 1851. 25 x 117 cm. © Victoria and Albert Museum, London.

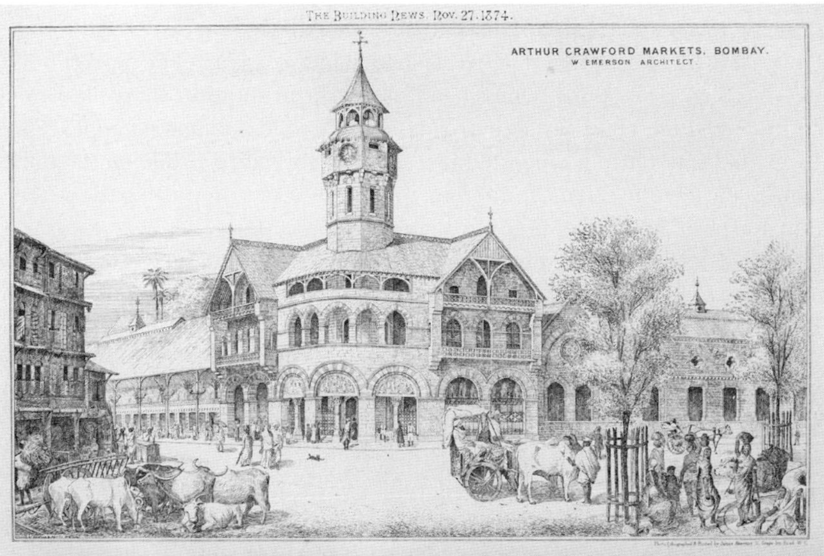

Figure 3.11. *Arthur Crawford Markets, Bombay*. Lithograph by Maurice B. Adams, reproduced in *Building News* 23 (November 27, 1874).

in exclusively Mussulman countries."[63] Andrew Leith, however, found the city's projecting domestic porches to be a menace to the safety and sanitation of Bombay's residences. He criticized the porches for encroaching on the street, depriving it of light, and noted that unstable wooden framing had caused many houses to collapse, resulting in sixty-nine deaths over the previous decade.[64]

Emerson's porches appear to respond to these critiques by abandoning the intricate carving common to the verandas; instead, Emerson focused on structural clarity by integrating the porches into the larger framework of the façade. The corbels supporting the porches are massive, made of the same local kurla stone as the rest of the wall, and run all the way up to the eaves. The woodwork supported by the brackets is dominated by a king-post truss supporting the upper porch, another example of rationally expressed structure in the verandas. Pointed arches set behind the trusses tie them to the rest of the structure, as do the Gothic portals that lead out to the porch (figure 3.11).

This focus on solidity and integration would have contrasted favorably with Indian verandas in the eyes of European critics such as Leith, who saw verandas in "Native Town" as tacked-on and insufficiently supported by over-carved brackets. Indeed, a drawing of the markets that appeared in the *Building News* in 1872 reinforced the contrast (figure 3.11). While most early images of the market tended to show the building standing alone on the Esplanade, this drawing was made from the perspective of Sheikh Memon Street and shows a few rickety buildings from that street, shaded in the corner. The market building, basking in the pure Bombay sun, is meant to stand in sharp, favorable contrast to those buildings, as it projects a more solid and unified appearance. Its verandas are firmly supported by the stone corbelling, while on the buildings on the left one can make out thin, narrow brackets supporting the porches that appear to be on the verge of collapse.

Clock towers were a staple of British market halls and served to inculcate efficiency as a moral virtue, as part of the market's larger moral regime.[65] In Bombay the Crawford Market took on added significance given the market's site in relation to the rest of the city. Standing on the corner of the entrance to Sheikh Memon Street from the Esplanade, the clock tower served as a dramatic punctuation to the end of the street, allowing it to serve its function as a beacon for patrons in "Native Town." As C. Thwaites, who replaced Russell Aitken as municipal engineer in 1869, noted from this "commanding situation" on the edge of "Native Town," "it ... [would] be the standard clock for the city of Bombay."[66] The *Bombay Builder* noted that the market faced the Jama Masjid, which sits three hundred meters down Sheikh Memon Street.[67] While the Crawford Market anchored one end of the street, the masjid's minaret anchored the other. The significance of these competing towers extends further, when one recalls the clock tower's function to introduce a more mechanical, abstract notion of work time to an industrializing society. Similarly, the minaret's purpose was to demarcate time through the call to prayer, structuring the daily lives of the city's Muslims. Crawford Market's new clock tower presented a challenge to the mosque's power to structure an individual's days around religion with the alternative secular structure of an abstract, rationalized system of hours.[68]

Emerson's design for the market was clearly based on his mentor Burges's unbuilt design for the Jamsetjee Jeejeebhoy School of Art, particularly in its central block, which takes Burges's scheme of a central stair tower flanked by pointed arcades and expressed corner eaves, shrinks that scheme, and bends it to fit the corner lot (figure 3.12). Emerson also adopted what Burges considered to be a twelfth-century French Gothic style. The use of Gothic motifs here was a multivalent attempt to imbue several layers of meaning into the building. On the one hand, since the writings of A.W.N. Pugin in the 1830s, the Gothic style had been associated with moral reform and thus reinforced the connection between sanitary and moral reform that drove the design of the markets.[69] Moreover, for the average Englishman, like Walter Crane, the early twentieth-century commentator we met in the introduction to this chapter, the building could be quickly read as "English Gothic," clearly demarcating it as a structure designed and constructed by the powerful, yet munificent British. T.

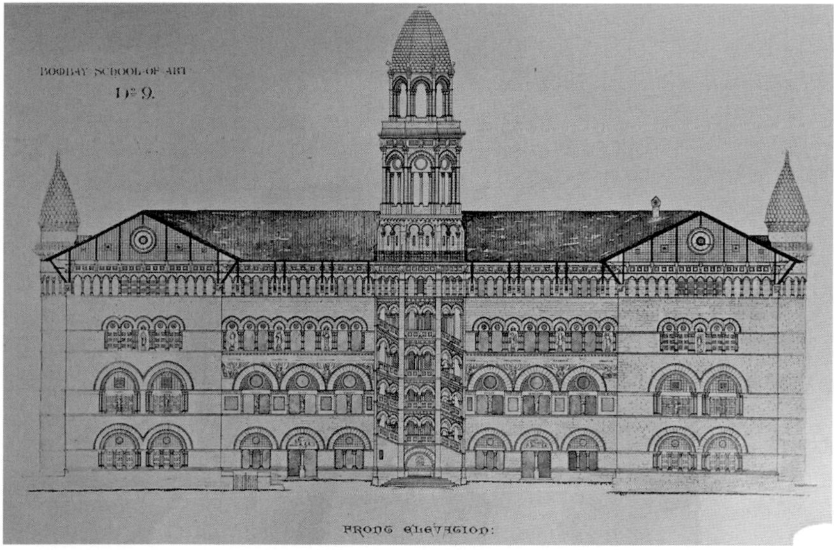

Figure 3.12. Elevation of the Bombay School of Art (unbuilt). William Burges, 1865. © Victoria and Albert Museum, London.

Roger Smith, who helped convince Frere to enshrine the Gothic as Bombay's style, argued that colonial buildings "ought to be European, both as a rallying-point for ourselves, and as raising a distinctive mark of our presence."[70]

While the market's ornament may have given the impression to the casual observer that the building was an alien British form transported to Indian soil, Emerson considered his choice of ornamental detail to be more subtle. In designing the market in the supposed early French Gothic, Emerson was following the lead of Burges, his mentor, who advocated the use of early French Gothic both for building in the "East" and for new building types spurred by industrialization.[71] Regarding the latter, Burges argued that "as to early French art, I believe it to be more suited to the requirements of the present day than any other phase of Medieval architecture. We live under very different conditions to our ancestors. They delighted in small pretty buildings … In French art everything is upon a large scale, and it is unusually suited for our large warehouses."[72] Further, in describing his unbuilt design for the Jamsetjee Jeejeebhoy School of Art, Burges "was careful to select [a style] which, without entailing any difficult stone-cutting, would admit of much or little ornament, and, above all, present those broad masses and strong shadows which go so far to make up the charm of Eastern architecture. The style of the end of the twelfth century appeared to fulfill these conditions better than any other, and to assimilate more with Eastern architecture, while it still retained a well-defined character."[73]

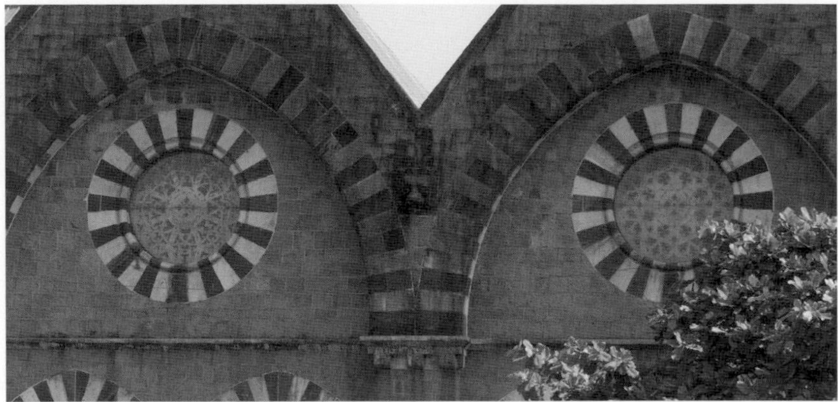

Figure 3.13. Detail of Crawford Market rosettes. Photograph by author, 2019.

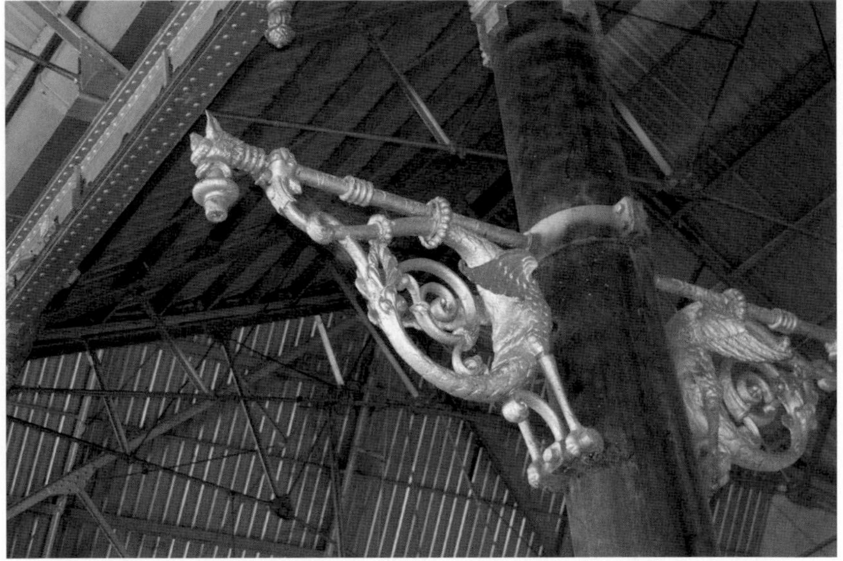

Figure 3.14. Detail of Crawford Market gas jets designed by William Emerson in the shape of a griffin. Photograph by author, 2019.

Emerson's blending of "Eastern" and Gothic motifs in his design is best seen in the rose lunettes, where traditional Gothic rose window motifs like quatrefoils are woven into delicate tracery patterns that are more common to the jali screens of India's Islamic tradition (figure 3.13). This fusion also appeared in the ornament that highlighted sanitary and technological improvements, like drainage spouts and ironwork. As Paul Dobraszyk has argued, the ornamental ironwork that appeared in British market halls was a way of taking the new technology of iron and familiarizing it for audiences.[74] At Crawford Market, Emerson designed iron gas jets so that they became fire-breathing, lithe griffins curled around iron Gothic colonettes (figure 3.14). As far back as the Roman period, griffins were believed to inhabit the lands of the "East," including India, where they guarded gold.[75] The gas-jet griffins were accompanied on the building's exterior by griffins that serve as waterspouts, designed by John Lockwood Kipling, Rudyard's father and head of the Jamsetjee Jeejeebhoy School of Art.[76]

The relationship between the "East" and the Gothic architecture may seem strained, but it was part of a larger ideological shift in Britain that began to see contemporary Indian culture as a relative of early medieval European society, a theory first voiced in Henry Somers Maine's 1863 *The Indian Village Community*.[77] As Clive Dewey succinctly put it, for Maine, "India was Europe's past." Maine's argument allowed its adherents to treat contemporary India as a window into their own historical past, while justifying British rule as a benevolent necessity, because of the metropole's more advanced state. The equation of Indian culture with a stagnant European medievalism can be found in many of the other ornamental features of the Crawford Market.

The centerpiece of its garden is a Gothic fountain designed by Emerson (figure 3.15). The fountain itself highlights and aestheticizes the connection of Crawford Market to other sanitary improvements by Crawford and the municipality, particularly reforms targeting clean water.[78] In its improvements to the city water supply, the municipality built on charitable work done by the city's Jain and Parsi merchants, who had donated to the foundation of several tanks and fountains throughout the city in the 1850s.[79] Indeed, a second, smaller fountain, placed directly behind the central entrance, was donated to Crawford Market by Cowasji Jehangir Readymoney (figure 3.2).[80]

Emerson's design for the central fountain relies heavily on an unbuilt one designed by Burges for Gloucestershire, England. Its sculptural motifs derived from the legend of Sabrina and were meant to tie Gloucester to a mythical medieval past. In Burges's rendering, his design is set in what he imagined Gloucester must have looked like during the medieval period, and places residents in thirteenth-century garb in the foreground.[81] The fountain was never built, but Emerson must have known the design, because his closely matches it.[82] Structurally, the Crawford Market fountain follows the Sabrina one by layering three tiers of grouped, stout medieval columns on top of each other. On the lower two levels, the columns support basins, while the topmost column support the fountain's crowning feature, from which the water was pumped. The Crawford Market fountain even appropriated the sculptural

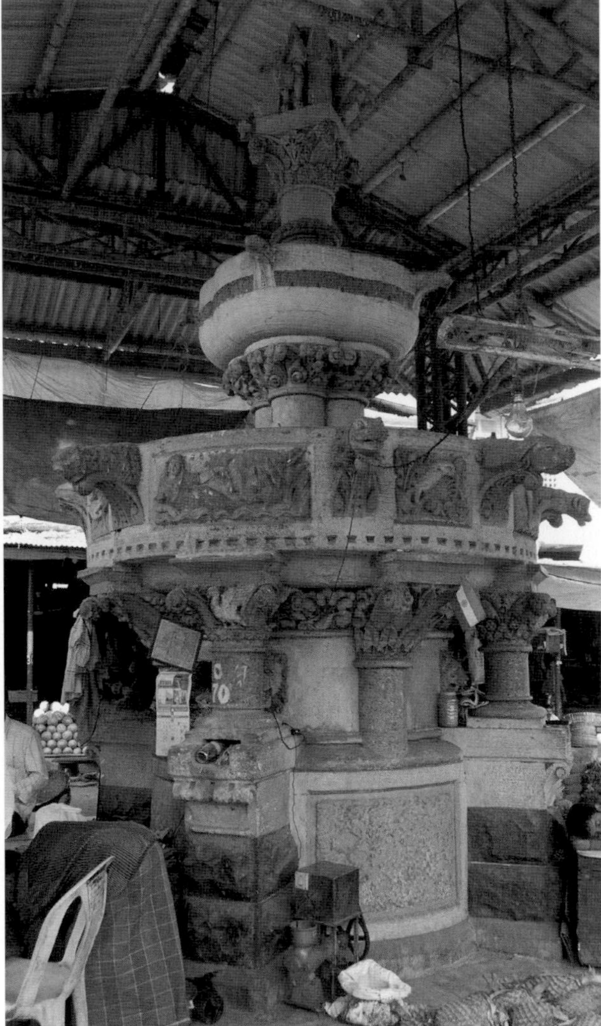

Figure 3.15. Crawford Market Fountain. William Emerson and John Lockwood Kipling. Photograph by author, 2010.

motifs of Burges's design and recast them for an Indian setting, executed by John Lockwood Kipling. The animals covering the Sabrina fountain were replaced with Indian animals. On bas-reliefs surrounding it, Crawford took the nude, reclining beauties who represented the water spirits that greeted the drowned Sabrina on the Gloucester fountain and clothed them in sarees as representatives of the four rivers of India. Here Maine's thesis becomes manifest, as British medievalisms become clearly linked to a British vision of timeless India, while linking the sanitary improvements of Bombay's water supply to a mythology of India's water ecology.

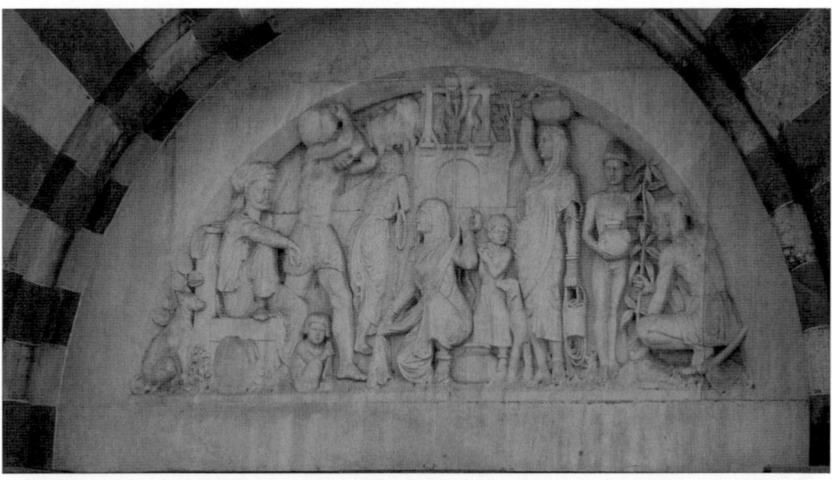

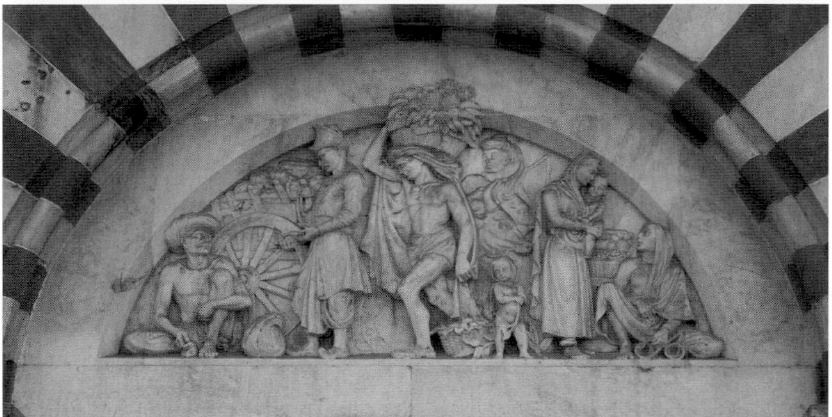

Figure 3.16. Tympana relief sculptures of Agrarian Scene (above) and Market Scene (below) on the Crawford Market, 1867. John Lockwood Kipling. Photograph by author, 2019.

Over the entrances to the market, John Lockwood Kipling designed two tympanum sculptures depicting an Indian market scene and an agrarian scene that further contradict the building's roots in rational, technical solutions to sanitary problems (figure 3.16).[83] In each sculpture, a tension exists between order and chaos. Based on the well that anchors the central axis, the themes of the right-hand scene were identified as irrigation and agriculture by an author in the *Building News*.[84] Around this well, Kipling depicts individuals engaged in the variety of activities and occupations associated with agriculture, from the cultivation of crops to the sale of food in the market. In terms of bilateral symmetry, the sculpture balances itself. Cultivation and selling anchor the corners of the sculpture and a female and male figure carrying lotas balance each other in a more central position. This balance is offset by a chaos of movement in the depth of the sculpture. Each figure moves in different directions, stuck in its own psychological space. A dog, a sheep, a crouching child, and a small girl wander through the scene. Nor is there any sign of the involvement of the technology that Crawford and Aitken championed as essential to sanitary reform.

The left-hand scene depicts a market scene and displays the same tension between an orderly bilateral symmetry of the figures in the foreground and a more chaotic scene in the middle ground. In the foreground, two sellers, seated on the ground, anchor the corners facing standing customers who balance each other on either side of the central axis. This central axis is dominated by a man in a dhoti. His muscles tense as he strides out of the background carrying a basket overflowing with fruit that breaks the frame of the sculpture and projects into our space. Like the lotas of the previous sculpture, baskets are placed at random throughout the scene. In the middle ground, a bullock cart, overflowing with melons, pushes through the scene, its massive wheel on the left side of the sculpture finding little to balance it on the right. Like its companion, the sculpture makes no reference to either the presence of the British or the systematic order and surveillance of the new markets. If Crawford saw the British technology of iron sheds and railway lines as essential for market reform, Kipling depicted the production and selling of food as primarily rural and preindustrial. Perhaps the market's designers believed these images were necessary to entice Bombay's population into a new building type by reminding them of the familiar chaos of the market and village well. Regardless, a nostalgic medieval front hid the technological innovations behind it.

Conclusion: Challenges to the Sanitary Regime

As the quotes from Crane and Davies at the beginning of the chapter suggest, Crawford Market ultimately became a successful landmark in the city. For the wealthy merchants of Bombay, the markets became a source of civic pride. As participants in the global economy, they were sensitive about the perception of inferiority toward Europe and considered the design of lavish public markets to be one of the staples of European cities. Thus, in a municipal meeting in April 1868, Dosabhoy Framjee moved that the markets officially take the name of Arthur Crawford, arguing that he had seen some of the best public markets in England and in the other countries of Europe and that "our public markets would not contrast unfavourably with some of the best public markets in Europe."[85]

Whether the market hall was the best building type to compete monumentally with European buildings was an open question for other observers, particularly the British authors and editors of the *Bombay Builder*. While they praised Emerson's architectural skills, they questioned whether the markets really deserved such elaborate treatment and the large sums of money that were required to make his vision a reality. They summed up what they perceived to be the misplaced priorities of the city's architecture by lamenting that "the weakness of the Commissioner for splendid markets continues; and from the plans and sections of the new general markets which are in course of erection on the esplanade, we perceive that this building will throw the now notorious Bombay Cathedral quite into the shade in point of architectural pretensions and beauty."[86]

They also were prescient in warning of the "exorbitant" costs of the market construction for the merchants and other native ratepayers in the town.[87] The municipality's tighter control, steeper rates, and disruption during construction led to widespread protests by the shopkeepers. Crawford initially sold rights to stalls in the new market via auction to maximize revenue. Like the butchers, the merchants' response was to supersede his authority and directly petition the government of the Bombay Presidency for relief. When they were rebuffed, some merchants attempted to set up an alternative private market, though that eventually failed. Despite these initial objections, Crawford argued in his autobiography that the shopkeepers were eventually won over, claiming "it was notorious … that they had on more than one occasion when he visited the markets given him quite an ovation."[88]

The actual sanitary benefits of the market were also challenged, not just by other citizens, but also by practical experience over time. On the one hand, the reorganization of the markets initially brought them under greater surveillance and control. On the other, other sanitary benefits of the market proved largely illusory. Crawford admitted as early as 1868 that attempts to control congestion had not worked out as hoped. As the crowds overwhelmed the market, the impression European visitors had was not one of sanitary order, as we have seen, but of an indoor version of the "exotic bazaar."

Further, Crawford's attempt to link sanitation solutions to imported British technology was only partially successful. The actual sanitary benefits of iron compared to tile roofs were never presented in a way that countered skeptics. The *Bombay Builder* dismissed his mania for "municipal novelties in the shape of wasteful iron sheds" that could not be "accounted for on sanitary grounds."[89] While the first municipal reports documented the success of the "meat train" through the collection of statistics about the amount of meat it brought into the Crawford markets per day, the expense of its operation led to its abandonment in the 1890s. It was replaced by transportation of meat by bullock cart. The 1890s also saw a new sanitary crisis that revealed the limits of the reforms of the 1860s: a massive plague outbreak that began a new round of urban sanitary measures in the city.[90]

As Dipesh Chakrabarty has documented, the cycle of sanitary reforms on display in the building of Crawford Market developed into a perennial occurrence in cities across India through the colonial and into the postcolonial period. Again and again, this included the rhetoric of disgust in documenting sanitary problems, proposed solutions rooted in modern civic bureaucracy, and resistance from targeted populations. As Chakrabarty notes, while this was initially framed as a colonial imposition of British values, by the independence period these reforms became framed as neutral modernization.[91] Crawford Market, then, reveals the limits of market hall design as a sanitary measure. In Bombay, market hall design became as much about the staging of sanitation reform as British munificence and bureaucratic control as it was about successfully alleviating sanitary conditions in the city.

Notes

1. Quotes taken from Walter Crane, "Crawford Market," in *The Charm of Bombay: An Anthology of Writings in Praise of the First City in India*, ed. R. P. Karkaria (Bombay: D. P. Taraporevala, Sons, 1915), 304; Philip Davies, *Splendours of the Raj: British Architecture in India, 1660 to 1947* (London: John Murray, 1985), 166.
2. The architecture of the Crawford Market has been described in passing in several secondary sources in addition to the above, including S. M. Edwardes, *Gazetteer of Bombay City and Island,* (Bombay: The Times India Press, 1910), 3: 53–55; J. H. Furneaux, *Glimpses of India: A Grand Photographic History of India, the Greatest Empire of the East* (1896; Reprint, New Delhi: Aryan Books International, 1992), 210; Christopher London, *Bombay Gothic* (Mumbai: India Book House, 2002), 62–66, derived from his dissertation, "British Architecture in Victorian Bombay" (D.Phil. Diss., Oxford University, 1987), 222–30; James Maclean, *A Guide to Bombay: Historical, Statistical, and Descriptive (*Bombay: Bombay Gazette Steam Press, 1880), 171–77; Thomas Metcalf, *An Imperial Vision: Indian Architecture and Britian's Raj* (Oxford: Oxford University Press, 2002); Jan Morris and Simon Winchester, *Stones of Empire: The Buildings of the Raj* (Oxford: Oxford University Press, 1983), 142–43; Dinshaw E. Wacha, *Shells from the Sands of Bombay: Being My Recollections and Reminiscences, 1860–1875* (Bombay: K. T. Anklesaria, 1920), 330–33.'Mariam Dossal has also briefly addressed market reform in Bombay in Mariam Dossal, *Imperial Designs and Indian Realities: The Planning of Bombay City, 1845–1885* (Oxford: Oxford University Press, 1991), 204–7.
3. Ananda Yang, *Bazaar India: Markets, Society, and the Colonial State in Bihar* (Berkeley: University of California Press, 1998), 2. It is important to note that the

equation of cast iron market interiors with the "exotic East" was also common in England, where the relatively new form of cast iron was so new that viewers reached for fantastical metaphors. See the discussion in Paul Dobraszyk, *Iron, Ornament and Architecture in Victorian Britain: Myth and Modernity, Excess and Enchantment* (London: Ashgate, 2014), 211.

4. One can find a similar response to the markets of New Orleans from the architect Benjamin Latrobe in 1819, as described in Helen Tangires, *Public Markets and Civic Culture in Nineteenth Century America* (Baltimore: Johns Hopkins Press, 2003), 56–57.
5. See for example, Russell Aitken's admission that "I did my best to produce an architectural building which would be an ornament to Bombay; yet I found that architecture is not a science which comes kindly to an engineer. As he is usually brought up to consider questions of utility only. You [Arthur Crawford] were therefore kind enough to relieve me of this duty, and call on Mr. Emerson, the architect, to design the elevation and other portions of the architectural work, leaving me to design the roofs and other parts of the building with which I am acquainted. The present commanding appearance of these markets, although they are only half finished seems to justify the correctness of your judgement in not having an engineer for an architect." In Russell Aitken, *Annual Report of the Municipal Engineer of Bombay for the Year 1867*, 7.
6. Russell Aitken, *Annual Report of the Municipal Engineer of Bombay for the Year 1867*, 12.
7. James Schmiechen and Kenneth Carls, *The British Market Hall: A Social and Architectural History* (New Haven: Yale University Press, 1999), 47–61.
8. On the centrality of this contradiction in British policy toward India after 1857, see Bernard S. Cohn, "Representing Authority in Victorian India," in *The Invention of Tradition*, ed. Eric J. Hobsbawm and Terence Ranger (Cambridge, UK: Cambridge University Press, 1983), 166. On the emergence of British racialist theories of Indian character, particularly after the 1857 rebellion, see Partha Chatterjee, *The Nation and its Fragments* (New Delhi: Oxford University Press, 1993), 16–22. See also David Cannadine, *Ornamentalism: How the British Saw Their Empire* (Oxford: Oxford University Press, 2001), 41–57.
9. The municipal corporation itself was the direct result of Andrew Leith's damning report on the sanitary conditions of Bombay. On the formation of the municipal corporation, see L. W. Michael, *The History of the Municipal Corporation of the City of Bombay* (Bombay: Union Press, 1902), 15, and Dinshaw E. Wacha, *Rise and Growth of Bombay Municipal Government* (Madras: G. A. Nateson.), 16–23.
10. For a full list of sanitary projects initiated by the municipal corporation in the 1860s, as well as illustrations, see T. G. Hewitt, *Annual Report of the Municipal Health Officer of Bombay for the Year 1866*, 1–22. For a secondary source that summarizes these reforms, see Dossal, 137–46.
11. Chatterjee, 19, and Maria Misra, *Vishnu's Crowded Temple: India since the Great Rebellion* (New Haven: Yale University Press, 2007), 3–12.

12. Arthur Crawford [T. C. Arthur], *Reminisces of an Indian Police Official* (London: Sampson Low, Marston, 1894), v.
13. Ibid.
14. As Swati Chattopadhyay has argued for colonial Calcutta, such clear distinctions between an Indian and British zone concealed a much more mixed reality. See Swati Chattopadhyay, "Blurring Boundaries: the Limits of 'White Town' in Colonial Calcutta," *Journal of the Society of Architectural Historians* 59, no. 2 (June 2000): 154–79.
15. On the building of "Frere Town" see Dossal, 192–202; London, 25–29, and Sharada Dwivedi and Rahul Mehrotra, *Bombay: The Cities Within* (Mumbai: Eminence Designs, 2001), 90–121. On the role of Indian businessmen, particularly Bombay's community of wealthy Parsis, in supporting major architectural projects in late nineteenth- century Bombay, see Preeti Chopra, *A Joint Enterprise: Indian Elites and the Making of British Bombay* (Minneapolis: University of Minnesota Press, 2011).
16. Stephen Halliday, "Death and Miasma in Victorian London: An Obstinate Belief," *BMJ: British Medical Journal* 323, 7327 (December 2001), 1469–71.
17. J. B. Harrison, "Allahabad: A Sanitary history," in *The City in South Asia: Premodern and Modern*, ed. Kenneth Ballhatchett and John Harrison (London: Curzon Press, 1980), 168–72.
18. H. Conybeare, *Report on the Sanitary State and Sanitary Requirements of Bombay* (Bombay: Bombay Education Society's Press, 1855), 5–6. Conybeare also makes explicit reference to the dangers of miasmas in the report. See also Dossal, 134. Interestingly, Conybeare not only wrote the city's first sanitary report, he also designed one of its first Gothic buildings, the Afghan Memorial church, between 1847 and 1858.
19. Andrew Leith, *Report on the Sanitary State of the Island of Bombay* (Bombay: Bombay Education Society's Press, 1864), 10. See also page 5: "No part of Bombay is exempt from fevers of the intermittent and remittent types, or such as are generally thought to be attributable to a cause of which the influence of marshy ground is an important element."
20. For a full description of the city's markets and their layout prior to the 1860s, see S. M. Edwardes, *Gazetteer of Bombay City and Island* (Bombay: The Times India Press, 1910), 3:53–55.
21. Leith, 26.
22. Sir Dinshaw E. Wacha, *Shells from the Sands of Bombay: Being My Recollections and Reminiscences, 1860–1875* (Bombay: KT. Anklesaria, 1920), 335.
23. Michael, 15.
24. Wacha, *Shells*, 25 and Wacha, *Rise and Growth*, 21, 95.
25. *Reform of the Bombay Municipality: Full Report of the Debates at the Bench of Justices* (Bombay: Times of India, 1871), 36. See also Christine Dobbin, *Urban Leadership*

in Western India: Politics and Communities in Bombay City, 1840–1885 (Oxford: Oxford University Press, 1972), 138, which noted that a petition of ratepayers and residents of Bombay demanding municipal reform referenced "alarming expenditure on items such as the Crawford Markets."

26. Arthur Crawford, *Annual Report of the Municipal Commissioner of Bombay for the Year 1867* (Bombay, 1868), 5.
27. Crawford, *Report of the Municipal Commissioner 1867*, 7.
28. See for example, Crawford, *Report of the Municipal Commissioner 1867*, 8 and 10.
29. Leith, 24.
30. Leith, 2; Edwardes, 3:58.
31. K. N. Kabraji, quoted in Edwardes, 3:54–55 n.5.
32. Wacha, *Shells*, 330.
33. Michael, 478.
34. Crawford, *Report of the Municipal Commissioner 1867*, 10.
35. Schmiechen and Karls, 56.
36. Edwardes 3:55 fn5.
37. Crawford, *Report of the Municipal Commissioner 1867*, 7.
38. *Building News* 13 (June 22, 1866): 421.
39. Ibid. For a description of the career of John Norton, see Alexander Graham, "The Late John Norton," *Journal of the Royal Institute of British Architects* 4 (1905): 63.
40. London, 20–25. On Jeejeebhoy's architectural patronage, see Chopra, 14–17.
41. The most complete biography of William Emerson can be found in H. D. Searles-Wood, "The Late Sir William Emerson, Past President," *Journal of the Royal Institute of British Architects* 24 (January 1925): 191–92.
42. "Responsibility versus Efficiency. Wanted, a Market for India," *Builder* 24 (March 17, 1866): 187.
43. "Responsibility versus Efficiency. Wanted, a Market for India," 188.
44. Aitken, 7.
45. Misra, 66-69.
46. Crawford, *Report of the Municipal Commissioner 1867*, 12.
47. Jonathan Haidt and Craig Joseph, "Intuitive Ethics: How Innately Prepared Intuitions Generate Culturally Viable Virtues," *Daedelus* 133, no. 1 (Fall, 2004): 55–66, and Paul Rozin, Jonathan Haidt, and Clark R. McCauley, "Disgust," in *Handbook of Emotions*, ed. Michael Lewis, J. M. Haviland-Jones, and L. F. Barrett (New York: Guilford Press, 2008), 757–71.
48. Rozin, Haidt, and McCauley, 763–64.
49. Rozin, Haidt, and McCauley, 764–65.
50. T. Roger Smith, "On Buildings for European Occupation," *Transactions of the Royal Institute of British Architects* 18 (1867-1868): 204.
51. Smith, 204.
52. Crawford, *Report of the Municipal Commissioner 1867*, 16

53. Crawford, *Report of the Municipal Commissioner 1867*, 16.
54. Proceedings of the Bombay Presidency, General Department, November 17, 1866.
55. *Bombay Municipal Record* (Bombay: Bombay Gazette Press, 1868), 4.
56. Aitken, *Report of the Municipal Engineer 1867*, 7.
57. Crawford, *Report of the Municipal Commissioner 1867*, 9.
58. *Bombay Builder*, 2 (April 5, 1867): 224.
59. *Bombay Builder*, 2 (April 5, 1867): 224
60. C. Thwaites, *Annual Report of the Municipal Engineer of Bombay for the Year 1870*, 3.
61. T. G. Hewitt, *Fourth Annual Report of the Health Officer of Bombay, 1870*, 39.
62. Sharada Dwivedi, "Homes in the Nineteenth Century," in *Bombay to Mumbai: Changing Perspectives*, ed. Pauline Rohatgi, Pheroza Godrej, and Rahul Mehrotra (Mumbai: Marg Publications, 2001), 154.
63. Louis Rousselet, "Mixture of Types in the Bazaar," in *Bombay: An Anthology*, 291.
64. Leith, 10– 11.
65. Schmiechen and Carls, 77.
66. Thwaites, *Report of the Municipal Engineer 1869*, 13.
67. *Bombay Builder*, 2 (April 5, 1867): 225.
68. For context on the significance of the introduction of clock time in reshaping industrial and urban populations, see E.P. Thompson's classic "Work, Time, and Industrial Capitalism," *Past and Present* 38 (1965): 56–96.
69. On the connection between "décor" and "decorum" in nineteenth-century market halls, see Paul Dobraszyk, *Iron, Ornament, and Architecture in Victorian Britain: Myth and Modernity, Excess and Enchantment* (London: Ashgate, 2014), 205.
70. Smith, 208.
71. William Burges, "Proposed School of Art at Bombay," *Transactions of the Royal Institute of British Architects* 18 (1867–1868): 85–87.
72. Burges, 85.
73. William Burges, "Our Future Architecture," *Bombay Builder* 2 (August 5, 1867): 67–68.
74. Dobraszyck, 211.
75. Adrienne Mayor, "Griffins," *Folklore* 104, 1 (1993): 44.
76. On Kipling's sculptural output in Bombay, as well as his role as an educator at the J. J. School of Art, see Julius Bryant, "Kipling as Sculptor," in *John Lockwood Kipling: Arts & Crafts in the Punjab and London*, ed. Julius Bryant and Susan Weber (New Haven: Yale University Press, 2018), 81–93.
77. As Clive Dewey succinctly put it, for Maine, "India was Europe's past." See Clive Dewey, "Images of the Village Community: A Study in Anglo-Indian Ideology," *Modern Asian Studies* 6, no. 3 (1972): 306. See also Ronald Inden, *Imagining India* (Bloomington: Indiana University Press, 2000), 137–40. For the connection between Maine's theories and the use of Gothic Revival in colonial India, see Misra, 10.

78. On Crawford's improvements to Bombay's water system in this period, see Sapna Doshi, "Imperial Water, Urban Crisis, a Political Ecology of Colonial State Formation in Bombay, 1850–1890," *Review (Fernand Braudel Center)* 37, no. 3–4 (2014). 202–3.
79. Chopra, 7–11.
80. Crawford, *Annual Report of the Municipal Commissioner of Bombay 1868*, 5.
81. J. Mourdant Crook, *William Burges and the High Victorian Dream* (Chicago: University of Chicago Press, 1981), 67–69.
82. London makes a similar connection, (2002) 64, 65 and (1986) 228–30. Nevertheless, London stops at a formal comparison without asking questions about what happens when the narrative scheme of the Sabrina fountain is mapped to the Bombay fountain. See also Bryant, "Kipling as Sculptor," 84–85.
83. Jan Morris provides an alternative reading of these sculptures, seeing in them "a paradigm of what a market ought to look like, in the dreams … of the Imperial British." See Morris and Winchester, 142.
84. Bryant, 82.
85. *Bombay Municipal Record 1867*, 101.
86. *Bombay Builder*, 3 (May 5, 1868): 383.
87. *Bombay Builder*, 3 (May 5, 1868): 383.
88. Crawford, *Reminisces*, 249–50. The third person construction is due to the fact that he originally wrote the book under the pseudonym T. C. Arthur. Thus, Crawford, writing as T. C. Arthur, refers to a "Mr. C---, the gentleman who, I believe was the first Municipal Commissioner of Bombay, the man who built the Markets called after his name." This bit of sophistry should raise some skepticism, given the self-serving nature of the passage.
89. *Bombay Builder* 2 (June 5, 1867): 271.
90. Sandip Hazareesingh, "Colonial Modernism and the Flawed Paradigms of Urban Renewal: Uneven development in Bombay, 1900–25," *Urban History* 28, no. 2 (August 2001): 239.
91. Dipesh Chakrabarty, "Of Garbage, Modernity, and the Citizen's Gaze," *Economic and Political Weekly* 27, no. 10/11 (March 1992): 541–47.

Archival Sources

India Office Records, British Library

Bombay City Corporation: Administration Report of the Municipal Commissioner for the City of Bombay, 1866–1867, IOR/V/24/2722: 1866–1867.

Bombay City Corporation: Administration Report of the Municipal Commissioner for the City of Bombay, 1868–1871, IOR/V/24/2722: 1868–1871, IOR/V/24/2723: 1868–1871.

Proceedings of the Government of Bombay, 1866–1867, IOR/P/442/19: 1866–1867

Newspapers and Journals

Bombay Builder
Builder
Building News
Journal of the Royal Institute of British Architects
Transactions of the Royal Institute of British Architects

Bibliography

Bryant, Julius, and Susan Weber (eds). *John Lockwood Kipling: Arts and Crafts in the Punjab and London*. New Haven: Yale University Press, 2018.

Burges, William. "Our Future Architecture." *Bombay Builder* 2 (1867): 66–70.

———. "Proposed School of Art at Bombay." *Transactions of the Royal Institute of British Architects* 18 (1867–1868), 85–90.

Caine, W. S. *Picturesque India: A Handbook for European Travelers*. London: George Routledge & Sons, 1890.

Cannadine, David. *Ornamentalism: How the British Saw Their Empire*. New York: Oxford University Press, 2001.

Chakrabarty, Dipesh. "Of Garbage, Modernity, and the Citizen's Gaze." *Economic and Political Weekly* 27, no. 10/11 (March 1992): 541–47.

Chatterjee, Partha. *The Nation and Its Fragments*. New Delhi: Oxford University Press, 1993.

Chattopadhyay, Swati. "Blurring Boundaries: The Limits of 'White Town' in Colonial Calcutta." *Journal of the Society of Architectural Historians* 59, no. 2 (June 2000): 154–79.

Chopra, Preeti. *A Joint Enterprise: Indian Elites and the Making of British Bombay*. Minneapolis: University of Minnesota Press, 2011.

Cohn, Bernard S. "Representing Authority in Victorian India." In *The Invention of Tradition*, edited by Eric J. Hobsbawm and Terence Ranger. Cambridge, UK: Cambridge University Press, 1983.

Collingham, E. M. *Imperial Bodies: The Physical Experience of the Raj, c. 1800–1947*. Cambridge, UK: Polity Press, 2001.

Conybeare, Henry. *Report on the Sanitary State and Sanitary Requirements of Bombay*. Bombay: Bombay Education Society's Press, 1855.

Crawford, Arthur. [T. C. Arthur] *Reminisces of an Indian Police Official*. London: Sampson Low, Marston, 1894.

Crinson, Mark. *Empire Building: Orientalism and Victorian Architecture*. London: Routledge, 1996.

Crook, J. Mordaunt. *William Burges and the High Victorian Dream*. London: John Murray, 1981.

Davies, Philip. *Splendours of the Raj: British Architecture in India, 1660 to 1947*. London: John Murray, 1985.

Dewey, Clive. "Images of the Village Community: A Study in Anglo-Indian Ideology." *Modern Asian Studies* 6, no. 3 (1972): 291–328.

Dobbin, Christine. *Urban Leadership in Western India: Politics and Communities in Bombay City, 1840–1885*. Oxford: Oxford University Press, 1972.

Dobraszyk, Paul. *Iron, Ornament and Architecture in Victorian Britain: Myth and Modernity, Excess and Enchantment*. London: Ashgate, 2014.

Doshi, Sapna. "Imperial Water, Urban Crisis, a Political Ecology of Colonial State Formation in Bombay, 1850–1890." *Review (Fernand Braudel Center)* 37, nos. 3–4 (2014): 173–218.

Dossal, Mariam. *Imperial Designs and Indian Realities: The Planning of Bombay City, 1845–1885*. Oxford: Oxford University Press, 1991.

Dwivedi, Sharada and Rahul Mehrotra. *Bombay: The Cities Within*. Bombay: Eminence Designs, 2001.

Edwardes, S. M. *The Rise of Bombay: A Retrospect*. Bombay: Times of India Press, 1902.

———. *Gazetteer of Bombay City and Island*. Vols. 1–3. Bombay: The Times India Press, 1910.

Evenson, Norma. *The Indian Metropolis: A View toward the West*. New Haven: Yale University Press, 1989.

Furneaux, J. H. (ed). *Glimpses of India: A Grand Photographic History of India, the Greatest Empire of the East*. 1896. Reprint, New Delhi: Aryan Books International, 1992.

Graham, Alexander. "The Late John Norton." *Journal of the Royal Institute of British Architects* 4 (1905): 63.

Haidt, Jonathan, and Craig Joseph. "Intuitive Ethics: How Innately Prepared Intuitions Generate Culturally Viable Virtues." *Daedelus* 133, 1 (Fall 2004): 55–66.

Halliday, Stephen. "Death and Miasma in Victorian London: An Obstinate Belief." *BMJ: British Medical Journal* 323, 7327 (December 2001): 1469–471.

Handbook of the Bombay Presidency with an Account of Bombay City. London: John Murray, 1881.

Harrison, J. B. "Allahabad: A Sanitary History." In *The City in South Asia: Premodern and Modern*, edited by Kenneth Ballhatchett and John Harrison, 167–96. London: Curzon Press, 1980.

Harrison, Mark, and Biswamoy Pati (eds). *Society, Medicine, and Politics in Colonial India*. New York: Routledge, 2018.

Hazareesingh, Sandip. "Colonial Modernism and the Flawed Paradigms of Urban Renewal: Uneven Development in Bombay, 1900–25." *Urban History* 28, no. 2 (2001): 235–55.

Herbert, George. *Pioneers of Prefabrication: The British Contribution in the Nineteenth Century*. Baltimore: Johns Hopkins University Press, 1978.

Inden, Ronald B. *Imagining India*. Bloomington: Indiana University Press, 2000.

Karkaria, Rustanji Pestanju (ed). *The Charm of Bombay: An Anthology of Writings in Praise of the First City in India*. Bombay: D. P. Taraporevala, Sons, 1915.

King, Anthony. *Colonial Urban Development*. London: Routledge and Kegan Paul, 1976.

Leith, Andrew. *Report on the Sanitary State of the Island of Bombay*. Bombay: Bombay Education Society's Press, 1864.

London, Christopher W. *Bombay Gothic*. Mumbai: India Book House, 2002.

———. "British Architecture in Victorian Bombay." PhD diss., Oxford University, 1986.

Maclean, James Mackenzie. *A Guide to Bombay: Historical, Statistical, and Descriptive*. Bombay: Bombay Gazette Steam Press, 1880.

Mayor, Adrienne. "Griffins." *Folklore* 104, no. 1 (1993): 40–53.

Metcalf, Thomas R. *An Imperial Vision: Indian Architecture and Britain's Raj*. New Delhi: Oxford University Press, 1989.

Michael, L. W. *The History of the Municipal Corporation of the City of Bombay*. Bombay: Union Press, 1902.

Misra, Maria. *Vishnu's Crowded Temple: India since the Great Rebellion*. New Haven: Yale University Press, 2007.

Morris, Jan and Simon Winchester. *Stones of Empire: The Buildings of the Raj*. Oxford: Oxford University Press, 1983.

Pevsner, Nikolaus. *A History of Building Types*. Princeton: Princeton University Press, 1967.

Richardson, Ruth, and Robert Thorne. *The Builder Illustrations Index: 1843–1883*. London: Builder Group and Hutton+ Rostron, 1994.

Reform of the Bombay Municipality: Full Report of the Debates at the Bench of Justices. Bombay: Times of India, 1871.

Rohatgi, Pauline, Pheroza Godrej, and Rahul Mehrotra (eds). *Bombay to Mumbai: Changing Perspectives*. Bombay: Marg Publications, 1997.

Rozin, Paul, Jonathan Haidt, and Clark R. McCauley. "Disgust." In *Handbook of Emotions*, edited by Michael Lewis, J. M. Haviland-Jones, and L. F. Barrett, 757–71. New York: Guilford Press, 2008.

Said, Edward. *Orientalism*. New York: Vintage Books, 1988.

Schmiechen, James, and Kenneth Carls. *The British Market Hall: A Social and Architectural History*. New Haven: Yale University Press, 1999.

Searles-Wood, H. D. "The Late Sir William Emerson, Past President." *Journal of the Royal Institute of British Architects* 24 (1925): 191–92.

Smith, T. Roger. "On Buildings for European Occupation." *Transactions of the Royal Institute of British Architects* 18 (1867/1868): 197–208.

Stamp, Gavin. "Victorian Bombay: Urb Prima in Indis." *Art and Archaeology Research Papers* (June 1977): 22–27.

Tangires, Helen. *Public Markets and Civic Culture in Nineteenth Century America*. Baltimore: Johns Hopkins University Press, 2003.

Tarapor, Marukh. "John Lockwood Kipling and British Art in India." *Victorian Studies* 24 (1980): 53–81.

Thompson, E. P. "Time, Work-Discipline, and Industrial Capitalism." *Past and Present* 38 (1965): 66–96.

Wacha, Sir Dinshaw E. *Rise and Growth of Bombay Municipal Government*. Madras: G. A. Nateson, 1913.

———. *Shells from the Sands of Bombay: Being My Recollections and Reminiscences, 1860–1875*. Bombay: K. T. Anklesaria, 1920.

Yang, Anand. *Bazaar India: Markets, Society, and the Colonial State in Bihar*. Berkeley: University of California Press, 1998.

CHAPTER 4

THE CENTRAL MARKET IN HONG KONG

Urban Amenities in a Speculative Field

Zhengfeng Wang

> Built for a century of service, and of a design and plan hitherto unknown in any local project of such magnitude, the new Central Market, over which members of the Press were taken on a special tour of inspection yesterday, created an extremely favorable impression.
> Not only is every modern facility and convenience, both for dealer as well as customer, incorporated in the general architecture, but nowhere else in the Far East, it may safely be said, is there another market which so thoroughly conforms to the highest standards of hygiene and public health.[1]
>
> — *Hong Kong Daily Press*, 1939.

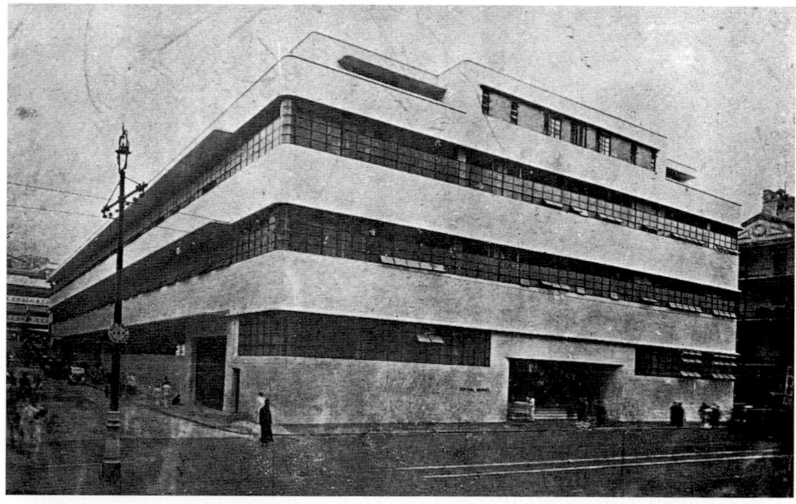

Figure 4.1. Central Market, Hong Kong. *Report on the Social & Economic Progress of the People of the Colony of Hong Kong for the Year 1939*. Courtesy of the University of Hong Kong Libraries.

Replacing a brick edifice in Italianate-inspired classicism with a reinforced concrete structure with strip glass walls, the Central Market of 1939 was one of the few modernist buildings erected in Hong Kong in the prewar period.[2] Its designer was Alfred Walter Hodges, a RIBA-qualified architect working in the colonial Public Works Department. Supervised by the Public Health Department, the project epitomized the implementation of sanitary bureaucracy across the British Empire. A regulative agent imposed on ordinary lives, it served to standardize commercial activities. The new structure, an efficient facility built in the context of the laissez-faire economic policy, proved to be a highly remunerative investment for the colonial government. The visually impressive architectural design drew from Shanghai precedents and embodied concepts of hygiene that were central to public health in the early twentieth century. The installation of the latest equipment supported by both local and foreign contractors advertised the supposed benefits of colonial rule and combined the idea of modern health with industrial amenities.

Bureaucratic Sanitation

During the 1830s, British reformers launched the public health movement to address sanitary issues exacerbated by rapid urbanization.[3] This empowered the local authorities to bring better facilities, improved housing, purer water, and healthier food to the increasing number of working-class people.[4] Thomas Osborne notes that by providing urban infrastructure, sanitary intervention ensured security within a liberal order, which emphasized "the *naturalism* of the progress to be regulated."[5] According to Dorothy Porter, the public health movement "interwove Victorian social science with Enlightenment political economy and was integrated into philosophical radicalism and the politics of social amelioration."[6]

In line with the practice at home, British authorities established the colonial sanitary administration, which served as "a tool of Empire" to cultivate the land and produce desired subjects.[7] As more expatriates spent large parts of their lives in the colonies and longevity rose in Britain itself, anxiety about the breakout of devastating epidemics and high mortality rates in foreign places began to grow. In the second half of the nineteenth century, the colonial municipalities enacted statutory regulations, conducted statistical investigations, and provided sewage, drainage, and water supply to the local population.[8] The instrumentality of hygiene embodied what David Scott has termed the "*political rationalities* of colonial power," which operated at microlevels.[9] At the same time, everyday implementation, often in the form of direct surveillance and social segregation imposed by Western-trained European and

Eurasian men neglecting Indigenous knowledge, encountered constraints and resistance from property owners and the lower class.[10] In short, these measures were more subject to economic factors than social impacts.[11] This history was not complementary but contemporaneous with and partly formative to the consolidation of British public health.[12]

In 1841, when the place could hardly be called a city, Britain took possession of Hong Kong for commercial purpose more than territorial gain and showed limited interests in investing in sanitary infrastructure and regulation restricting economic prosperity.[13] The colonial Governor's Council served as the administrative body that planned urban facilities to support trade stability. In the first forty years of Hong Kong's colonial period, hygiene management was far from sound. Malaria caused high mortality amongst the military and civilian populations and the overcrowded accommodation of the working class aggravated hygiene problems.[14] To address the deteriorating conditions, London dispatched the royal engineer Osbert Chadwick to Hong Kong, who submitted a thorough sanitary report based on substantial fieldwork. This in turn prompted the setting up of a permanent Sanitary Board composed of government officers and nonofficial members in 1883 and the promulgation of the 1887 Public Health Ordinance. However, these efforts failed to prevent a cholera breakout in the Chinese neighborhood of Taipingshan in 1894. Hong Kong recalled Chadwick along with the disease expert W. J. Simpson and enacted the Public Health and Buildings Ordinance in 1903. It was in effect until 1936, when the Urban Council took shape following the suggestion of sanitary officer A. R. Wellington. Led by public health practitioners working in Britain and its overseas territories, bureaucratic sanitation provided the institutional framework and technical apparatus supporting the colonial administration.[15]

From the beginning of British rule, the establishment of public markets represented the local authority's approach to urban order and its promotion of commercial services. The earliest town planning ensued after the first land sale held in 1841 and the construction of the Central Road along the coast.[16] On the thoroughfare, several private marketplaces and bazaars were built with government permission to provide food and other necessities for the Chinese and European populations.[17] Among them, the Upper and Lower Bazaars consisting of rows of shops contributed to the formation of the earliest officially endorsed Chinese settlements.[18] Meanwhile, prevalent hawking and peddling in the urban area aroused health and safety concerns, and sanitary legislation termed the encroachment of the street as a public nuisance.[19] In 1842, one year before the foundation of the Crown colony, the first Central Market was completed near the two aforementioned bazaars. Situated on Queen's Road and occupying a central position in the burgeoning city (figure 4.2), the

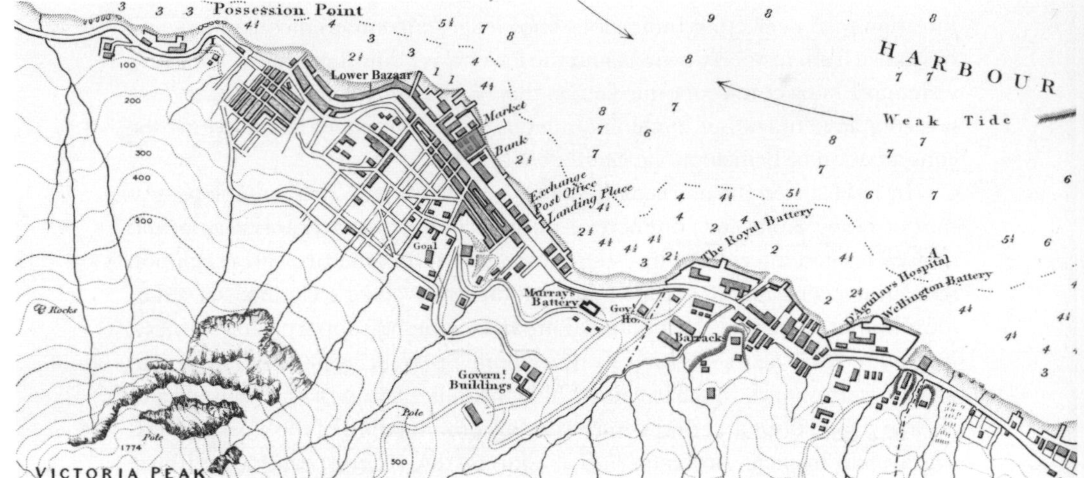

Figure 4.2. *Ordinance Map of Hong Kong* (with the "Market" shown in the center and author annotations), 1846. Thomas Collinson. Courtesy of the National Library of Scotland.

orderly trading venue was composed of four or five mat-covered sheds housing meat, poultry, salt fish, fresh fish, fruits and vegetables and provided a weighing and money-changing service.[20] The earliest market ordinance in 1847 required all markets to be licensed and supervised by the chief magistrate of police.[21] The 1857 ordinance first entitled the Governor to appoint the inspector of markets and a subsequent bylaw set up positions for the "Market Porters" and "Market Scavengers."[22] In 1867, the Registrar General in charge of Chinese affairs took over the market duties from the Surveyor General, except for construction, alteration, and maintenance.[23]

Though early supervision of markets focused on registration and fee collection, the British increasingly viewed urban amenities as a means of health control. The Local Government Act of 1858 first empowered local authorities, elsewhere than in London, to establish markets, and the Public Health Act of 1875 included a provision for slaughterhouses. Aware of the problems caused by private franchise, from 1858 onward the Hong Kong government directly auctioned the stalls.[24] The 1887 Public Health Ordinance authorized the Sanitary Board to license markets and to regulate food sanitation.[25] In 1903, the new Public Health and Buildings Ordinance, a comprehensive legislation pertaining to markets, slaughterhouses, factories, and workshops, integrated building codes with hygiene requirements. The Veterinary Surgeon of the Sanitary Department was charged with inspecting meat, the Medical Officer of Health was responsible for cleanliness, and each market was under the supervision of the inspector of the district.[26] Despite objections by the Registrar General, the Sanitary Department eventually took charge of the rental of market stalls.[27] Under this administrative reform, market regulation joined the urban sanitation agenda.

During the interwar period, the Hong Kong authority increased its attention to public works and social legislation and welfare.[28] In 1935, when nearly one million residents lived in the city, the Buildings Ordinance introduced higher structural and hygienic standards. By this time, more than thirty markets were scattered across Hong Kong Island and the Kowloon Peninsula.[29] The Public Works Department supervised the construction of buildings and city facilities. The Public Health (Food) Ordinance placed the Sanitary Department in charge of slaughterhouses, markets, dairies and milk shops, food factories, food shops, eating houses, and restaurants and was entitled to expel from any market any person convicted of contravening any regulation. Though not administered by a municipality as in other colonial cities, Hong Kong upheld similar standards of sanitary governance.

As early as 1887, the bylaws prescribed each stallholder to keep the markets clean and local newspapers reported violations.[30] The bylaws required the butchers, fishmongers, and poultry sellers to wash their fittings and utensils on a regular basis daily, while all sellers were ordered to clean the stalls before the reception. Stallholders had to furnish portable dust bins for all garbage and empty them at a specific location.[31] Keeping dogs inside the market was prohibited. Nobody was allowed to sleep, hawk, beg, or spit in the market, nor to sit, stand, or lie on any slab or counter intended for the display of foodstuffs for sale, or to wash or bathe in any fish tank or receptacle used for the storage of food.[32] The signboards and blinds set by shops or stalls could not impede traffic and the tenants only could operate a business within their own premises; throwing offensive matters to the passageways was forbidden.[33] The cleanliness of the environment and free and orderly movement were of utmost importance.

Deborah Lupton argues that "the practices and discourses of public health are not value-free or neutral, but rather are highly political and socially contextual, changing in time and space."[34] Under British influence, the sanitary administration in Hong Kong introduced scientific knowledge and bureaucratic control, becoming a powerful tool for the strengthening of state authority. Quoting an early twentieth-century bureaucrat, Alison Bashford declares that imperial cleanliness entailed "colonizing by means of the known laws of cleanliness rather than by military force."[35] The regulation of space and the provision of urban infrastructure extended government management of daily life, and this discipline was exemplified in the design of market buildings.

The Clean Machine

In an attempt to tame urban chaos, modern European market buildings became vehicles for expressing social progress as well as increasing food supplies.[36] Their metal structures left unexposed on their façades, the market halls were among the most prominent new buildings in British towns, regularly used by large numbers of the working class.[37] In France, Victor Baltard's redesign of Les Halles, a showcase of Second Empire Paris, replaced stone walls with ventilated iron ones. The new "umbrellas" sheltered spaces that facilitated both surveillance and circulation.[38] Following the British and French models, more European countries adopted the new building type until reinforced-concrete technology provided an alternative for large-span structures.[39] The Markthalle (1908) in Breslau (Wrocław) supported by parabolic arches was an early example with a civic appearance, while the Grossmarkthalle in Munich (1912) and Frankfurt (1928) were more utilitarian structures serving the modern city.[40]

New British market halls that took advantage of the possibilities created by the widespread availability of iron and glass inspired change in the colonies. For instance, sanitary concerns prompted the Singapore government to reorganize the city and rebuild the Telok Ayer Market as a metal structure in

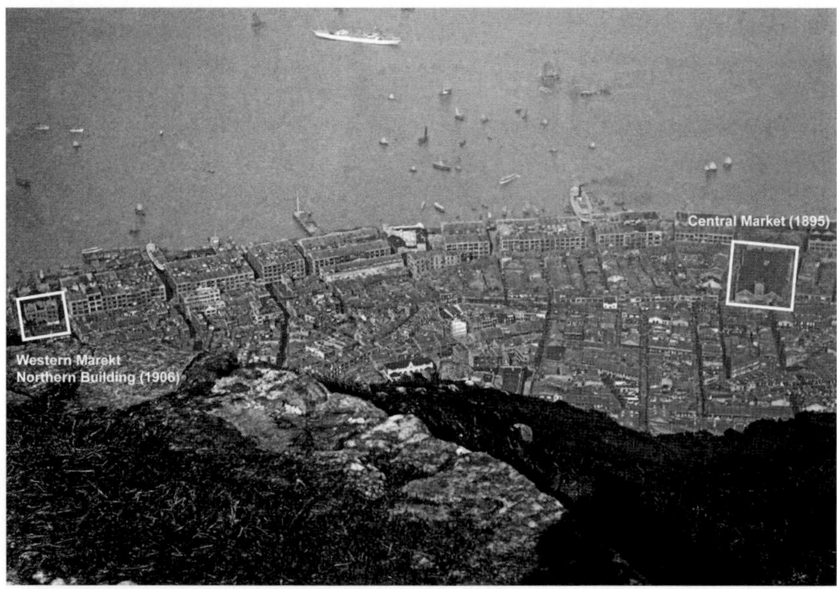

Figure 4.3. Aerial view of Central and Sheung Wan (with author annotations), Hong Kong, 1908. Photograph by Dezső Bozóky. Ferenc Hopp Museum of Asiatic Arts, Budapest, F 2004.89. © Museum of Fine Arts, Budapest, 2020.

1894.[41] Arthur Crawford, the first municipal commissioner of Bombay and a key advocator of sanitary reform, created public markets for all classes and castes. He believed these would "compete favorably with those to be found in any place in England or elsewhere."[42] In his report for the Hong Kong government, Osbert Chadwick proposed reconstructing the Central Market as an iron structure with impervious floors and pointed out that masonry stalls and pillars inhibited proper cleansing.[43] The 1887 market ordinance did not take into account these recommendations on building materials but noted that "the stalls shall be fitted with stone or wooden counters."[44] However, Chadwick's proposal foresaw the completion of the two-story Central Market in 1895 (figures 4.4 and 4.5), for which the ironwork and steel was imported from England and which set an example for the public markets that followed.[45] The Western Market Northern building (1906) was supported by cast iron columns and steel beams, and the roof was covered with double pan and roll tiling on steel trusses and purlins (figures 4.6 and 4.7). Though equipped with a light gallery above stalls and electric lamps over the passages, the 1895 Central Market was dark inside. After opening to the public, it had to increase the window heights on the ground floor; dealers were allowed to use oil lamps to save costs.[46] The Western Market South Building (1913) had large openings on the walls in addition to the circular dormer windows in the cement roof and the glass louvers in the gables.

With the creation of treaty ports in mainland China, the municipal governments in the foreign settlements erected civic buildings, including modern market halls that changed local practices. The Chinese were used to procuring necessities from traditional fairs held at particular times and places and shopping for food from the open-air stalls along streets and rivers.[47] By the end of the nineteenth century, the medical and sanitary infrastructure in the International Settlement in Shanghai was nearly on par with the best in urban areas of Europe and America, and the Chinese embraced the projects of public health inspired by Western progress.[48] The Municipal Council erected the steel-framed Maloo Market in 1899 and remodeled the Hongkew Market into a three-story concrete structure in 1923.[49] The fireproof mushroom slab system saved construction and maintenance costs and established a new paradigm in the region (figure 4.8).[50] In Tientsin, the British Municipal Council intended to build the most hygienically advanced neighborhood among the settlements that represented eight foreign countries.[51] Its public market, supported by tall parabolic arches, provided open space and introduced ample light and air through the clerestory windows (figure 4.9), which evoked a similar practice in the City Market in Nairobi and the Lawrence Hall in London. Characterized by modernist abstract purity, these urban amenities proclaimed the modern and hygienic presence of foreign power.

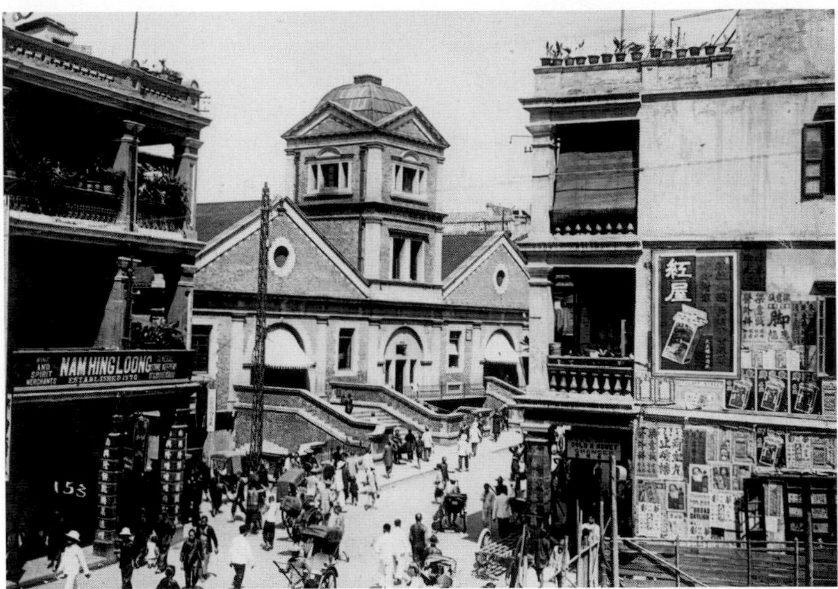

Figure 4.4. Central Market, Hong Kong, ca. 1922-1925. Frank and Frances Carpenter Collection, Prints and Photographs Division, LC-USZ62-120790. Courtesy of the Library of Congress.

Broadly following the Shanghai examples, the 1939 Central Market had strip windows wrapping around the facade and a courtyard in the center, reflecting a simplified building program to facilitate control. Ronald Ruskin Todd, the first chairman of the Urban Council, and Alfred Water Hodges, the municipal architect, carried out a field trip to Shanghai to study precedents.[52] According to the 1857 and 1867 Hong Kong Market Ordinances, there were stalls, houses, shops, Lan (the local term for wholesale business), and depots, as well as tenements in the markets. After 1887 all stalls were numbered and set apart for different kinds of foodstuffs.[53] No food, with a few exceptions enumerated in the bylaws, could be sold outside the public market. The 1939 project hosted retail space with 285 stalls, service areas, and offices. The wholesale business was relocated to Kennedy Town in the northwest extremity of the island and away from the city center. This market was a one-story concrete shelter for trade in fresh and saltwater fish and vegetables, and each department had its own entrance and exit for vehicles. It was located in a district "little devoted to residential purposes" and had easy access to the waterfront and the main public abattoir, which was constructed in 1895.[54] Based on early experience, the most recent Central Market epitomized up-to-date design strategies in pursuit of good health.[55]

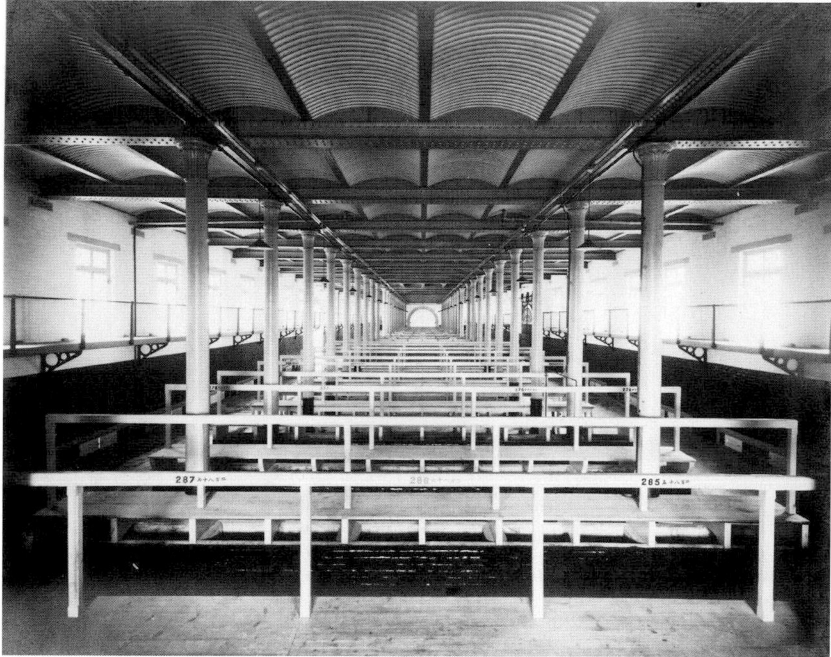

Figure 4.5. Central Market, Hong Kong, 1895. This photograph shows the ground floor of the northern block containing 150 stalls. The vegetable stalls were fitted with tiers of receding shelves, the pork stalls with iron rails and hooks, and some fish stalls with water tanks. Courtesy of the National Archives, London, CO 1069/446 (27).

The rational layout of the 1939 Central Market featured a rectangular plan and the well-organized circulation further improved its spatial efficiency. Occupying an advantageous position and covering the entire block, the 1895 project provided two main entrances, one from Queen's Road, and the other from Praya, which commanded a sea view (figure 4.10). Reconstructed on the same site, now one block away from the coastline, the new market still took advantage of the sloping site and was approached from both the ground and first floors. The customers were guided in by the grand double staircases facing the courtyard. A passenger lift with a capacity of twenty persons was installed beside the Des Voeux Road entrance. Foodstuffs entered from the other two sides of the building in a layout that did not cross paths with shoppers. Fish supplies entered from Jubilee Street and the poultry from Queen Victoria Street. At the southwest corner of the first floor, an unloading platform lifted meat to the first floor, while fruit and vegetables were carried up through a dedicated stair to the upper level. The courtyard was lined with foodstuff stalls and service rooms connected by a twenty-foot-wide passageway.

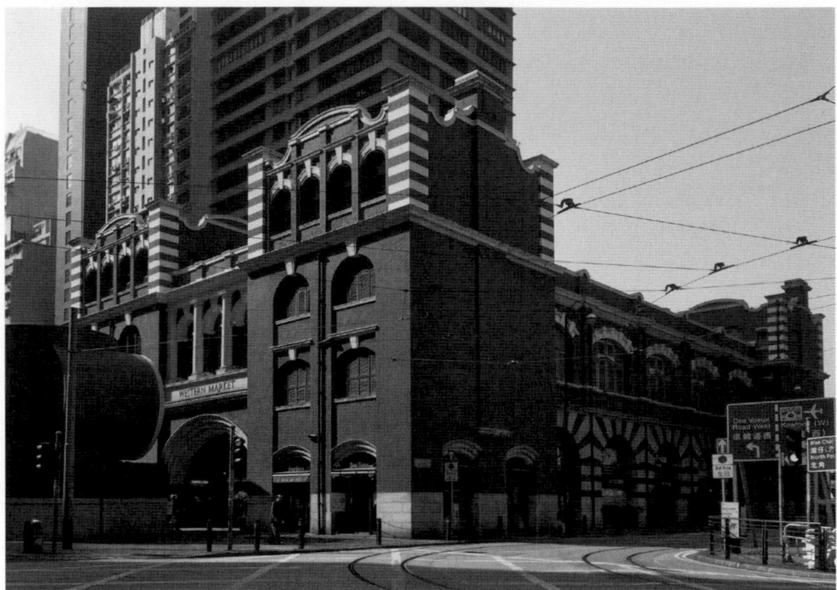

Figure 4.6. Western Market Northern Building, originally built in 1906, Hong Kong. It operated as a food market until 1988 and was transformed into a shopping center after refurbishment. Photograph by author, 2019.

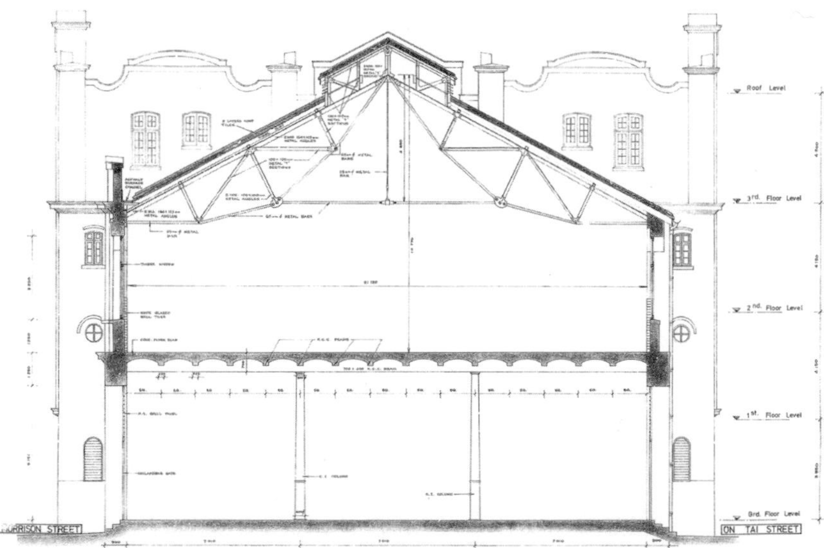

Figure 4.7. Western Market Northern Building Cross Section, Hong Kong, 1986. Courtesy of the Architectural Services Department, Hong Kong. When first completed, it contained poultry shops on the ground floor and sales of fish on the upper level.

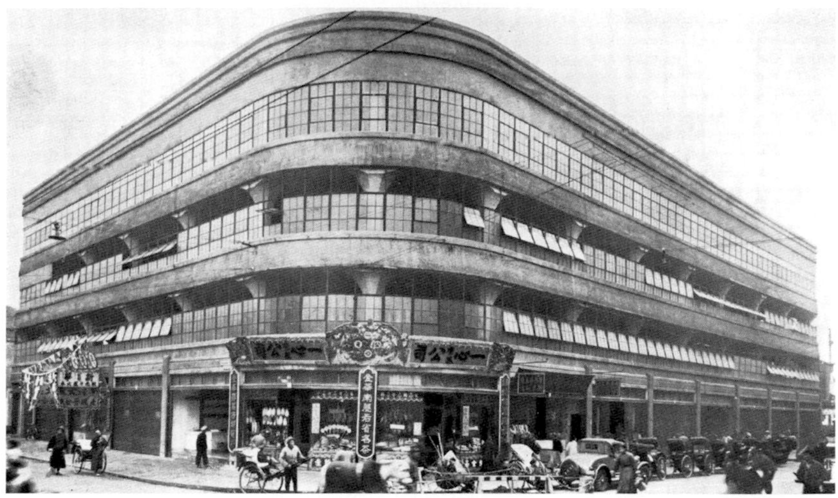

Figure 4.8. Foochow Road Market, Shanghai, 1930. *Report for the Year 1930 and Budget for the Year 1931*, Shanghai Municipal Council. Courtesy of the Virtual Shanghai Project. Located in the Central District of the International Settlement, Foochow Road Market was built to relocate the dealers from the old Maloo Market. The building was equipped with a lift, cold storage in the basement, and water-flushed latrines for both sexes.

In the commercial area, the foodstuff sections consisted of standardized and well-equipped concrete stalls serving classified activities. The vegetable and fruit sections allowed the customers free entry to the stalls (figures 4.12 and 4.13). The pyramid-shaped fruit stalls had raised edges that prevented the commodities from rolling off and cluttering up the frontage. Fitted with hanging bars, the meat stalls had a concrete counter at the front and a small platform at the back. The poultry and fish sections exhibited live animals. The poultry stalls installed grooved counters so that air could pass beneath. There were specific rooms for killing and plucking the birds as well as for the storage and preparation of chicken feed. At the back of each fish stall, there were two storage cisterns with aerated water. In front of each stall, the flooring of the lanes inclined from center to gutter. The interior wall was covered with terrazzo to facilitate cleansing. Separate service areas were devoted to the storage of baskets, electrical controls, and administration. Linking different floors, the refuse chutes allowed a lorry to collect rubbish on the ground floor. These detailed designs helped specify how to use the space, which normalized individual behaviors and maintained order.

The municipal markets in Hong Kong commonly provided accommodation and workspace. The top floor of the new building housed a portion of the Sanitary Department on one side and living quarters for the market officials

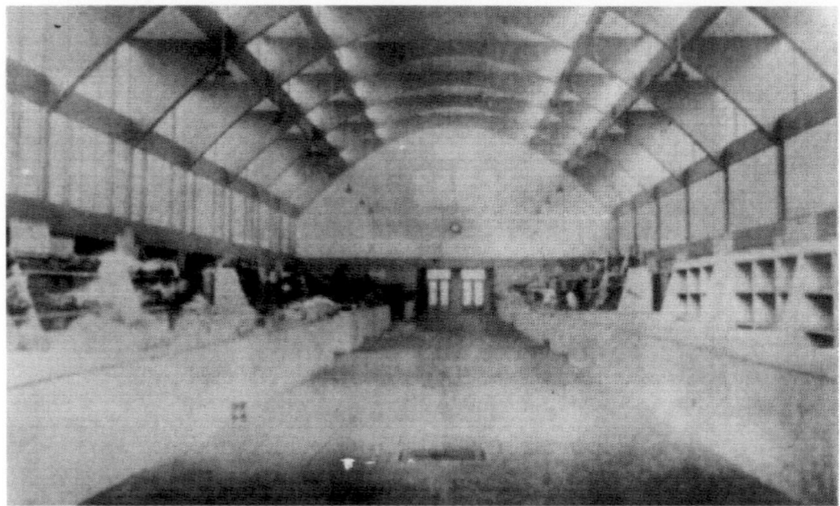

Figure 4.9. British Municipal Market, Tientsin, 1928. Courtesy of *Jindai Tianjin tuzhi* (Tianjin: Tianjin guji chubenshe, 2004).

and workers on the other (figure 4.14). The Central and Western Market Offices contained desk space for twelve market inspectors, two subinspectors, eleven interpreters, and two clerks. The European inspectors had their own living quarters. Six Chinese foremen shared a community kitchen, the cleaners lived in a dormitory of thirty bunks fitted with a mess room and clothes chamber, and there was a special section for ten meat porters. In the 1895 Central Market, the inspector's quarters were located in the tower over the central avenue between the two blocks. This facilitated his free access to every part of the building at all times, as mandated by the regulations.

Espousing modernist openness and transparency, the new Central Market replaced the "old, dank, dark, dismal building" with its accumulated dirt, refuse, and smells with one that adhered to the principles of efficiency and standardized construction.[56] At the same time, introducing the latest sanitary standards regarding light, ventilation, and other aspects of hygiene also promoted British colonial control over the shopping experiences and business practices of Hong Kong's Chinese inhabitants.

Mundane Pragmatism

Built as a rational structure embracing functionality, the 1939 Central Market broke away from the aesthetic of classicism and stood out from contemporary government-sponsored projects in the colony.[57] In the 1930s, Hong Kong had

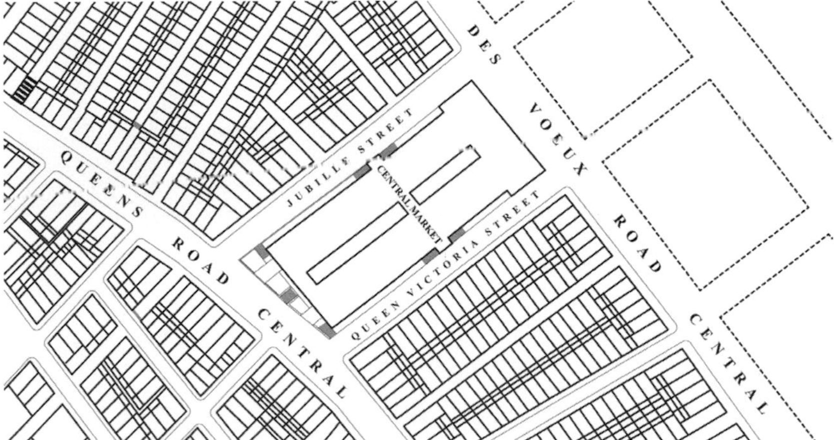

Figure 4.10. Site plan of the 1895 Central Market. Drawing by the author. It is based on "Plan of Victoria," 1901. Government Records Service, Hong Kong, HKRS 209-1-1.

little connection with the International Style, which was also slow to be accepted in Britain. While institutional buildings conveyed strength and created an aura of stability and permanency, Art Deco was a popular choice for commercial buildings in the city. It signified wealth and conveyed a modern urban lifestyle favored by both the British and Chinese who could afford it. Meanwhile, Hong Kong benefited from the global transfer of construction technology and adopted the latest building equipment. Beginning in 1903, surveyors and army engineers could register as "Authorized architects."[58] The Public Works Department gained support from local Chinese contractors and collaborated with companies based in industrialized countries.[59] Fostered by a free-port policy, Hong Kong could not impose customs duties. The colonial authority, which was financially independent of the British Treasury, had to generate adequate income, such as land rent and licensing fees for local trade, to cover its expenditure. In this context, the Central Market was an urban amenity that displayed the authority's embrace of utilitarian rationalism.

Under the influence of the worldwide trade depression and deep uneasiness about the Civil War in mainland China, the Hong Kong government largely curtailed its expenditure on public works in the 1930s and selectively invested in infrastructure to fund its activities. The operation of sanitary facilities depended on the income they could generate, and even hospital development was only partially funded by the government.[60] In 1931, when speaking about the desirable items to be deferred, the Colonial Secretary stated that "the programme … represents the best effort of the Government after very careful consideration of detail to fashion its coat according to the attenuated

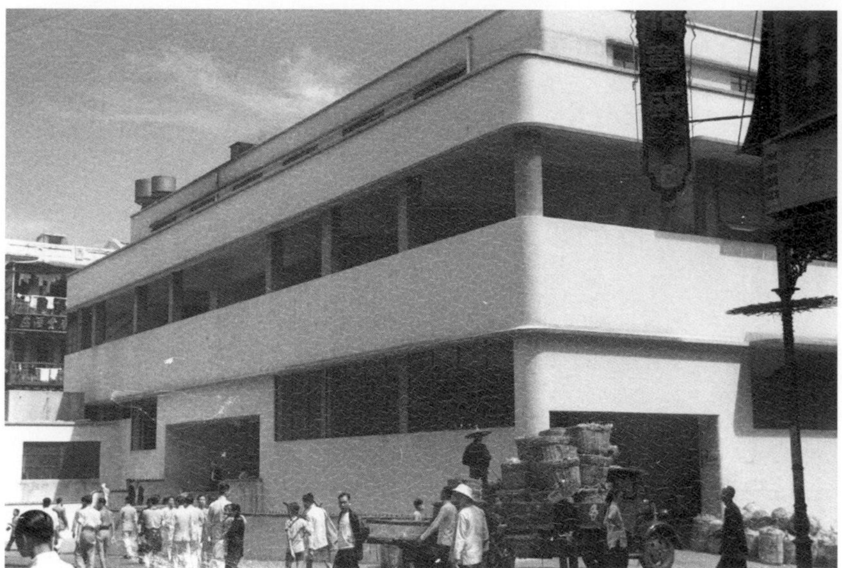

Figure 4.11. Central Market, view from Queen's Road Central and Queen Victoria Street, Hong Kong, ca. 1941. Amid the hustle and bustle of the city and occupying the whole block, the massive building with smooth white wall was intended to sanitize the environment and showcased its cleanliness. Courtesy of the University of American Geographical Society Library, Wisconsin-Milwaukee Libraries, Harrison Forman Collection, fr200228.

supply of cloth available. It will be no party dress, but it is hoped it will prove a useful working garment."[61] However, the provision of markets was regarded as "necessary for the properly ordered life of the community" and the projects for the Sanitary Department accounted for a fair portion of municipal expenses.[62] The fund for the Central Market came from the Dollar Loan enacted in 1934. The scheme was revised annually to measure the need of eight listed items, which also received credits from their profitable projects.[63] For instance, the Central Market benefited from the sale of plants in the Aberdeen and Shing Mun Valley Water Schemes and the earnings from Air Port Development.[64] It was the only large-scale project realized during this period of financial stringency, after the 1937 Queen Mary Hospital.

Abiding by the laissez-faire policy, the 1939 Central Market earned a quick return at the cost of Chinese stallholders' interest. By the 1930s, statistics showed that government's revenue from property rent largely depended on the markets, with the Central Market consistently contributing half. In the proposal for the new projects, the colonial government confidently anticipated that the Central Market and the wholesale market would bring in much more

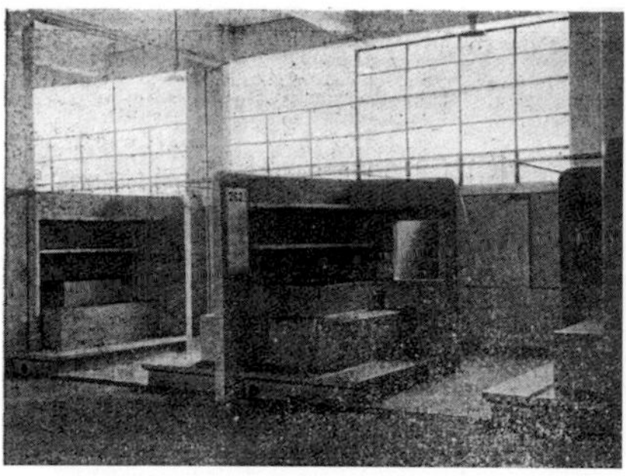
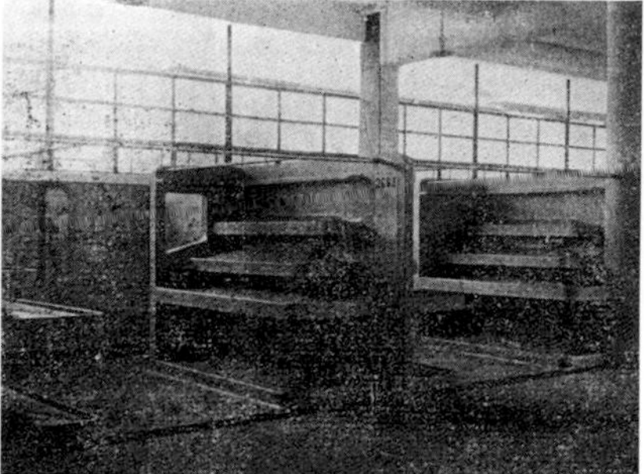

Figures 4.12 & 4.13. Vegetable and Fruit Stalls. *Report on the Social & Economic Progress of the People of the Colony of Hong Kong for the Year 1939*. Courtesy of the University of Hong Kong Libraries.

income.[65] They valued the municipal markets for their ability to provide stable food supply and their potential to keep down living costs, employ a large number of laborers, and drive economic growth.[66] However, the local government rarely reined in those who overcharged for food, and local businesses deemed the high rents economically unsound.[67] Still, despite the loss, the stallholders suffered due to unjust competition in the preferential tenders, the authority prioritized revenue.[68] The 1939 statistics showed that the Central Market achieved first-year rental of HK$348,315 accounting for more than one-third of the investment.[69]

As explained by Peter Scriver, the production of utilitarian buildings and infrastructure was in line with a "parsimonious cognitive economy" of India under early British rule. However, with more monumental structures completed by the Public Works Department, "the phantasm of permanent Raj" replaced the provisional "scaffold of Empire."[70] In Hong Kong, the representation of colonial authority was still varied enough to be fragile.[71] The public markets of brick walls with granite stone dressings showed no real stylistic ambition but adopted pragmatic decor derived from European historicism. In the debate over the design of the 1895 Central Market, the Governor preferred the Surveyor General's less "pretentious" and economical solution, which was "good enough for the purpose" and would not be "a discredit to the town."[72] Free from symbolic decorations, the 1939 project simply conveyed newness to a public audience.[73] The off-center entrances cast dark shadows on the façade and broke the symmetry, which differentiated from stripped classicism prevailing among institutional buildings at that time. The random openness of the awning windows captured the rhythm of everyday use and eliminated the dullness of the flat curtain walls. The ribbon windows under the sun-shade ledges added a sense of lightness. Its austere functionalism lacked,

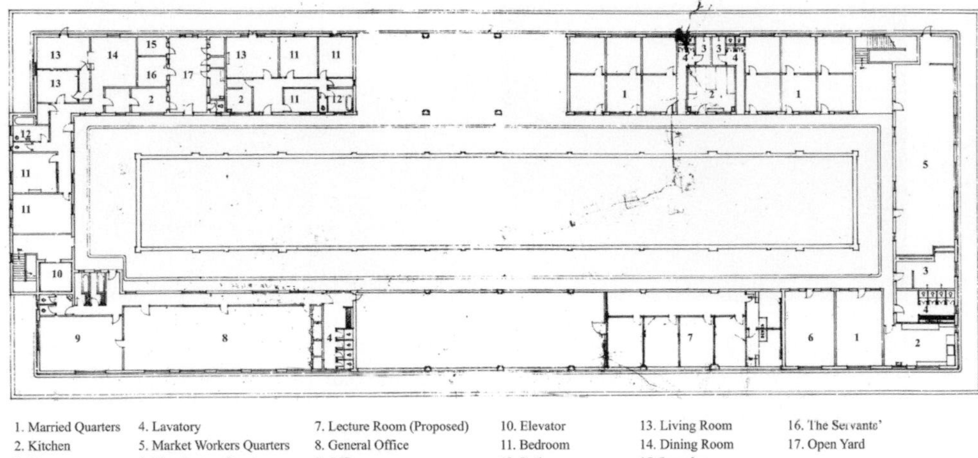

Figure 4.14. Top floor plan (with author annotations), Hong Kong, 1953. It proposed to add a new lecture room and convert part of the existing inspectors' living quarter into office space, as the original design allowed future expansion. See "Central Market: Additions, Alternations and Repairs," HKRS565-7-1, Government Records Service, Hong Kong. Courtesy of the Architectural Services Department Hong Kong.

as well, the playful glamour of the slightly earlier streamlined steel-framed Wanchai Market (Figure 4.15) whose pronounced horizontality it shared.

Though there were few discussions about architectural modernism in Hong Kong in the 1930s, demands for sanitation and comfort were high. Modern structures that combined with new mechanical systems created an "architecture of well-tempered environment."[74] The installation of cold storage in the basement of the Wanchai Market was a breakthrough, for it was impossible for most markets to enjoy "such luxuries."[75] When the construction of the Central Market was completed, the bimonthly *Hong Kong and South China Builder* gave an overall presentation of the project and listed ten participating contractors.[76] It identified the local construction firm Tak Hing, directed by Sun Kwong as the general contractor, and elucidated the techniques of other suppliers, such as the Vibro Piling Company and the General Electric Company of China.[77] The Central Market project became an advertisement broadcasting new achievements in the construction industry.

Exposing people from different origins to diverse ranges of foodstuffs, markets in cosmopolitan cities also became the site of multicultural interaction.[78] In Shanghai's Hongkew Market, the supply right before Christmas included everything from an owl to an omelet.[79] As noted by the Registrar General, at the end of the nineteenth century, more European residents began

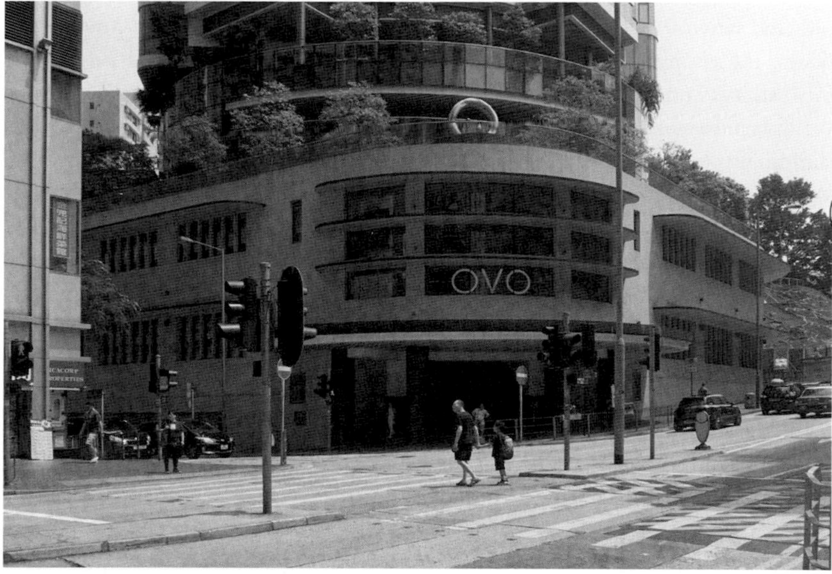

Figure 4.15. Wanchai Market, Hong Kong. This was originally built in 1937, and the renovation project maintains the building's exterior. Photograph by author, 2019.

to regard Hong Kong "more as a permanent home."[80] The government's regulations on behaviors, for instance, altered the eating choices of native Chinese.[81] Despite the colonial policy that encouraged residential segregation and privileged access to city facilities, the discourses on sanitation and health reflected specific interests-based collaboration and contestation between Chinese and European communities.[82] The government officers, sanitary inspectors, market porters, stallholders, and Chinese, British and foreign customers shared the public markets.[83] In the case of the 1895 Central Market, the living condition of the European quarters atop the building was far from satisfactory, and the assistant inspector A. Waston and his family moved out.[84] The 1939 project fostered social mixing through improvements in the facilities on offer. For instance, it provided a European-type women's lavatory for visitors and tourists with an attendant on duty, and the roof terrace connected the accommodation for colonial officers and market workers.[85]

Aware of its economic and social impact, the colonial authority rebuilt the Central Market to improve public services. After the Japanese attacks on the Mainland in 1937, an unprecedented number of refugees inevitably placed intense pressure on Hong Kong's environment, which prompted the government to switch to more interventionist policies.[86] The new market represented the improvement in public health administration and "the transition between old and new of the Hong Kong society."[87] Accompanied by the sanitary officers, the chairman of the Urban Council carried out a special inspection tour after its opening.[88] The splendid modern market drew crowds, and the vendors hosted a three-hour firecracker celebration.[89] As one of the earliest buildings pictured through photography in the report by the Director of Public Works (figure 4.1), the Central Market was an impressive project that brought government agency into daily life.

In the colonial context, sanitary infrastructure offered a symbolic gesture of "imminent modernity."[90] On the one hand, the rational architectural design met the demand for urban sanitation and created an orderly and disciplined retail environment ensuring convenience and safety. It embraced the latest technology for the benefit of the public. On the other hand, under financial pressure the Hong Kong authority expected the project to be a profitable investment that would bring immediate returns, which created tensions between the colonial government and the local Chinese vendors. The adoption of a modernist aesthetic offered an expedient indication of pragmatic governance. By removing what had long been a danger and disgrace and replacing it with something clearly both modern and functional, the government was able to display itself as progressive and forward-looking.

"A Century of Service"

Designed following economic rationality of the colonial rule in Hong Kong, the latest Central Market revealed how the urban amenities were employed by the British authorities as a social instrument. Its history in food supply is traced back to the founding of the colony and evolved with the consolidation of sanitary bureaucracy. Complying with the latest Public Health Ordinance, the project allowed effective official surveillance and educated the populace to act in public in a new manner. Learning from Shanghai precedents and adapting to the local climate conditions, it functioned as a clean machine that offered light and air and evoked industrial efficiency. The application of scientific knowledge and up-to-date technology was consistent with the building's functional requirements, but it also shaped the bodily experience of individual users, while informing their perception of the new.

As the local authority succeeded in attracting Chinese to participate in the business, the project proved to be highly rewarding. This prominent piece of urban infrastructure indicated that the government, though restrained by limited financial resources, strategically funded its activities and accepted increased responsibility to foster public well-being. In the 1930s, the Public Works Department designed and built more everyday buildings for social service in addition to colonial administration. The 1939 medical report expressed concerns about food safety in relation to sanitation and pointed out that the recently completed Central Market was a "sanitary measure of major importance." The project played a role in safeguarding public health and was conceived as part of modernizing the environment, which in the eyes of the colonial authorities doubled as a civilizing mission and, for the "present generation and for many generations to come," a commitment to urban stability under political and economic uncertainty.[91]

In the past decades, continuous refurbishments on the Central Market have been carried out, though the 1939 project failed to keep up with Hong Kong's rapid development that brought about gentrification of the neighborhood. In 2003 all the food stalls were relocated. During the closure, it was listed as a Grade III historic building in 2009. Reopened to the public in August 2021, the revitalized Central Market under the jurisdiction of the Urban Renewal Authority aims to provide cultural and retail facilities to enhance the environmental quality of the Central District, now part of Hong Kong's Central Business District. The adaptive reuse scheme emphasizes sustainability in architectural heritage and explores the social agenda of modernist design beyond the conservation of architectural aesthetic value.

Acknowledgments

The publication of this chapter was generously supported by the Paul Mellon Centre for Studies in British Art.

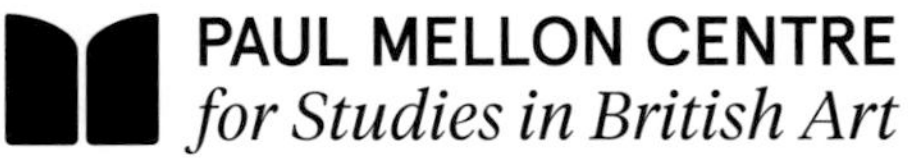

Notes

1. "H.K Will be Proud of its New Market," *Hong Kong Daily Press*, March 17, 1939.
2. In 1842 the first Central Market (Government Market no.1) was constructed at the Marine Lot 16. To ensure the local authority a stable income with minimal management cost, the Hong Kong government sold the market franchise two years later to the highest bidder, who then charged rents from the stallholders. The second Central Market was built in 1858 when the farming system ended. In 1887 the colonial government acquired Marine Lot 18 to form a rectangular-shaped site to construct the third Central Market. This project was completed in 1895 and was replaced by the fourth one in 1939. Gary Chi-hung Luk,

"Occupied Space, Occupied Time: Food Hawking and the Central Market in Hong Kong's Victoria City during the Opium War," *Frontiers of History in China* 11, no. 3 (2016): 406–8; Ma Koon-Yiu, *Xianggang Gongcheng Kao II: Sanshiyi Tiao Yi Gongchengshi Mingming de Jiedao* (Hong Kong: Joint Publishing [Hong Kong] Company, 2014), 166–70; "Plan of Proposed New Market (Central)," CO-129-231, Government Records Service.

3. For industrialism and the sanitary reform in Britain and its influence on the other European countries and the United States, see George Rosen, *A History of Public Health* (New York: MD Publications, 1958), 192–293.
4. Anthony S. Wohl, *Endangered Lives: Public Health in Victorian Britain* (Cambridge, MA: Harvard University Press, 1983).
5. Thomas Osborne, "Security and Vitality: Drains, Liberalism and Power in the Nineteenth Century," in *Foucault and Political Reason: Liberalism, Neo-Liberalism, and Rationalities of Government*, ed. Andrew Barry, Thomas Osborne, and Nikolas S. Rose (Chicago: University of Chicago Press, 1996), 116.
6. Dorothy Porter, *Health, Civilization, and the State: A History of Public Health from Ancient to Modern Times* (London: Routledge, 1999), 63.
7. Daniel R. Headrick, *The Tools of Empire: Technology and European Imperialism in the Nineteenth Century* (New York: Oxford University Press, 1981).
8. See for instance, Mark Harrison, *Public Health in British India: Anglo-Indian Preventive Medicine, 1859–1914*, Cambridge History of Medicine (Cambridge, UK: Cambridge University Press, 1994); and Lenore Manderson, *Sickness and the State: Health and Illness in Colonial Malaya, 1870–1940* (Cambridge, UK: Cambridge University Press, 1996).
9. David Scott, "Colonial Governmentality," *Social Text*, no. 43 (1995): 191–220. Employing modern scientific knowledge to preserve colonial hegemony, it involved environmental regulation and affected behavior and manners.
10. See, for instance, Veena Talwar Oldenburg, *The Making of Colonial Lucknow, 1856–1877* (Princeton, NJ: Princeton University Press, 2014); Brenda S. A. Yeoh, *Contesting Space: Power Relations and the Urban Built Environment in Colonial Singapore* (Kuala Lumpur: Oxford University Press, 1996).
11. Robert K. Home, *Of Planting and Planning: The Making of British Colonial Cities* (London: Spon, 1997), 85–95.
12. Alison Bashford, *Imperial Hygiene: A Critical History of Colonialism, Nationalism and Public Health* (New York: Palgrave Macmillan, 2004), 9–10.
13. Though not uninhabited, Hong Kong was described as "a barren island with hardly a house upon it" by the then–British Foreign Secretary Lord Palmerstone in a private letter. Later authors often quote this depiction in writing the city's colonial history.

14. Lennox A. Mills, *British Rule in Eastern Asia: A Study of Contemporary Government and Economic Development in British Malaya and Hong Kong* (London: Oxford University Press, 1942), 484–89.
15. For the development of the public health system in Hong Kong, see Moira MW Chan-Yeung, *A Medical History of Hong Kong: 1842–1941* (Hong Kong: Chinese University of Hong Kong Press, 2018) and Robin Gauld and Derek Gould, *The Hong Kong Health Sector: Development and Change* (Hong Kong: Chinese University Press, 2002), 33–42.
16. For the city planning of early Hong Kong, see Charlie Q.L. Xue et al., "The Shaping of Early Hong Kong: Transplantation and Adaptation by the British Professionals, 1841–1941," *Planning Perspectives* 27, no. 4 (2012): 549–68; and Pui-yin Ho, *Making Hong Kong* (Cheltenham, UK: Edward Elgar Publishing, 2018): 6–14.
17. Luk, "Occupied Space," 405–8.
18. To build the "European town," the Upper Bazaar was relocated to Taipingshan in 1844. Dafydd Emrys Evans, "Chinatown in Hong Kong: The Beginnings of Taipingshan," *Journal of the Hong Kong Branch of the Royal Asiatic Society* 10 (1970): 69–71; John M. Carroll, *Edge of Empires: Chinese Elites and British Colonials in Hong Kong* (Cambridge, MA; London: Harvard University Press, 2005), 23–32.
19. In 1844, Hong Kong formulated the first act on urban sanitation, "An Ordinance for the Preservation of Order and Cleanliness," which prohibited any negative impacts on the street environment.
20. Luk, "Occupied Space," 418–19.
21. "An Ordinance for Licensing Markets, and for Preventing Disorders Therein," Hong Kong, 1847.
22. "The Market Ordinance, 1857," *Hong Kong Government Gazette*, September 12, 1857; "Bye-laws, Made and Notified by His Excellency the Governor in Executive Council, Pursuant to the Market Ordinance, 1858," *Hong Kong Government Gazette*, June 22, 1858.
23. "The Market Ordinance, 1867," *Hong Kong Government Gazette*, May 18, 1867.
24. Dafydd Emrys Evans, "The Origins of Hong Kong's Central Market and the Tarrant Affair," *Journal of the Hong Kong Branch of the Royal Asiatic Society* 12 (1972): 150–51.
25. The market ordinance introduced a standard registration form for stallholders. All markets were open to sanitary inspection and conspicuously posted copies of the regulations governing them. See "The Cattle Diseases, Slaughter Houses and Markets Ordinance," *Hong Kong Government Gazette*, June 25, 1887; "Bye-laws Made under Section 16 of the Public Health and Building Ordinance, 1903," *Hong Kong Government Gazette*, October 8, 1909.
26. "The Central Market Amenities," *Hong Kong Telegraph*, May 26, 1909.

27. Hong Kong Legislative Council Meeting Report, May 20, 1909; "A Bill Entitled an Ordinance to Amend the Public Health and Buildings Ordinance 1903," *Hong Kong Government Gazette*, April 2, 1909.
28. John M. Carroll, *A Concise History of Hong Kong* (Lanham, MD: Rowman & Littlefield, 2007), 107–9.
29. For the full list, see "Ordinance no.13 of 1935. (Public Health [Food])," *Hong Kong Government Gazette*, May 14, 1937.
30. "The Market Ordinance, 1887."
31. "Bye-laws, 1909."
32. "Public Health (Food) Ordinance, 1935."
33. The design of the Smithfield Market in London reflected similar concerns, and relevant restrictions could be seen in the municipal code of British towns, such as Manchester. See Patrick Joyce, *The Rule of Freedom: Liberalism and the Modern City* (London: Verso, 2003), 83–87.
34. Deborah Lupton, *The Imperative of Health: Public Health and the Regulated Body* (London: Sage Publications, 1995), 2.
35. Bashford, *Imperial Hygiene*, 1.
36. Thomas A. Markus, *Buildings & Power: Freedom and Control in the Origin of Modern Building Types* (London; New York: Routledge, 1993), 300–306.
37. James Schmiechen and Kenneth Carls, *The British Market Hall: A Social and Architectural History* (New Haven: Yale University Press, 1999), 160–81.
38. Christopher Curtis Mead, *Making Modern Paris: Victor Baltard's Central Markets and the Urban Practice of Architecture* (University Park: Pennsylvania State University Press, 2012), 10–18.
39. Manuel Guàrdia i Bassols, and José Luis Oyón, ed., *Making Cities through Market Halls: Europe, 19th and 20th Centuries* (Barcelona: Ajuntament de Barcelona, Museu d'Història de Barcelona, 2015); Nikolaus Pevsner, *A History of Building Types* (Princeton, NJ: Princeton University Press, 1976), 235–56.
40. Kathleen James-Chakraborty, *German Architecture for a Mass Audience* (London: Routledge, 2000), 31–32; Bundesverband der Deutschen Zementindustrie e.V., Cologne, *Concrete Construction Manual* (Basel: Edition Detail, 2002), 19.
41. Cast iron columns and beams also had the advantage of easy assembly. The cast iron work was imported from Glasgow and the erection was done by a local firm. For its historical evolution, see Kip Lin Lee, *Telok Ayer Market: A Historical Account of the Market from the Founding of the Settlement of Singapore to the Present Time* (Singapore: Archives & Oral History Dept, Singapore, 1983).
42. L. W. Michael, *The History of the Municipal Corporation of the City of Bombay* (Bombay: Union Press, 1902), 19. Before the creation of the Bombay Municipal Corporation in 1865, the 1862 Markets and Fairs Acts concerning the establishment permission were intended to solve disputes between landowners.

43. Osbert Chadwick, *Mr. Chadwick's Reports on the Sanitary Condition of Hong Kong* (London: George E. B. Eyre and William Spottiswoode, 1882), 40.
44. "The Cattle Diseases, Slaughter Houses and Markets Ordinance, 1887." The 1847 ordinance first prescribed markets be built of stone or brick according to the approved plan.
45. According to *the Report of the Director of the Public Works for 1895*, the upper floor of concrete finished in cement was supported by cast iron columns and wrought iron girders with steel joists and corrugated steel decking.
46. Hong Kong Legislative Council Meeting Report, July 15, 1901; "Reports Relative to the Lighting of the Central Market," *Hong Kong Weekly Press*, July 29, 1901. Those who required additional light in their stalls were only allowed to use electric lamps or smokeless oil lamps of an approved pattern. See "Additional Bye-Law," *Hong Kong Government Gazette*, October 19, 1901.
47. Yanxiang Tang and Xiaoqi Zhu, *Jindai Shanghai Fandian Yu Caichang* (Shanghai: Shanghai Cichu Chubanshe, 2008), 270–350.
48. Kerrie L. Macpherson, *A Wilderness of Marshes: The Origins of Public Health in Shanghai, 1843–1893* (Hong Kong: Oxford University Press, 1987), 259–75.
49. "Hongkew Market," U1-14-1801, 1912/11/29, Shanghai Municipal Archive. On the Maloo Market, see Edward Denison, *Modernism in China: Architectural Visions and Revolutions* (Chichester, UK: John Wiley, 2008), 61.
50. Xiaoming Zhu, "Original Construction: A Comparative Study of the Original Shanghai Municipal Council Chushan Road Public Market," *Time+Architecture*, no. 2 (2015): 110–17.
51. Ruth Rogaski, *Hygienic Modernity: Meanings of Health and Disease in Treaty-Port China* (Berkeley: University of California Press, 2004), 193–224. From 1860 to 1902, Britain, France, Japan, Germany and Russia, Austria-Hungary, Italy, and Belgium established their self-contained concessions in Tientsin.
52. "Cankao shanghai zhuangkuang," *Kung Sheung Daily News*, November 1, 1936.
53. "The Cattle Diseases, Slaughter Houses and Markets Ordinance, 1887."
54. "Central Market: Proposed Rebuilding," CO 129/559/20, The National Archives.
55. On modernist design and sanitation, see Margaret Campbell, "What Tuberculosis Did for Modernism: The Influence of a Curative Environment on Modernist Design and Architecture," *Medical History* 49, no. 4 (2005): 463–88; Paul Overy, *Light, Air & Openness: Modern Architecture between the Wars* (London: Thames & Hudson, 2007); Beatriz Colomina, *X-Ray Architecture* (Zürich: Lars Müller Publishers, 2019).
56. "The New Central Market in Hong Kong," *Hong Kong and South China Builder* 4, no. 2 (1939), 9.
57. The Central Market is regarded as one of the earliest examples of the International Style in Hong Kong. Man Han, "The Characteristics of Modern

Architecture in Hong Kong, 1930s–1970s" (PhD diss., Hong Kong, Chinese University of Hong Kong, 2016), 48–51; Daqing Gu, Vito Bertin, and Peiling Hu, "The Greatest Form Has No Shape: The Case Study of Hong Kong Modern Architecture The Central Market," *Time+Architecture*, no. 3 (2015): 128.

58. Hong Kong University first founded the architectural department in 1950 and it was not until 1957 that architects and engineers were shown separately in the A.A. List. Haoyu Wang, "Mainland Architects in Hong Kong after 1949: A Bifurcated History of Modern Chinese Architecture" (PhD diss., Hong Kong, University of Hong Kong, 2008), 113.
59. Peiran He, *Becoming Hong Kong: Development History of Construction Industry 1840–2010*, (Hong Kong: Commercial Press HK, 2010), 121–31.
60. Gauld and Gould, *Health Sector*, 39.
61. Hong Kong Legislative Council Meeting Report, October 2, 1930.
62. Hong Kong Legislative Council Meeting Report, September 22, 1932. According to the annual report of the Director of Public Works in the 1930s the provision of latrines, bathhouses, markets, and hospitals accounted for around half budget for "Buildings" in the "Public Works Extraordinary."
63. "The Hong Kong Dollar Loan Ordinance, 1934" granted the government to raise a loan of 25 million that would be "payable out of the revenue and assets of the Colony." It included Aberdeen Valley Water Scheme, Shing Mun Valley Water Schemes, Vehicular Ferry, New Gaol at Stanley, Tytam Tuk Catchwaters, Air Port Development, Redemption of Hong Kong 3.5% Inscribed Stock 1918/43, and Other Public Works. The Estimates of Expenditure for 1937 increased the schedule of Other Public Works from $10,338 to $1,025,000 to build the new Central Market and the Wholesale Market at Kennedy Town. See Hong Kong Legislative Council Meeting Report, May 28, 1937.
64. Hong Kong Legislative Council Meeting Report, September 29, 1937; Hong Kong Legislative Council Meeting Report, July 7, 1938.
65. "Central Market," National Archives.
66. Hong Kong Legislative Council Meeting Report, September 27, 1934; "Weishengju zuihou huiyi: zhuxi tuote baogao." *Shun Pao*, December 21, 1938.
67. When questioned about the overcharges that made food unaffordable to low-income people, the colonial secretary insisted on free competition. "Rent too High in Market: Many Stallholders to Cease Business," *Hong Kong Telegraph*, May 13, 1939; and "Central Market Difficulties," *China Mail*, June 5, 1939.
68. "Central Market Mystery: Preference in Calling of Tenders," *Hong Kong Telegraph*, April 17, 1939; and "Zhonghuan jieshi tanfan lianqing dangju jianzu," *Ta Kung Pao*, April 18, 1939.
69. Some of the stall-holders prepaid two months' rent but had to quit their business before the lease ended. The colonial authority rejected the application for rent reductions and simply withdrew stalls and put on new tender. Thanks to the

higher rentals in the new Central Market, rent of Government Property was two hundred thousand dollars in excess of the estimate. See *The Financial Report for the Year 1939*; "Sanshi jia tanwei zhunbei tingye qianchu," *Ta Kung Pao*, June 3, 1939, and "At Cheaper Rentals: Reletting of Stalls in Central Market," *Hong Kong Telegraph*, June 29, 1939.

70. Peter Scriver, "Empire-Building and Thinking in the Public Works Department of British India," in *Colonial Modernities: Building, Dwelling and Architecture in British India and Ceylon*, ed. Peter Scriver and Vikramaditya Prakash, The Architext Series (London; New York: Routledge, 2007), 69–92.
71. G. A. Bremner, "Fabricating Justice: Conflict and Contradiction in the Making of the Hong Kong Supreme Court, 1898–1912," in *Harbin to Hanoi: The Colonial Built Environment in Asia, 1840 to 1940*, ed. Laura A. Victoir and Victor Zatsepine, Global Connections (Hong Kong: Hong Kong University Press, 2013), 151–80.
72. "The Gap Rock Lighthouse and the Central Market," *China Mail*, February 12, 1890. Also, the Hong Kong authority rejected the design made by an architect sent from London. See Ma, *Gongcheng Kao*, 167–77.
73. Some said that the approach taken in the Central Market followed that of the 1933 China Emporium, one of the most popular department stores in Hong Kong. See "Zhongshi tuze huijiu," *Chinese Mail*, December 19, 1937.
74. Reyner Banham, *Architecture of the Well-Tempered Environment* (Chicago: University of Chicago Press, 1984).
75. "New Market at Wanchai: Up-to-Date Structure Being Built," *Hong Kong Sunday Herald*, September 27, 1936.
76. With its publisher representatives and correspondents located in various Asian cities including Tsingtao, Kobe and Manila, the journal brought about practical information targeting the architects, developers, and contractors in mainland China, Macao, the Philippine Islands, and Malaya.
77. Sun later became the chairman of the Hong Kong Building Contractors' Association, and its members worked in close partnership with the government.
78. Su Lin Lewis, *Cities in Motion: Urban Life and Cosmopolitanism in Southeast Asia, 1920–1940* (Cambridge, UK: Cambridge University Press, 2016), 65–68.
79. "A Specialized Aspect of Christmas," *North-China Herald and Supreme Court & Consular Gazette*, December 31, 1926.
80. Robert Peckham, "Introduction: Panic: Reading the Signs," in *Empires of Panic: Epidemics and Colonial Anxieties*, ed. Robert Peckham (Hong Kong: Hong Kong University Press, 2015), 1; and Hong Kong Census Report 1891.
81. Shuk-Wah Poon, "Dogs and British Colonialism: The Contested Ban on Eating Dogs in Colonial Hong Kong," *Journal of Imperial and Commonwealth History* 42, no. 2 (March 15, 2014): 308–28.

82. Lawrence W. C. Lai, "Discriminatory Zoning in Colonial Hong Kong: A Review of the Post-War Literature and Some Further Evidence for an Economic Theory of Discrimination," *Property Management* 29, no. 1 (2011): 50–86; Cecilia Chu, "Combating Nuisance: Sanitation, Regulation, and the Politics of Property in Colonial Hong Kong," in *Imperial Contagions: Medicine, Hygiene, and Cultures of Planning in Asia*, ed. Robert Shannan Peckham and David M. Pomfret (Hong Kong: University Press, 2013), 17–36.
83. Reports on market violation related to European customers focus mainly on bag snatching and profanity.
84. During his visit, the colonial vice-president remarked that it was not suitable for Europeans to inhabit and "might do for a colored man or a Chinese." "The European Quarters at the Central Market," *Hong Kong Daily Press*, October 21, 1898.
85. It was clean, well-equipped, frequently-used, and became exclusive to Europeans in the later forties. "Zhonghuan jieshi yijian gaiwei xiren zhuanyong," *Overseas Chinese Daily News*, June 25, 1949.
86. According to the *Annual Medical Report for 1939*, Hong Kong's population had almost doubled as a result of the influx of refugees since the start of the Sino-Japanese Incident in July 1937. See also Margaret Jones, "Tuberculosis, Housing and the Colonial State: Hong Kong, 1900-1950," *Modern Asian Studies* 37, no. 3 (2003): 653–82; and Leo F. Goodstadt, "The Rise and Fall of Social, Economic and Political Reforms in Hong Kong, 1930–1955," *Journal of the Royal Asiatic Society Hong Kong Branch* 44 (2004): 57–81.
87. "H. K. Will be Proud of Its New Market: Modern Building with Every Facility and Convenience"; and "Xin zhonghuan jieshi poushi chongjing," *Shun Pao*, March 18, 1939.
88. "Inspection of New Central Market," *Hong Kong Daily Press*, April 26, 1939; and "Gangdu canguan," *Kung Sheung Daily News*, April 19, 1939.
89. "Mei lun mei huan zhi xin zhonghuan jieshi zuochen kaishi yingye," *Kung Sheung Daily News*, May 4, 1939.
90. Awadhendra Sharan, "In the City, Out of Place: Environment and Modernity, Delhi 1860s to 1960s," *Economic and Political Weekly* 41, no. 47 (2006): 4906.
91. "The New Central Market in Hong Kong," 9.

Archival Sources

Architectural Services Department, Hong Kong
Government Records Service, Hong Kong
The National Archives, London
Museum of Fine Arts, Budapest

Library of Congress, Washington
National Library of Scotland, Edinburgh
Shanghai Municipal Archive
American Geographical Society Library, University of Wisconsin Milwaukee Libraries

Journals and Newspapers

China Mail
Hong Kong and South China Builder
Hong Kong Daily Press
Hong Kong Government Gazette
Hong Kong Sunday Herald
Hong Kong Telegraph
Hong Kong Weekly Press
Kung Sheung Daily News
North-China Herald and Supreme Court & Consular Gazette
Ta Kung Pao
Overseas Chinese Daily News
Shun Pao

Government Records

Report on the Social & Economic Progress of the People of the Colony of Hong Kong for the Year 1939

Bibliography

Awadhendra, Sharan. "In the City, Out of Place: Environment and Modernity, Delhi 1860s to 1960s." *Economic and Political Weekly* 41, no. 47 (2006): 4905–11.

Barry, Andrew, Thomas Osborne, and Nikolas S. Rose (eds). *Foucault and Political Reason: Liberalism, Neo-Liberalism, and Rationalities of Government*. Chicago: University of Chicago Press, 1996.

Bashford, Alison. *Imperial Hygiene: A Critical History of Colonialism, Nationalism and Public Health*. New York: Palgrave Macmillan, 2004.

Bundesverband der Deutschen Zementindustrie e.V., Cologne. *Concrete Construction Manual*. Basel: Edition Detail, 2002.

Campbell, Margaret. "What Tuberculosis Did for Modernism: The Influence of a Curative Environment on Modernist Design and Architecture." *Medical History* 49, no. 4 (October 2005): 463–88.

Carroll, John M. *A Concise History of Hong Kong*. Lanham, MD: Rowman & Littlefield, 2007.

———. *Edge of Empires: Chinese Elites and British Colonials in Hong Kong*. Cambridge, MA: Harvard University Press, 2005.

Chadwick, Osbert. *Mr. Chadwick's Reports on the Sanitary Condition of Hong Kong*. London: George E. B. Eyre and William Spottiswoode, 1882.

Chan-Yeung, Moira M. W. *A Medical History of Hong Kong: 1842–1941*. Hong Kong: Chinese University of Hong Kong Press, 2018.

Colomina, Beatriz. *X-Ray Architecture*. Zürich: Lars Müller Publishers, 2019.

Denison, Edward. *Modernism in China: Architectural Visions and Revolutions*. Chichester, UK: John Wiley, 2008.

Evans, Dafydd Emrys. "Chinatown in Hong Kong: The Beginnings of Taipingshan." *Journal of the Hong Kong Branch of the Royal Asiatic Society* 10 (1970): 69–78.

———. "The Origins of Hong Kong's Central Market and the Tarrant Affair." *Journal of the Hong Kong Branch of the Royal Asiatic Society* 12 (1972): 150–60.

Gauld, Robin, and Derek Gould. *The Hong Kong Health Sector: Development and Change*. Hong Kong: Chinese University Press, 2002.

Goodstadt, Leo F. "The Rise and Fall of Social, Economic and Political Reforms in Hong Kong, 1930-1955." *Journal of the Royal Asiatic Society Hong Kong Branch* 44 (2004): 57–81.

Gu, Daqing, Vito Bertin, and Peiling Hu. "The Greatest Form Has No Shape: The Case Study of Hong Kong Modern Architecture The Central Market." *Time+Architecture* no. 3 (2015): 128–36.

Guàrdia i Bassols, Manuel, and José Luis Oyón (ed.). *Making Cities through Market Halls: Europe, 19th and 20th Centuries*. Barcelona: Ajuntament de Barcelona, Museu d'Història de Barcelona, 2015.

Gullick, J. M. "Kuala Lumpur, 1880–1895." *Journal of the Malayan Branch of the Royal Asiatic Society* 28, no. 4 (1955): 1–172.

Han, Man. "The Characteristics of Modern Architecture in Hong Kong, 1930s–1970s." PhD diss., Chinese University of Hong Kong, 2016.

Harrison, Mark. *Public Health in British India: Anglo-Indian Preventive Medicine, 1859–1914*. Cambridge, UK: Cambridge University Press, 1994.

He, Peiran. *Becoming Hong Kong: Development History of Construction Industry 1840–2010*. Hong Kong: Commercial Press HK, 2010.

Headrick, Daniel R. *The Tools of Empire: Technology and European Imperialism in the Nineteenth Century*. New York: Oxford University Press, 1981.

Ho, Pui-yin. *Making Hong Kong*. Cheltenham, UK: Edward Elgar, 2018.

Home, Robert K. *Of Planting and Planning: The Making of British Colonial Cities.* London: Spon, 1997.

James-Chakraborty, Kathleen. *German Architecture for a Mass Audience.* London: Routledge, 2000.

Jones, Margaret. "Tuberculosis, Housing and the Colonial State: Hong Kong, 1900–1950." *Modern Asian Studies* 37, no. 3 (July 2003): 653–82.

Joyce, Patrick. *The Rule of Freedom: Liberalism and the Modern City.* London: Verso, 2003.

Lai, Lawrence W. C. "Discriminatory Zoning in Colonial Hong Kong: A Review of the Post-War Literature and Some Further Evidence for an Economic Theory of Discrimination." *Property Management* 29, no. 1 (January 2011): 50–86.

Lam Chung-Wai, Tony. "From British Colonization to Japanese Invasion: The 100 Years Architects in Hong Kong 1941–1941." *Hong Kong Institute of Architects Journal* 45 (2006): 44–55.

Lee, Kip Lin. *Telok Ayer Market: A Historical Account of the Market from the Founding of the Settlement of Singapore to the Present Time.* Singapore: Archives & Oral History Dept, Singapore, 1983.

Lewis, Su Lin. *Cities in Motion: Urban Life and Cosmopolitanism in Southeast Asia, 1920–1940.* Cambridge, UK: Cambridge University Press, 2016.

Luk, Gary Chi-hung. "Occupied Space, Occupied Time: Food Hawking and the Central Market in Hong Kong's Victoria City during the Opium War." *Frontiers of History in China* 11, no. 3 (2016): 400–430.

Lupton, Deborah. *The Imperative of Health: Public Health and the Regulated Body.* London : Sage Publications, 1995.

Ma, Koon-Yiu. *Xianggang Gongcheng Kao II: Sanshiyi Tiao Yi Gongchengshi Mingming de Jiedao.* Hong Kong: Joint Publishing (Hong Kong) Company, 2014.

Macpherson, Kerrie L. *A Wilderness of Marshes: The Origins of Public Health in Shanghai, 1843–1893.* Hong Kong; New York: Oxford University Press, 1987.

Manderson, Lenore. *Sickness and the State: Health and Illness in Colonial Malaya, 1870–1940.* Cambridge University Press, 1996.

Markus, Thomas A. *Buildings & Power: Freedom and Control in the Origin of Modern Building Types.* London: Routledge, 1993.

Mead, Christopher Curtis. *Making Modern Paris: Victor Baltard's Central Markets and the Urban Practice of Architecture.* University Park: Pennsylvania State University Press, 2012.

Michael, L. W. *The History of the Municipal Corporation of the City of Bombay.* Bombay: Union Press, 1902.

Mills, Lennox A. *British Rule in Eastern Asia: A Study of Contemporary Government and Economic Development in British Malaya and Hong Kong.* London: Oxford University Press, 1942.

Oldenburg, Veena Talwar. *The Making of Colonial Lucknow, 1856–1877*. Princeton, NJ: Princeton University Press, 2014.

Overy, Paul. *Light, Air & Openness: Modern Architecture between the Wars*. London: Thames & Hudson, 2007.

Peckham, Robert (ed). *Empires of Panic: Epidemics and Colonial Anxieties*. Hong Kong: Hong Kong University Press, 2015.

Peckham, Robert Shannan, and David M. Pomfret, (ed.). *Imperial Contagions: Medicine, Hygiene, and Cultures of Planning in Asia*. Hong Kong: University Press, 2013.

Pevsner, Nikolaus. *A History of Building Types*. Princeton, NJ: Princeton University Press, 1976.

Poon, Shuk-Wah. "Dogs and British Colonialism: The Contested Ban on Eating Dogs in Colonial Hong Kong." *Journal of Imperial and Commonwealth History* 42, no. 2 (March 2014): 308–28.

Porter, Dorothy. *Health, Civilization, and the State: A History of Public Health from Ancient to Modern Times*. London: Routledge, 1999.

Rogaski, Ruth. *Hygienic Modernity: Meanings of Health and Disease in Treaty-Port China*. Berkeley: University of California Press, 2004.

Rosen, George. *A History of Public Health*. New York: MD Publications, 1958.

Schmiechen, James, and Kenneth Carls. *The British Market Hall: A Social and Architectural History*. New Haven: Yale University Press, 1999.

Scott, David. "Colonial Governmentality." *Social Text*, no. 43 (1995): 191–220.

Scriver, Peter, and Vikramaditya Prakash. *Colonial Modernities: Building, Dwelling and Architecture in British India and Ceylon*. London: Routledge, 2007.

Tang, Yanxiang, and Xiaoqi Zhu. *Jindai Shanghai Fandian Yu Caichang*. Shanghai: Shanghai Cichu Chubanshe, 2008.

Victoir, Laura A., and Victor Zatsepine. *Harbin to Hanoi: The Colonial Built Environment in Asia, 1840 to 1940*. Hong Kong: Hong Kong University Press, 2013.

Wang, Haoyu. "Mainland Architects in Hong Kong after 1949: A Bifurcated History of Modern Chinese Architecture." PhD diss., University of Hong Kong, 2008.

Wohl, Anthony S. *Endangered Lives: Public Health in Victorian Britain*. Cambridge, MA: Harvard University Press, 1983.

Xue, Charlie Q.L., Han Zou, Baihao Li, and Ka Chuen Hui. "The Shaping of Early Hong Kong: Transplantation and Adaptation by the British Professionals, 1841–1941." *Planning Perspectives* 27, no. 4 (October 2012): 549–68.

Yeoh, Brenda S. A. *Contesting Space: Power Relations and the Urban Built Environment in Colonial Singapore*. Kuala Lumpur: Oxford University Press, 1996.

Zhu, Xiaoming. "Original Construction: A Comparative Study of the Original Shanghai Municipal Council Chushan Road Public Market." *Time+Architecture*, no. 2 (2015): 110–17.

CHAPTER 5

NAIROBI CITY MARKET

The Versatile Afterlife of a Colonial-Era Building in a Postcolonial World

Nkatha Gichuyia

Place, Setting and Postcolonial Conceptions of the Built Environment

Nairobi City Market is a populous, lively complex. Its hum and bustle are evident today to anyone who walks along Muindi Mbingu[1] and Koinange Streets,[2] which abut its main entrances (figures 5.1 and 5.2). The sounds of "Fish *hapa*," "Porkchop chunks for you, my lady?," "Exchange dollars?," "*Mama* beautiful, some jewellery for you," and many more trader callouts are synonymous with the market, as various merchants tout their diverse wares. It is the only location in Nairobi's Central Business District (CBD) where you can get ready-made funeral flower arrangements, and it is also one of the few places where authentic *Nyama choma* is available at any time of the weekday.[3]

The complex's main space—the market hall—with its vaulted ceilings and Art Deco features gives the market a bold presence (figure 5.2). What truly stands out, however, is that it is a relatively untouched colonial-era building. Yet despite its age and colonial legacy, it is replete with life and activity, qualities shared by few surviving colonial buildings around it and across Nairobi.

Most colonial architecture in African cities has a static, isolated presence in the ever-changing urban contexts. There are existential vulnerabilities imposed on buildings and cities that were built and planned in settler colonies.[4] Under colonialism, urban centers were planned with somewhat policed social and racial borders that preserved the identity of the foreign settler population. As for buildings, "colonial architecture was an insignia of colonial authority and symbols of colonial desire, exploitation, oppression, dominance and discipline."[5] Today, many postcolonial cities like Nairobi are places of immense and rapid urban transformation. As such, their colonial buildings and urban plans raise difficult questions about the past and what should be preserved.

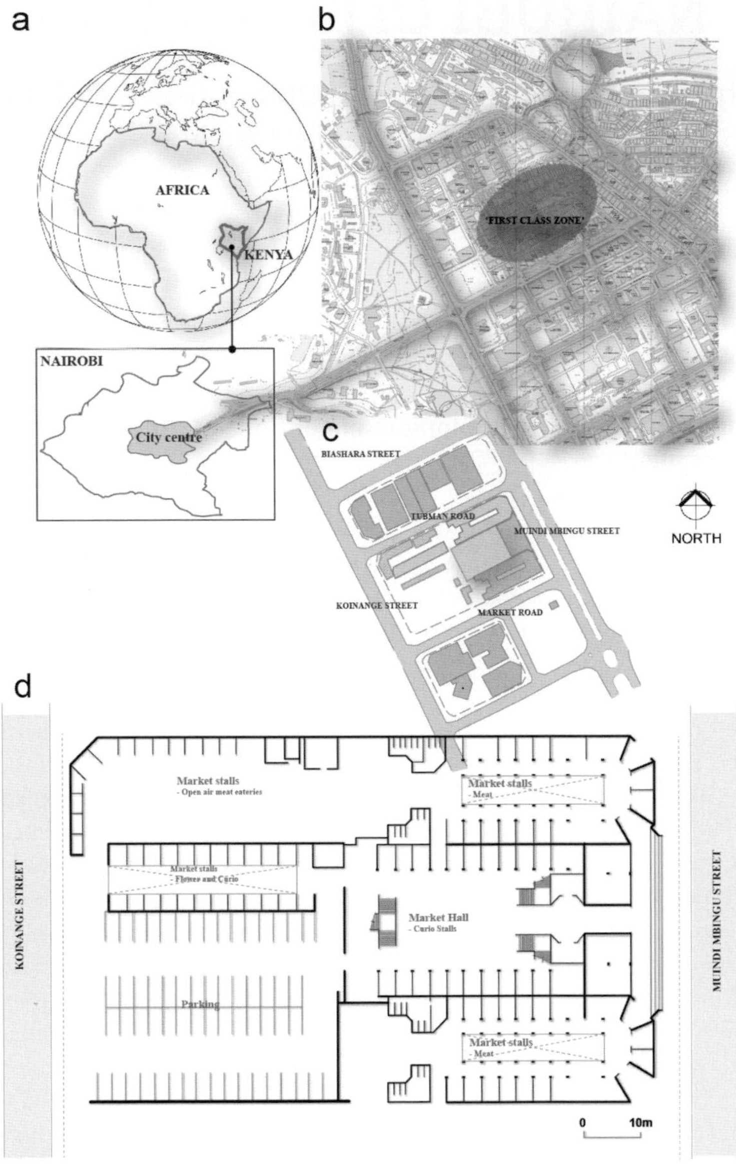

Figure 5.1. Maps and plans. (a, b): Location maps of Africa, Kenya, Nairobi, and Nairobi's Central Business District. (c): Site plan of the Nairobi City Market. (d): Ground floor layout of City Market. All traced maps and drawn plans by author, 2020.

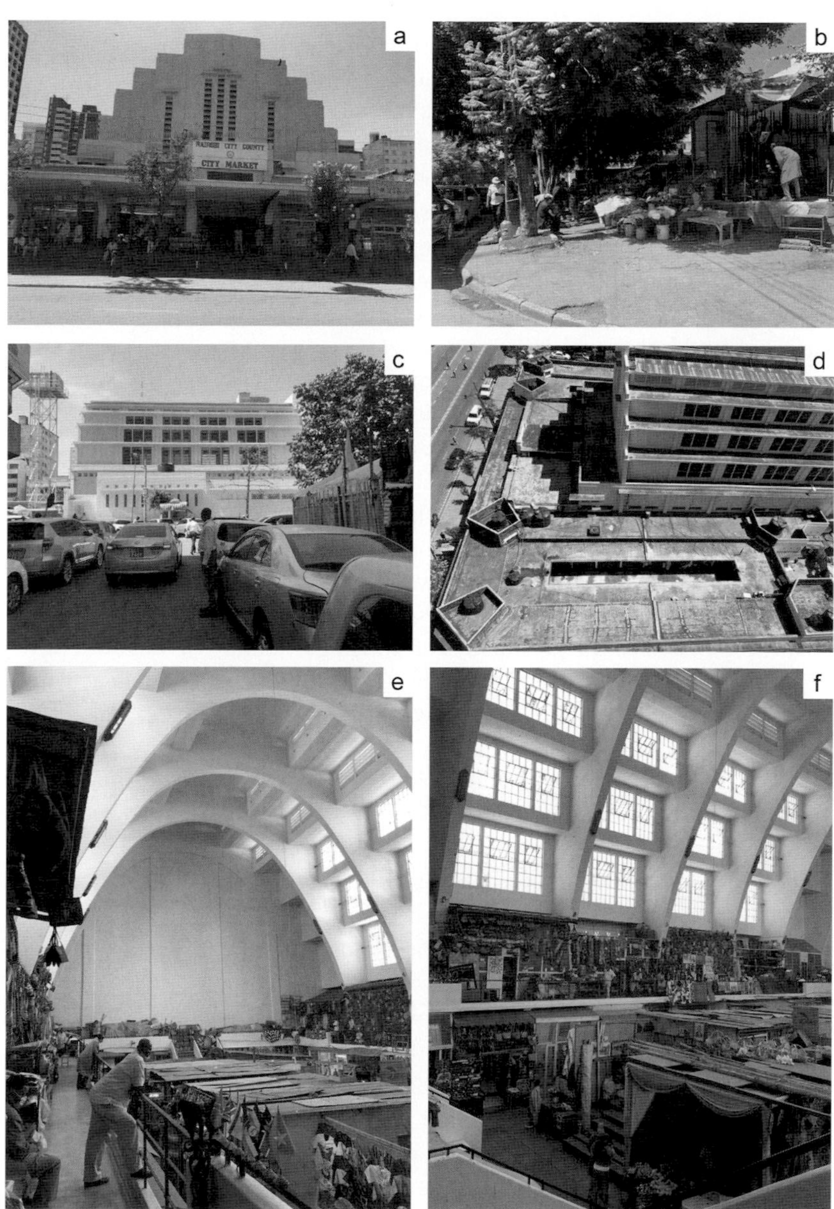

Figure 5.2. City Market from different vantage points. (a): view from Muindi Mbingu Street; (b): view from Koinange Street; (c): view from Market Road; (d): Aerial view from Tubman Road; (e, f): internal views of the market hall. Photographs by author, 2020.

Along with this conflict between urban change and heritage is a lingering, persistent question: What properties should a building embody to characterize the African genius loci of postcolonial Nairobi?[6] A closer look at the legacy of colonial architecture in Kenya's capital indicates that few buildings from that period have stood the test of time in a postcolonial, politically independent and globalized Nairobi.[7] Understandably, some colonial-era ones have been challenged by market pressures and changing times. As a result, such buildings have been wholly reinterpreted, changed their use, or undergone modification of their architectural forms or spatial configuration. That is not the case for Nairobi City Market, which is an anomaly.

The market is a large, important landmark in the city, one that was architecturally ahead of its time. It was designed and constructed to bring order to Nairobi's mercantile and colonial culture during the 1930s. Despite its colonial legacy, it portrays an impressive ability to persist and endure even in present-day Nairobi. The market complex has managed to withstand the effects of time and urban transformation, and continues to be exceptionally well-known and thoroughly used. Its history, however, has not been widely documented or shared. In this chapter, City Market is presented as a vehicle to describe the challenges as well as the possibilities of studying colonial-era buildings in the present day. Acknowledging the afterlives of such buildings as an issue within the study of architecture is relevant beyond Nairobi, as these cases can serve as valuable narrators of the past.

This chapter embarks on a discussion of City Market: a municipal market in the heart of Nairobi's CBD that predominantly sells meat in its covered stalls, souvenirs in its main market hall, authentic Kenyan food in its food court, and flowers in its street-front shops. For close to ninety years, the market complex has stood witness to Nairobi's urban development and the attendant social, economic, political, and infrastructural changes. The reciprocities between City Market's physical form and the evolving street character, socioeconomics, and cultural compositions are reviewed to explore the qualities allowing City Market to hum, bustle and persist in a dynamically changing Nairobi.

The discussion begins with an architectural description of the market, its historic setting as well as its position in the transformation of Nairobi over the last century. The social, economic, and political conditions surrounding Nairobi's formative years are used as a backdrop to discuss the context in which City Market was built. The contrasting and divergent conditions in Nairobi's postcolonial setting are progressively traced to examine City Market's ability to thrive in a versatile way. City Market's spatiotemporal versatility contrasts with most colonial-era buildings that face decimation as a result of the modification of spaces by developers hoping to keep up with changing times. This study ultimately overturns a shared scholarly claim that most colonial architecture has a static relationship to the passage of time in an ever-changing urban context.

The Architecture of Nairobi City Market

City Market, which was known as Nairobi Municipal Market pre-independence,[8] was designed by the city's council architects and its construction was completed in 1932. Based on contemporary reports in the *Architects' Journal*, the consulting architects were Rand Overy and S. L. Blackburne, both of whom were well-known in Nairobi and involved in other building projects.[9] City Market consists of a main, covered market hall that is flanked on both sides by one-level stalls arranged around two courtyards. Larger, closable shop spaces face the market's main podium entrance along Muindi Mbingu Street, while the flower shops—a combination of open-air and covered stalls—face Koinange Street. A customer parking lot with sixty spaces takes up at least a third of the market's street length along Koinange Street, leaving only one entry point to City Market from this end via the floral shops (figures 5.1 and 5.7). The market is two blocks north of Nairobi's central business thoroughfare, Kenyatta Avenue.

While many other colonial-era institutional buildings in the city were inspired by the Classical tradition, City Market is an Art Deco masterpiece, and its distinctive architectural characteristics give it prominence in Nairobi's skyline. This is especially evident in early aerial photographs of the city that show the market standing tall and overshadowing its neighbors; its profile is always easy to discern (figure 5.6). In fact, throughout the mid-twentieth century, City Market remained one of the most imposing structures in the city (figure 5.5). An outstanding aspect of the complex is the main covered hall. Here, a set of four soaring concrete parabolic arches form high vaulted ceilings in the interior. In the exterior, a series of stepped-back tiers support four rows of clerestories that increase in size down to the lower ends of the arches (figure 5.2). The massive, exposed arches create 17.5-meter high internal ceilings that meet the one-level stalls flanking them on either side. The resulting form facing the main Muindi Mbingu and Koinange Streets is a stepped façade consisting of extrusions at different heights.[10] With the street-front shops that accommodate a covered walkway canopy on the ground level, a layered façade effect is created on all elevations.

The overall effect of this complex on the city streetscape cannot be underestimated: its bold, sleek aerodynamic interior and clean, bright exterior distinguishes it from the surrounding urban fabric.

Large-Span Hall Typologies of the Interwar Period

Importantly, a closer look at the market hall's layout, structure, massing, and proportions reveals its close connection with concrete vault and parabolic arch typologies of large-span spaces in Britain, Germany, Poland, and France that were designed and built between the interwar periods of 1919 and 1940. So far, no studies concerning the history of concrete architecture have included Nairobi's City Market. Nonetheless, it is evident that this building sits within the global development of large-span concrete buildings. One of Andrew

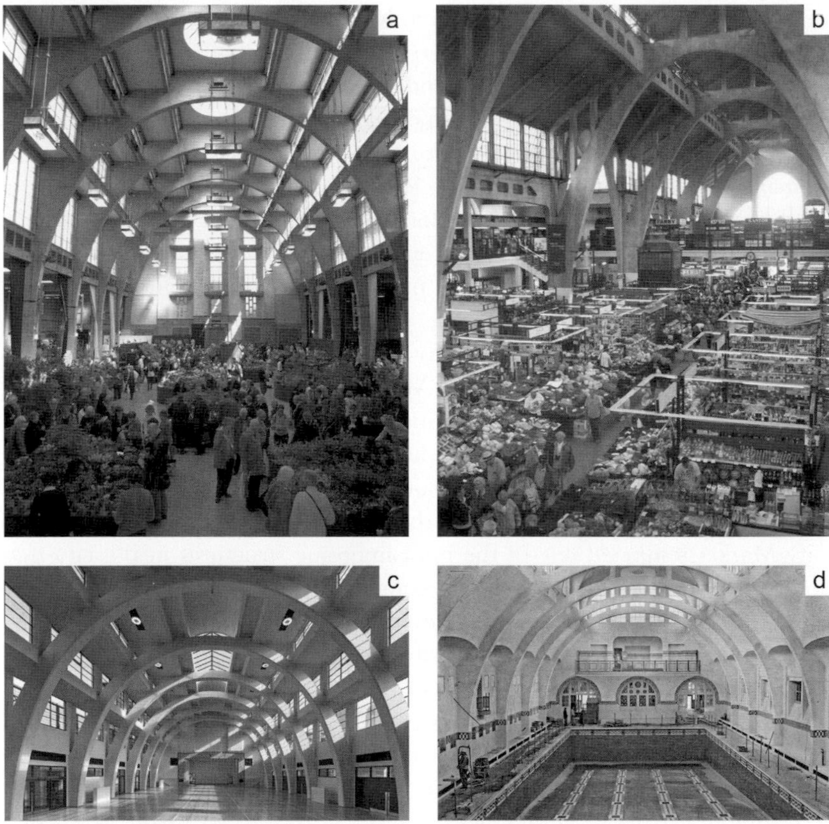

Figure 5.3. Examples of hall types in England, Poland and France that could be said to have influenced the form of the Nairobi City Market hall. (a): Lawrence Hall, London, England. Patche99z, Public domain, via Wikimedia Commons. (b): Wrocław Market Hall, Poland. Pkc mckinsey, CC BY-SA 3.0 via Wikimedia Commons: (c): Poplar Baths, London, England. Courtesy of Clarkson Alliance. (d): Baths at Butte-aux-Cailles, France. Bibliothèque nationale de France, EI-13 (1088).

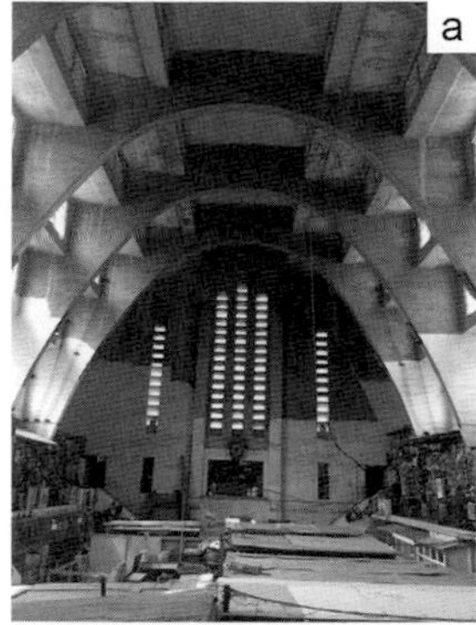

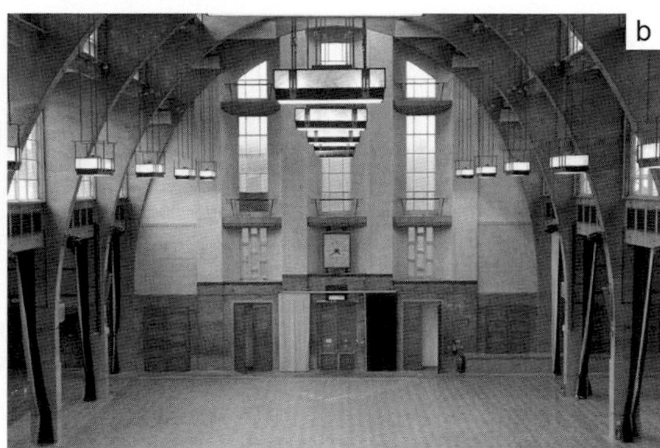

Figure 5.4. Comparison of City Market, Nairobi and Lawrence Hall, London. Note the close similarities between the parabolic arches and stepped fenestration of the two buildings. (a): Photograph of City Market by Samantha Martin, 2019. (b): Photograph of Lawrence Hall reproduced by kind assistance of the Governing Body of Westminster School.

Saint's studies of concrete architecture offers an overview of parabolic and elliptically arched buildings, an assemblage that reads like an extended family of the Nairobi market (figure 5.3).[11] Globally, in the early 1900s the development of reinforced concrete transformed its structural possibilities. The expressiveness of concrete was seen not only in engineering projects like bridges and dams but also in large-span buildings, including offices, schools, markets, factories, and hangars.

Saint's discussion on the advent and development of reinforced concrete after 1900 offers examples of large-span buildings.[12] Some of these are predecessors of Nairobi City Market, based on structural resemblances and through their use of large concrete arches as structural elements (figure 5.3). In France, for instance, the Voirin-Marinoni Factory in Montataire, built between 1920 and 1921 and designed by the Perret brothers, has characteristic clerestory windows along its stepped arches that resemble those of City Market. Other projects located in Paris integrated concrete arches or vaults akin to those of the concrete arch design of the Esders clothing factory by the Perret brothers (constructed in 1919 and since demolished), or the baths at Butte-aux-Cailles by Louis Bonnier (built between 1921 and 1923). In Britain, the parabolic arch structure of Lawrence Hall (figure 5.4)—one of the Royal Horticultural Halls in Westminster—designed by Murray Easton and Howard Robertson and built between 1927 and 1928, has strong similarities to Nairobi City Market's hall. All the designs have a similar interior expression of a full-height hall with stepped clerestory windows on elliptical concrete arches. The main difference is that one does not appreciate the expressive nature of Lawrence Hall's structure from the outside of the building.

From the street level, Lawrence Hall's structural system is not noticeable. The brick and stone plinth surrounding its street elevation tucks it away, presumably to make the hall blend in with and respect the nearby domestic buildings.

Structurally, a close relative to the Nairobi City Market hall can be seen in Poland's Breslau (Wrocław) Market Hall (see figure 5.3b), designed by Heinrich Küster (architect) and built by Karl Brandt (contractor) between 1906 and 1908. The Wrocław Market Hall has elliptical concrete arches that support stepped clerestories, resembling the Nairobi City Market hall structure. The ramped back clerestories of the Wrocław Market made an appearance in Stuttgart, Germany, in 1927, with the Heslach baths, built by E. Züblin, a specialist contractor. Poplar Baths, designed by Poplar Borough Engineers Department and built between 1932 and 1934 in Britain had similar characteristics (see figure 5.3c). Other buildings constructed outside Europe also embody design traits akin to those of the Nairobi market. An example is the market built by the British Municipal Council in the British concession in Tientsin.[13] Overall, the expressive potential of a combination of exposed arches, vaults, ribs, buttresses, and undivided spaces free of columns provided for large-scale openness. The apex of this form of large-span building construction was reached between the interwar periods of 1919 and 1940, when Nairobi's market emerged.

City Market's Pivotal Role in Urban Development

Modern architecture arrived in East Africa in the 1930s.[14] As the first modernist building in Kenya, Nairobi City Market instigated an important conversation between architecture in East Africa and developments much further afield, both in Europe and other cities that were part of the British Empire. Between 1920 and 1940 Nairobi witnessed an increasing population of British government officials, Indian merchants, and local settlers.[15] It was during this time that it was officially named the Colony and Protectorate of Kenya, and as a result, intense and more permanent building development occurred. Additionally, the effects of World War I altered power relations among different groups residing in Nairobi. City Market was then, and continues to be, pivotal to Nairobi's urban development.

For a present-day visitor to appreciate City Market fully, they must understand the market's role and meaning within colonial-era city planning, which reveal how the British used urban design to construct social, economic, and political control. In fact, Nairobi has come a long way since its establishment as a colonial capital in 1905, and as the capital of independent Kenya since

1963, in terms of demography, city planning, politics, transport, economy, housing, education, health, and culture.

City Market was built to be more than an Art Deco landmark. During the colonial era, it was not only central to the urban development of Nairobi, it was also an imperial symbol. The colonial government devised urban plans that embodied and enforced social and political order. Retail was the most conspicuous function in the capital's central area.[16] Commercial land use occupied 60 percent of the city center.[17] Beyond the civic buildings of law courts, the town hall, railway headquarters, a library, and religious facilities, City Market was central to the first-class shopping district, given that it was the only fruit and vegetable outlet in this zone.[18] Surprisingly for that time, City Market was open to all races and attracted both Indian and African retailers.[19] It is not clear whether it allowed buyers from all races, especially at a time when the colonial segregationist agenda was enforced. Segregation divided the city into racial zones, consisting of European, African, and Indian socioeconomic and political compartments.[20]

Postcolonial times continue to pose a challenge for African cities like Nairobi, a city that still struggles to adjust to an enduring spatial legacy of colonial segregationist urban planning. Today, Nairobi is a "characteristic blend of modernism and traditionalism."[21] It is a city that enjoys a dynamic mix of cultures, opinions, beliefs, enterprises, heritage, histories, and implications of globalization. The spatial manifestation of these changes across time in the city's architecture, urban form, and spatial extent is quite conspicuous (figure 5.4). In both colonial and postcolonial Nairobi backdrops, however, City Market continues to thrive and accommodate these transitional forces of change.

Nairobi City Market's Design and Calculated Versatility over Time

The Changing Urban Morphology of Nairobi

Since its establishment as a colonial capital in 1905, Nairobi has been in an almost constant state of systematic morphological transformation. The streets and blocks surrounding City Market have changed to such a degree that it is sometimes difficult to recognize earlier renditions in archival photographs (figure 5.5). Through all this change, however, the market itself has held fast, maintaining its singular form of expression. The interplay of its design features makes it a versatile and dynamic structure that can accommodate urban change. While it is no longer tall enough to be a part of the city's skyline, its design—in particular its relationship to the street—has enabled it to remain an

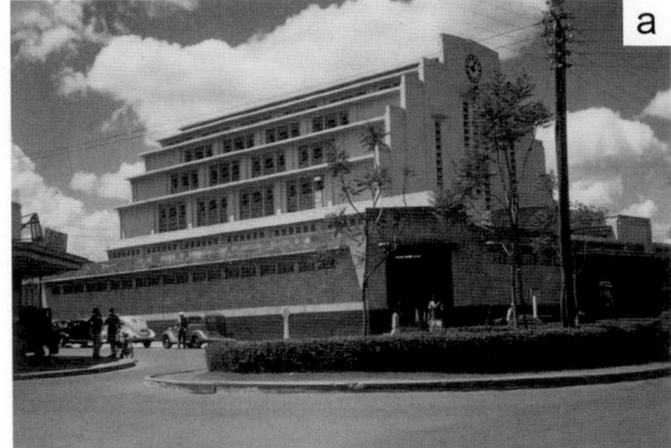

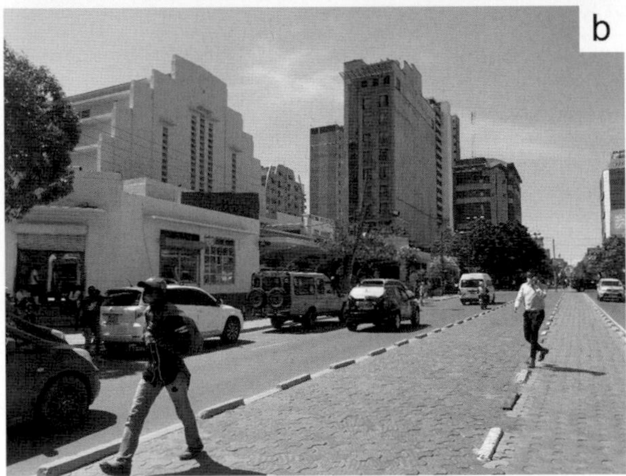

Figure 5.5. City Market over time. (a): ca 1950. R.E. Bruce photograph collection, reproduced courtesy of Patricia Worth. (b): 2020, photograph by author.

important and practical landmark in the everyday urbanism of Nairobi. Figures 5.5 and 5.6 illustrate how the City Market has always contributed to a coherent urban context, even as a stand-alone building. This contradicts a shared view that most colonial architecture has a static, isolated presence in the ever-changing urban context of African cities.[22]

Versatility in Public Health and Wellbeing Concepts

Another significant preconfigured potential of City Market may be seen in how it has accommodated public health and wellbeing concepts over time. The colonial policies shaping public health in the 1900s, not only in Kenya, but across the British Empire, emphasized sanitation planning, waste management, and the regulation of congestion.[23] In today's globalized and postcolonial world, public

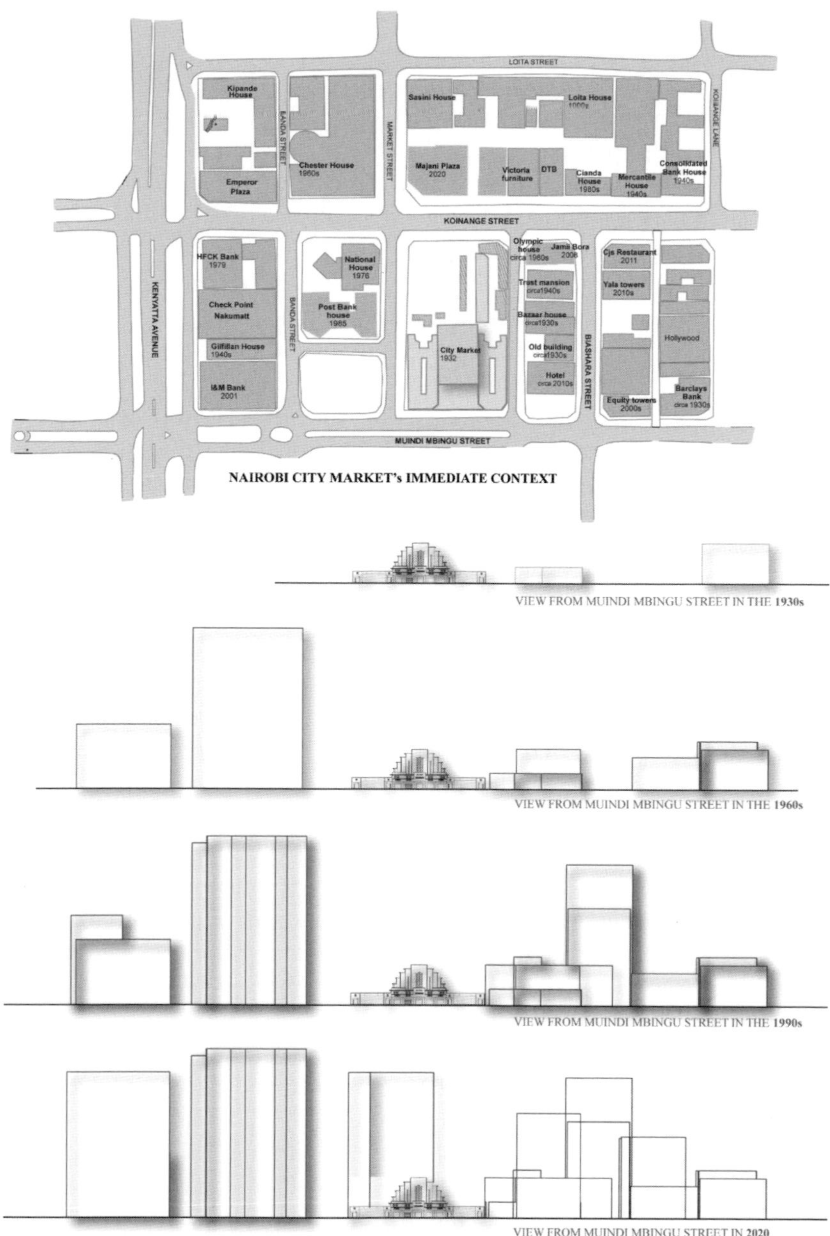

Figure 5.6. Site context plan of city market and elevation drawings from Muindi Mbingu Street across time—1930s, 1960s, 1990s, and 2020. This depicts the kinetic urban context that has formed City Market's backdrop for decades. Drawings by author, 2020.

health trends, efforts, and solutions focus on connecting health, wellbeing, sustainability, and energy neutrality.[24] In many ways, City Market has and continues to fit into these evolving public health goals, but it is important to consider in more detail the particular context in which the market was constructed.

The historical backdrop of the public health ecosystem in Nairobi's formative years has been discussed by several scholars.[25] At an urban level, public health conditions deteriorated during early colonial rule. A 1900 report by Colonel T. Gracey of the Whitehall-based Railways Committee called for "the improvement of the housing, sanitation and drainage of Indian residential areas."[26] This was an early basis of aligning race to hygiene and public health that led to racial segregation in Nairobi's urban plan. In 1929, Nairobi established its own municipal Public Health Department (PHD) that was responsible for vital statistics, sanitary administration, rodent and vermin control, public health education, and licensing business premises (particularly food markets, which were known to be sources of communicable diseases).[21] The PHD developed sanitation regulations and had oversight and enforcement roles in buildings. Sanitation requirements ran the gamut of measures, from the provision and location of toilets and sinks to types of floor finishes that are easy to clean; they also included wider measures like drainage regulations. When it opened, City Market complied fully with the 1929 regulations and was a model for the PHD implementation, albeit not without challenges in later years.[27] As a model, the market offered a new, formal and easily overseen space to organize and control the sale of food. The design conformed to sanitation measures and ensured sellers and vendors followed specific guidelines.

Beyond public regulations that anchored the market's existence in its early years, the design of City Market addresses today's existing global energy and consumption concerns, which emphasize holistic human comfort, public health and wellbeing. Design and space utilization strategies have diverged from water- and sanitation-central design seen during the colonial era, and from energy use reduction to the current design emphasis on occupants' thermal, visual, and acoustic comfort, productivity, health, and general wellbeing. Passive design and space utilization strategies that achieve cross-cutting sustainability in tropical climates have been proposed and discussed by scholars over the years. These include built form orientation, internal heat gain minimization, as well as façade design, solar control, and ventilative cooling strategies.[28] City Market was ahead of its time because its design incorporated passive thermal comfort, daylighting comfort, and indoor air quality maintenance that saves energy consumption.

The continued significance of the market's environmental design strategies almost a century later is hard to overstate. In tropical climates like in Kenya, heat and its mitigation are the dominant factors for comfort.[29] As discussed by Loki and Njoroge in their respective theses investigating the state of City Market's indoor thermal comfort, the market boasts of a myriad of passive design features that makes it a unique building, while affording its indoor users sustained levels of thermal comfort even in the hottest months of February and March.[30] The market hall, for instance, has a rectangular floor plate with longitudinal façades facing north and south. Its shorter eastern- and western-facing façades ensure that the hot morning sun and even hotter afternoon sun have a shorter façade surface area that would let the radiant heat into the spaces. Additionally, the market hall's stepped tiers support clerestory windows that occupy 30 percent of the building envelope. Each window is inset and protected by horizontal concrete projections running along the stepped façades, and these maintain the horizontal sun-shade device, a typology of sun-shading devices (figure 5.2). This reduces the transmittance of radiant heat waves through the clear glass panes.

Indoor thermal cooling is enhanced further by two top-stepped tiers that have permanently open louvre windows for ventilation cooling via a constant stack air movement to the interior market spaces below. Additionally, the market stalls that flank the hall on either side (figures 5.1d and 5.2d) are organized around a series of open courtyards that ensure cross-ventilative cooling. This is further complemented by entrance canopies with deep eaves for extra sun shading.[31]

As the world becomes warmer, mitigating indoor overheating risk levels in tropical buildings is key for public health and wellbeing. Studies undertaken by Gichuyia[32] on non-residential buildings in Nairobi show that the market's passive architectural features may keep the market complex at minimal risk of overheating even in the worst-case climate scenario of A2 in 2080 projected by the Intergovernmental Panel on Climate Change (IPCC).[33] To maintain minimal indoor overheating risk, the market's percentage of openable window area would have to be increased. More of the fixed clerestory windowpanes must be operable. Other than that, no other major structural reconstructions are likely needed to maintain healthy indoor thermal comfort levels even in the hottest climate projected by the IPCC.

City Market's passive environmental design also stands out due to the visual comfort of its spaces.[34] Daytime visual comfort is emphasized by the stepped nature of the market hall, which ensures the even spread of indoor natural light through the clerestory window system. This minimizes glare in interior spaces and emphasizes constant ventilation through its stack effect. The open courtyards assist not only with natural ventilation but also with the provision and propagation of natural light (figure 5.1d).

In addition, the market complex's ability to accommodate diverse use over time is supported by these environmental design strategies for the provision of natural light, passive thermal comfort, and ventilation. The market's passive design features show that its preconfigured environmental adaptability allows for several user-driven changes around its immutable infrastructure. In this way, City Market is a sustainable space, as buildings should be, that will adapt with minimal demolition and restructuring of the built form and its spatial configurations.

The Ability to Diversify without Changing Its Main Use

City Market was thc main retail outlet in Nairobi selling fruits and vegetables in the 1930s. In those early years, the main market hall used to hold boxing tournaments and other sporting activities.[35] It was even suggested during its opening in 1932 that the hall could be used to hold Kenya Defence Force army drills. However, in 1937, the use of the market hall for sports and entertainment was banned, lest its primary purpose be lost. Importantly, the facility was carefully planned in relation to the railway line that ran along present-day Loita Street, which is located one block west of the market.[39] Over the years, the market has housed several types of businesses. While in the beginning it was entirely dedicated to fruits and vegetables, it gradually changed over the decades to accommodate a meat market, flower sellers, arts and crafts vendors, and now ready-made food outlets.[36]

The gradual change in use is permitted by the versatility of the design. City Market today comprises four types of vending spaces that maintain physical independence as business units (figure 5.7). The shops fronting the adjoining streets, and the lockable stalls around the inner courtyards may be considered formal and house diverse activities, like meat and butcher shops, foreign exchange bureaus, art galleries, and convenience stores. These spatial modules have housed different users over time with minimal interior design restructuring. In comparison, the market hall outlets and hawker stands along the corridors that lead to the shops, the market voids, and the courtyards are informal. All these vending areas are linked. The walkways leading to the lockable butcher shops, for instance, are lined with small-scale sellers who operate from rented fridges that flank the accesses to the meat stalls. The open-air florists and food court stalls similarly occupy the market voids and courtyards that abut covered shops, offering complementary goods. In this way, they operate symbiotically with alongside lockable stalls. Some of these informal open-air enterprises operate at certain times of the day, not necessarily throughout all business hours. Thus, the building's functions extend and contract at various times of the day.

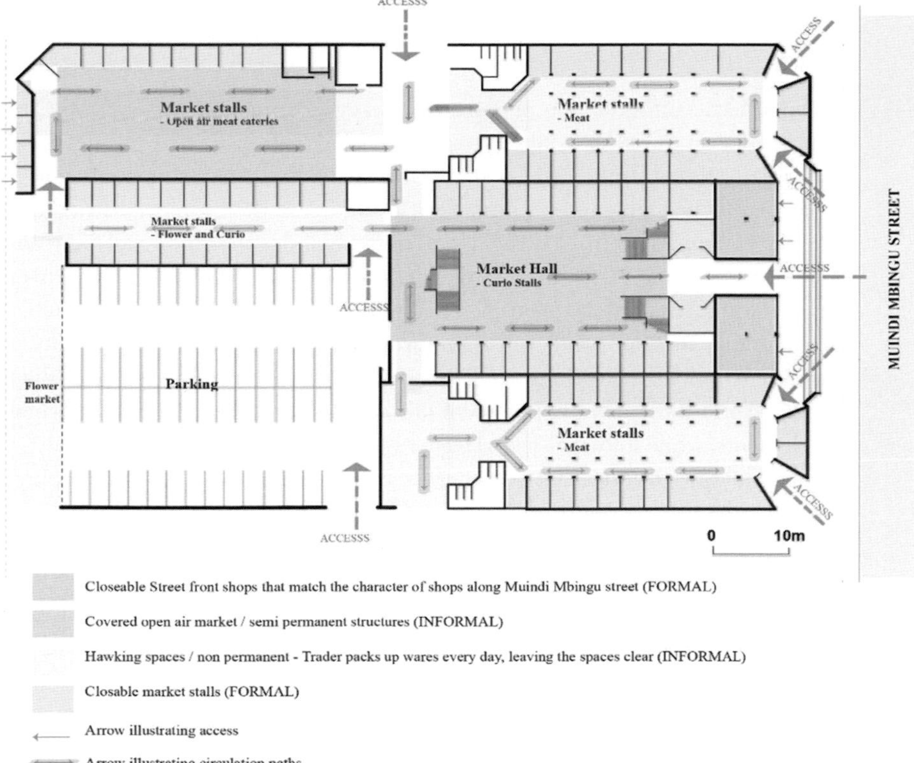

Figure 5.7. Spatial configuration and flow of movement in City Market. Drawn by author, 2020.

The market's flexibility allows for the covered market hall to host several businesses under one roof. The hall's footprint and structure allow for refitting and customizability. For example, the plan of the covered market permits trader-defined stall spaces where circulatory flow is facilitated by corridors that weave through the market hall and eventually link with the market's courtyards and voids (figure 5.7). Each stall consists of temporary timber frames that are easily dismountable, extendable, and collapsible without affecting the market hall's structure (figures 5.2e and 5.2f). These spatial aspects allow the changing activities that the market hosts over time.

Versatility in Accommodating a Continuum of Formal and Informal Businesses

Beyond its accommodation of diversity of use over time, another reason City Market has endured is its ability to accommodate both formal business and informal vending. In its early years, it provided only formal shopping experiences; street hawking and vending were forbidden in the business district during the colonial period.[37] Yet the design of the building was ultimately amenable to change, and in the present day, it accommodates a hybrid economy of several formal and informal businesses that interlace and evolve together, albeit not always without conflict. It is important to underscore that informality is persistent both in the working and living conditions in Nairobi today. According to the World Bank, about 60 percent of the city's population lives in informal settlements, while informal sector businesses contribute 34 percent of Kenya's gross domestic product and account for 77 percent of the country's employment.[38] The urban context of Nairobi's CBD, where City Market stands, was originally a formal space (figures 5.1b and 5.1c). However, today it combines both formal and informal businesses.[39]

Some scholars affirm that "there is no formality without informality."[40] The often-unacknowledged symbiotic relationship between formal and informal processes has partly led to the lack of a real bridge between these two processes in Nairobi's rigid urban planning, urban design, architecture, and building, and more so in a regulatory sense. Today, the city's inflexible land-use zoning separates formal and informal settlements and businesses, and architecture has been purely aligned to formal responses.[43] Thus market spaces and buildings in Nairobi house either formal businesses or informal ones but rarely a combination of the two. Because of the high percentage of informal businesses in the country, spaces are needed that acknowledge the hybrid nature of Kenya's economy: ones that allow for the formal/informal continuum in varying but sensitive ratios.

City Market's architecture has allowed for the mutual existence of formal and informal businesses in three ways. First, its external boundary, interior edges, and spatial boundaries delineate formal and informal businesses in such a way that one activity, either formal or informal, complements and minimally obstructs the other (figure 5.7). The same physical edges in its internal spaces allow for the layering of activities, such that informal businesses progressively pitch camp through accretion and decamp when they need to move, depending on daily business cycles or yearly businesses changes. Second, City Market's internal design arrangements delineate spaces that maintain the hierarchical flow of informal spaces, which are mostly open-air, while formal businesses mainly occupy closable shops. Their permeability is reinforced by visual edges and entryways to the formal shops and the flexible areas right outside these shops where informal businesses can stack up. Third, City Market boasts numerous voids, courtyards, and arcades that open to walkways leading to single-banked shops. Although not originally intended, these areas have adequately accommodated a flux of informal traders and hawkers, allowing an infill of varying sizes and logistical needs.

City Market accommodates more than it was planned for. Its ability to host a formal/informal continuum without losing its architectural character is what gives it an added advantage. With this ability, it can readjust to multiple renditions presented by the city of Nairobi. In this way, the building resists the homogenizing process of imposed modernization often reflected by formal processes.[41] City Market shows that formal and informal businesses can mutually exist and thrive. The spatial representation and understanding of this coexistence as presented by City Market's preconfigured adaptability could inform the current need to integrate informal businesses into the formal fabric of the city.

Versatility in a Changing Socioeconomic and Cultural Landscape

Beyond its versatility in use, City Market has continued to thrive through Nairobi's economic transitions. Trade liberalization, information, and communication advancements, market geographic expansion, changing trade regulation, and broadening resource allocation have fostered economic changes in the consumer, retailer, and market space globally. In Nairobi, the combined effect of these forces in varying magnitudes, frequencies, and ranges over time has resulted in changes to the consumer and market landscape reciprocated by corresponding commercial building design styles proposed and built over time. While markets in Nairobi have come and gone, City Market is exceptional in that it has undergone only superficial upgrades, such as painting, over the years.

In Nairobi's early years, Kenya's consumer trends were underpinned by the need to buy and sell goods for basic human existence and community survival. This early commerce was a neat transition from barter trade that was practised by cultural communities long before colonization. Buying and selling goods for essential existence required basic shop architecture referred to as "odd one-storey structures for shops" during the interwar period when City Market was built.[42] Some consisted of a basic countertop that divided the stored goods for sale and the trader on one side, and the buyer on the other side who could see the goods on display and purchase what was necessary. These simple shop designs worked for one-product vendors. The construction of City Market brought many goods under one roof in an organized fashion, which corresponds to present-day markets.

Moreover, the market facilitated social integration in Nairobi over the years. Racial, ethnic, socioeconomic, and political segregation were significant factors that underpinned the establishment of Nairobi as a railway town in 1899.[43] Containment and social exclusion in those early years secured the British imperial government's control and ability to impose colonial rule.[44] Given this segregationist context of Nairobi as a colonial capital, City Market stood out as a contravention to the prevailing rule. It was in the heart of a secluded first-class shopping zone, an exclusive *European zone*. However, City Market was open to all races, including Indian and African traders.[45]

Almost six decades after independence, the city is still organized around segregationist urban practices despite the end of colonial rule.[46] Accordingly, and perhaps without deliberation, some aspects of Nairobi's built form and urban practices today still entrench socio-spatial segregation. In Nairobi's CBD, for instance, the spatial manifestation of socio-exclusion can be seen through the physical organization and design of the built form. Examples include intentionally erected physical barriers around some buildings or armed guards manning fences and barriers, as well as nonintentional exclusionary spaces caused by imposing office blocks, commercial and institutional buildings. Several buildings in Nairobi today may not have been designed to align and reconcile with the impact of the social statements they make. Instead, the design of the buildings is attributed to development control guidelines and the assertion of their visual prominence in Nairobi's skyline. Additionally, market forces have a way of defining how space is produced, exchanged, and appreciated by the public.[47] As Mike Davis points out, even though people are legally free to enter all areas in the city, subtle and not so subtle aspects may signal that some people of a particular gender, age, race, or income bracket might not be welcome.[48] Some of these buildings and spaces project a sense of social control, which does not acknowledge the inherent heterogeneity of the individual(s) who occupy them.

City Market's architecture continues to accommodate these emergent sociocultural compositions in various ways: through its indoor/outdoor encounter that encourages uninterrupted access to the market; its indoor spatial configuration that allows for porosity and the free flow of pedestrian traffic into and across the market; and via indoor market spaces that allow for the four types of vending spaces (i.e., an open-air market, market stalls, covered shops, and hawking spaces as illustrated in figure 5.7) to mutually exist. From Muindi Mbingu Street, the market boasts five pedestrian access points: a centrally placed main entrance via a podium and four other entrances located in chamfered corners to create side entries. Additionally, each of the street-front shops have independent access off the main street. These multiple entry points ease the sense of a *policed access* as experienced by similar establishments. Multiple access points, including the one from Koinange Street, and the patterns of permeability and interconnectedness formed within spaces in City Market, give it an inclusive social quality. The diversity of activities in the market increases the presence of different people in the building. The reality of working as a trader—meat, curios, flowers—or using the space as a buyer illustrates that the market spaces offer an increased frequency of meetings: encounters across the trader-trader, trader-customer and customer-customer dyads (see figure 5.7).

City Market's spatial qualities respect human participation across several levels. The market's expression of boundary, spatial edges, and spatial continuity, and its control of space enhances the interdependence between different demographic sectors of the community without discrimination. It is almost as if the market has a complementary layer that connects people as they move into, through, and beyond the building into the rest of the urban fabric. Overall, this makes it an inclusive urban platform for exchange that accommodates the evolving societal and cultural dynamics of Nairobi.

Conclusion

This chapter tells a story of a timeless market complex and the implication of time: moments that have the potential of changing the functional and physical demands placed on buildings during their service life. The City Market building is a rarity due to its versatility, which has allowed it to fit into a postcolonial world despite it having been designed and built at the height of the colonial hegemony in Nairobi. The market has continued to reinvent itself within the prevailing socio-cultural, economic, environmental, cultural, and urban morphological conditions without any changes to its architectural structure and form. Its adaptability stands out notably in a context where other colonial-era buildings in the city have had to be wholly reinterpreted, change their use, or undergo modification of their architectural forms or spatial configuration to keep up with market pressures and changing times.

Scholarly interpretation of colonial architecture within a postcolonial world has indicated that existing colonial-era buildings face extinction as they attempt to keep up with change in rapidly urbanising and politically independent countries.[49] However, Nairobi City Market is one of the few such buildings that has maintained its relevance throughout the years. This is despite it being a commercial building, a typology that is prone to obsolescence given changing demands to accommodate spaces for buyers, sellers, and products. Even with its colonial legacy, City Market continues to thrive decades after it opened its doors as a fruit and vegetable market hub for the colonial capital, without any alterations to its original architecture.

When it was built, City Market belonged to a global architectural language that offered large-scale openness by exploring the expressive potential of combining exposed arches, vaults, ribs, buttresses, and undivided spaces free of columns; a language that can be traced across France, Poland, Britain, and Germany. In the 1930s, it stood as an imperial symbol for a European-centric first-class zone (figure 5.1) and was pivotal to Nairobi's urban development, as one of the first modernist buildings in Kenya. In addition, it was built to adhere to the controversial public health regulations of 1929, which largely led to racial segregation. Even with the market's existence anchored in colonial hegemony, it is surprising that it still thrives, almost nine decades on. Following the different conditions of today's postcolonial Nairobi as traced in this chapter, City Market has a high level of adaptive capacity.[50] The building is progressive and egalitarian despite its colonial urban design setting, which was deeply flawed and unjust from the beginning. A combination of its historical factors and present-day abilities makes City Market an exception. Indeed, it is as if the market has a series of complementary layers that keep reinventing themselves in a loose-fitting, long-life formwork because of its persistence through immense urban changes without adjustments to its structure and spatial design.

This study of City Market's afterlife illuminates the broader challenge of existential vulnerability that is not only experienced by colonial-era buildings. It also speaks to whether we can fully anticipate and design for the unforeseen. In architecture and related fields, flexibility and adaptability are terms that have been used interchangeably to maximize the value of the built environment in changing circumstances over time.[51] However, this preconfigured potential seems to have less to do with the building's modularity, edges, and components, in terms of flexibility and adaptability, and more to do with spatial connection and interfacial properties coupled with reserve capacity and passive design features. The underpinning properties of City Market that ensure its timelessness are less about its construction method and more about the relationship of its architecture to the prevailing context, be it urban morphology, socioeconomic and cultural composition or ambient microclimate. Thus, City Market resists obsolescence and continues to accommodate heterogeneous and emergent needs over time.

The lessons learned from this in-depth study of City Market could be used for critical dialogues on the versatility of stand-alone buildings or building complexes and to complement urban discussions for more inclusive and time-conscious cities. To support what Appadurai quite rightly identifies as "the locality of a space by what it has evolved from, against, in spite of and in relation to" is to conquer the existential vulnerability of space as expressed by Christian Norberg-Schulz in his book, *Genius Loci*. Nairobi City Market is truly a market and urban experience with an understanding of time.[52]

Acknowledgments

This chapter received financial support for editing purposes from Toronto Metropolitan University.

Notes

1. Muindi Mbingu Street was formerly known as Stewart Street up until 1964 when Kenya gained independence.
2. Koinange Street was formerly known as Sadler Street up until 1964 when Kenya gained independence.
3. This barbecued meat slow roasted in large chunks over an open fire (select charcoal from specific trees) brought to you in cut pieces is one of the most popular dishes in Kenya. It is served with Ugali (cornmeal) and green vegetables.
4. A typology of colonialism, distinct from exploitation/plantation colonialism. Using the description by Veracini (2010, p. 4), settler colonialism can be defined as "the domination imposed by a foreign minority, racially (or ethnically) and culturally different, acting in the name of a racial (or ethnic) and cultural superiority dogmatically affirmed, and imposing itself on an indigenous population constituting a numerical majority but inferior to the dominant group from a material point of view."
5. Fassil Demissie, *Colonial Architecture and Urbanism in Africa: Intertwined and Contested Histories* (Burlington, VT: Ashgate, 2012).
6. This draws on Norberg-Schulz's description of genius loci as "the spirit of a place." See Norberg-Schulz, Christian, *Genius Loci: Towards a Phenomenology of Architecture* (New York: Rizzoli, 1979).
7. See in particular T. Muhoro, G. Munala, and N. Mugwima, "Reflections on Architectural Morphology in Nairobi, Kenya: Implications for Conservation of the Built Heritage," in *Conservation of Natural and Cultural Heritage in Kenya*, ed. A. Deisser and M. Njuguna (London: UCL Press, 2016), 75–92.
8. Before 1963.
9. See O. Faber, "Building Structures," *Architects' Journal* 77 (March 22): 391–92. Following the Nairobi municipal regulations published on April 16, 1900 (see Smart 1950, p. 17; Ibid, 35.), a municipal committee was created to manage the city's development. It later grew into a council, and it is believed that the council architects sat on this advisory group. The council architects made substantial contributions to the city's architecture during the colonial period. See also: S. Longair, "Visions of the Global: The Classical and the Eclectic in Colonial East African Architecture," *Les Cahiers D'Afrique de L'est/The East African Review* 51 (2016): 161–78.

be modified through natural and ambient energy sources in the natural environment. (See Yeang 1999, 202)

35. J. Smart, *A Jubilee History of Nairobi* (East African Standard, 1950).
36. The future, as indicated in Nairobi County Council's 2018–2022 strategic plan, points to a mix of variegated market activities. Given the historic importance of the building and its prime central location in the city, the council intends to expand the remit of the site to include additional activities: operationalizing a tourist information center, an art gallery, a cultural night selling food, entertainment, and flowers. These uses could increase the number of local and international tourists, boost trade at the market and include more fun night activities that promote Nairobi's CBD as a secure tourism destination. See Nairobi City Council. *Nairobi City County Integrated Development Plan* (2018).
37. This included hawking activity. Legally, no hawking was allowed in the high-class "European zone." See M. A. Achola, "Colonial Policy and Urban Health: The Case of Colonial Nairobi," *AZANIA: Journal of the British Institute in Eastern Africa* 36, no. 1 (2001): 119–37.
38. World Bank, *Combined Project Information Documents*, Kenya Informal Settlements Improvement Project 2, vol. 1.
39. Informal businesses in the country are not registered and are based on individual effort and small enterprise. They mainly remain unprotected by labor-related regulations and mostly lack social security. There is a shared scholarly view that both informal settlements and informal businesses often fill the void left by the failure of formal urbanization processes. The spatial forms associated with informality are shanty structures erected without the support from any built environment professionals.
40. T. Anyamba, "Nairobi's Informal Modernism." Paper presented at the N-Aerus Conference, 2005. https://www.uonbi.ac.ke/openscholar/sites/default/files/tomanyamba/files/n-aerus_workshop_paper_2005.pdf.
41. These processes have mostly ignored the existence of 60 percent of Nairobi's informal settlement population and 34 percent of Nairobi's businesses, which remain informal.
42. A. K. Nevanlinna, *Interpreting Nairobi: The Cultural Study of Built Forms* (Helsinki: Finish Literature Society, 1996).
43. S. O. Owuor and T. Mbatia. "Post Independence Development of Nairobi City, Kenya." Paper presented at Workshop on African Capital Cities, Dakar, September 22–23, 2008.
44. The essence of how Nairobi's colonial urban plan and buildings embodied social segregation between the African, European, and Indian populations has been exhaustively discussed by Salm and Falola 2005; Demissie 2012; Greenwood and Topiwala 2020; Ogilvie 1946; and Myers 2003.

45. M. A. Achola, "Colonial Policy and Urban Health: The Case of Colonial Nairobi," *AZANIA: Journal of the British Institute in Eastern Africa* 36, no. 1 (2001): 119–37.
46. See Anyamba, 2005.
47. E. W. Soja, "The Spatiality of Social Life: Towards a Transformative Retheorisation," in *Social Relations and Spatial Structures*, ed. D. Gregory and J. Urry (London: Palgrave, 1985), 90–127.
48. M. Davis, "Planet of Slums," *New Perspectives Quarterly* 23, no. 2 (2006): 6–11.
49. See in particular Demissie (2012); F. Demissie, "Representing Architecture in South Africa," *International Journal of African Historical Studies* 30, no. 2 (1977): 349–55; and T. Muhoro, M. Gerryshom, and M. Njuguna, "Reflections on Architectural Morphology in Nairobi, Kenya: Implications for Conservation of the Built Heritage," *Conservation of Natural and Cultural Heritage in Kenya* (London: UCL Press, 2016), 19.
50. Sinclair et al. (2012) have defined adaptive capacity of a building as the ability "to cope with future changes with minimum demolition, cost and waste and with maximum robustness, mutability and efficiency, and which leads to building agility and resilience."
51. Of course, the term flexibility itself embodies many qualities and conditions, such as adaptability and the latitude for accommodating change. Sinclair et al. (2012) have defined spatial flexibility in a building as "the capacity of change in a spatial structure."
52. Ibid, 6.

Bibliography

Achola, Milcah Amolo. "Colonial Policy and Urban Health: The Case of Colonial Nairobi." *AZANIA: Journal of the British Institute in Eastern Africa* 36, no. 1 (2001): 119–37.

Anyamba, Tom. "Nairobi's Informal Modernism." *Oslo School of Architecture and Design, Maridalsveien 29, N-0175 Oslo*, 2004.

Baker, Nick V. *Passive and Low Energy Building Design for Tropical Island Climates.* Commonwealth Secretariat, 1987.

Baker, Nick, and Koen Steemers. *Healthy Homes: Designing with Light and Air for Sustainability and Wellbeing.* London: Routledge, 2019.

Bigon, Liora. "Sanitation and Street Layout in Early Colonial Lagos: British and Indigenous Conceptions, 1851–1900." *Planning Perspectives* 20, no. 3 (2005): 247–69.

Cole, Festus. "Sanitation, Disease and Public Health in Sierra Leone, West Africa, 1895–1922: Case Failure of British Colonial Health Policy." *Journal of Imperial and Commonwealth History* 43, no. 2 (2015): 238–66.

Cooper, Nicola. "Urban Planning and Architecture in Colonial Indochina." *French Cultural Studies* 11, no. 31 (2000): 75–99.

Davis, Mike. "Planet of Slums." *New Perspectives Quarterly* 23, no. 2 (2006): 6–11.

Demissie, Fassil. *Colonial Architecture and Urbanism in Africa: Intertwined and Contested Histories*. Burlington, VT: Ashgate, 2012.

———. "Representing Architecture in South Africa." *International Journal of African Historical Studies* 30, no. 2 (1997): 349–55.

Free, Melissa. "Settler Colonialism." *Victorian Literature and Culture* 46, no. 3–4 (2018): 876–82.

Gichuyia, Linda. "Indoor Overheating Risk: a Framework for Temporal Building Adaptation Decision-Making." PhD diss., University of Cambridge, 2017.

Givoni, Baruch. *The Passive and Low Energy Cooling of Buildings*. New York: John Wiley & Sons, 1994.

Greenwood, Anna, and Harshad Topiwala. "Visions of Colonial Nairobi: William Simpson, Health, Segregation and the Problems of Ordering a Plural Society, 1907–1921." *Social History of Medicine* 33, no. 1 (2020): 57–78.

Halliman, Dorothy, and William Thomas Wilson Morgan. "The City of Nairobi." In *Nairobi: City and Region*, edited by William Thomas Wilson Morgan. Oxford: Oxford University Press, 1967.

Hirst, Terry, and Davinder Lamba. "The Struggle for Nairobi." Mazingira Institute, 1994, 64–83.

IPCC. "The Physical Science Basis: Working Group I Contribution to the Fourth Assessment Report of the IPCC." In *Climate Change 2007*, 2007.

Ken Yeang. *The Green Skyscraper: The Basis for Designing Sustainable Intensive Buildings*. Munich: Prestel, 1999.

Koenigsberger, O. H., T. G. Ingersoll, A. Mayhew, and S. V. Szoklay. "Manual of Tropical Housing and Building: Climatic Design Part 1." London: Orient Longman, 1974.

Loki, David. "Passive & Low Energy building Design in Nairobi: Building Design Strategies for Thermal Comfort, Day-Lighting & Natural Ventilation in Nairobi's Tropical Upland Climate." Undergraduate dissertation, University of Nairobi, 2009.

Murunga, Godwin Rapando. "The Cosmopolitan Tradition and Fissures in Segregationist Town Planning in Nairobi, 1915–23." *Journal of Eastern African Studies* 6, no. 3 (2012): 463–86.

Myers, Garth Andrew. *Verandahs of Power: Colonialism and Space in Urban Africa*. Syracuse, NY: Syracuse University Press, 2003.

Nairobi City Council. Nairobi City County Integrated Development Plan (2018).

Nevanlinna, Anja Kervanto. *Interpreting Nairobi: The Cultural Study of Built Forms.* Helsinki: Suomen historiallinen seura, 1996.

Njoroge, Bob. "Nairobi Architecture in a Climate of Change: A Study of the Evolution of the Carbon Footprint of Buildings in Nairobi CBD and Upper Hill Area." Undergraduate dissertation, University of Nairobi, 2012.

Norberg-Schulz, Christian. *Genius Loci: Towards a Phenomenology of Architecture.* New York: Rizzoli, 1979.

Ogilvie, Gordon C W. *The Housing of Africans in the Urban Areas of Kenya.* Kenya Information Office, 1946.

Owuor, Samuel O., and Teresa Mbatia. "Post Independence Development of Nairobi City, Kenya." Paper presented at Workshop on African Capital Cities, Dakar, September 22–23, 2008.

Saint, Andrew. "Some Thoughts about the Architectural Use of Concrete." *AA Files*, 1991, 3–12.

Salm, Steven J., and Toyin Falola. *African Urban Spaces in Historical Perspective.* Rochester, NY: University Rochester Press, 2005.

Sharp, Dennis. "The Modern Movement in East Africa." In *Otto Koenigsberger Festschrift: Action Planning and Responsive Design. Aspects of Housing, Building, Planning And Development in the Third World in Spéc*, edited by W. Aldhous, S. Groak, B. Mumtaz, and M. Safier, 7:1–394. Pergamon Press, 1983.

Smart, James. *A Jubilee History of Nairobi.* East African Standard, 1950.

Soja, E. W. "The Spatiality of Social Life: Towards a Transformative Retheorisation." *Social Relations and Spatial Structures*, 1985, 90–127.

Swanson, Maynard W. "The Sanitation Syndrome: Bubonic Plague and Urban Native Policy in the Cape Colony, 1900–1909." *Journal of African History*, 1977, 387–410.

Szokolay, Steven V. *Introduction to Architectural Science: The Basis of Sustainable Design.* London: Routledge, 2004.

Teckla, Muhoro, Munala Gerryshom, and Mugwima Njuguna. "Reflections on Architectural Morphology in Nairobi, Kenya: Implications For Conservation of the Built Heritage." In *Conservation of Natural and Cultural Heritage in Kenya*, 19. London: UCL Press, 2016.

Veracini, Lorenzo. *Settler Colonialism.* Houndmills, UK: Palgrave Macmillan, 2010.

White, Leonard William Thornton, Leo Silberman, and Peter Ronald Anderson. *Nairobi, Master Plan for a Colonial Capital: A Report Prepared For the Municipal Council of Nairobi.* HM Stationery Office, 1948.

World Bank. "Kenya Informal Settlements Improvement Project 2: Combined Project Information Documents." Vol. 1, 2018.

CHAPTER 6

THE ST. LAWRENCE MARKET, TORONTO

Changes and Continuity

Leila Marie Farah

The St. Lawrence Market in downtown Toronto, Canada, is a place entwined with the city's history. Butchers, farmers, and other vendors have been selling goods in this market area for over two hundred years. The buildings on the site have been contributing their particular character to the neighborhood despite, or perhaps because of, a series of construction, demolition, mobilization, and revitalization phases. This chapter investigates the evolution of the spaces the market occupies and their infrastructural and sanitary context. While the relationship between public health and its architecture is important to its development, existing scholarship about the market does not specifically address such links, and even thorough architectural studies of it present a fragmented picture. Hence, to better understand how the market transformed, this work pieces together information from maps and orthographic drawings in archives, bylaws, and newspaper articles as well as from diaries, letters, and autobiographies. The complexity of these physical transformations over time is further visualized in many of the illustrations for this chapter. What emerges is a rich picture of both change—in composition, form, size, program, experiences and public health measures—and continuity, given the market's perennity and centrality.

Establishment

While the history of the area within "the traditional territory of many nations including the Mississaugas of the Credit, the Anishnabeg, the Chippewa, the Haudenosaunee and the Wendat peoples and [...] now home to many diverse First Nations, Inuit and Métis peoples"[1] goes much farther back in time, and despite preexisting trade activity between Indigenous peoples and European settlers, the establishment of a permanent open public market can be traced to 1803, when the Lieutenant Governor of the Province of Upper Canada specified its location in the Town of York.[2]

Situated close to the lakefront, on the northeastern coast of Lake Ontario, the site was originally five and a half acres, bordered by King, Church, Market, and New Streets.[3] Initially scheduled to operate only on Saturdays, this was the place for selling "cattle, sheep, poultry, and other provisions, goods and merchandize" to support the growing town.[4] A modest wooden structure known as the Old Market House was constructed in 1820. According to Robertson, it measured forty-five by thirty-five feet, and a public well was dug three years later.[5] The small building was disassembled in 1831, and in December 1832 its material was offered for sale at auction.[6] Until 1834, this site was also used for public punishment.[7]

New Market House

The "New" Market House was designed by James Cooper in 1830, roughly four years before an expanding Town of York would become incorporated as the City of Toronto, adopting an earlier Mohawk name.[8] It was built between 1831 and 1833, on a portion of the lot previously dedicated to the market. This larger two-story complex encompassed the urban block bordered by King, West Market Place, Front, and Nelson Streets.[9] The main north façade ran along King Street, a key commercial route, and the south elevation, along Front Street, faced the waterfront. A quadrangular courtyard, known as the Market Place, was central to the composition in plan (figure 6.1).

The ground floor of this new building was dedicated mainly to commercial activities, with shops along the north and south street-facing façades. The main volume facing King Street was marked by its height, reaching above the two stories of the rest of the complex, and the town hall was housed on top of the three arched openings.[10] In addition, before it moved into a different building south of Front Street in the mid-1840s, the first City Hall of Toronto and municipal offices were also located in parts of the New Market House.[11] The rest of the upper level housed a newsroom, printing offices, and a number of storage areas—some serving as granaries and others occasionally used as meeting spaces or for other temporary functions.[12] Hence, besides storing goods, its mixed-use upper floor also hosted spaces of civic decision making, news publishing, and cultural and political gatherings. Even at this early date, the market's uses were diverse and extended beyond food.

The paved courtyard at the heart of this complex was in rubble stone and was accessed from the street through openings.[13] Besides the three aforementioned archways along King Street, another one fronted the lakeside. Further, as depicted in the map, figure 6.1, three passages on each of the longitudinal elevations enabled the movement of vehicles as well as the flow of people and

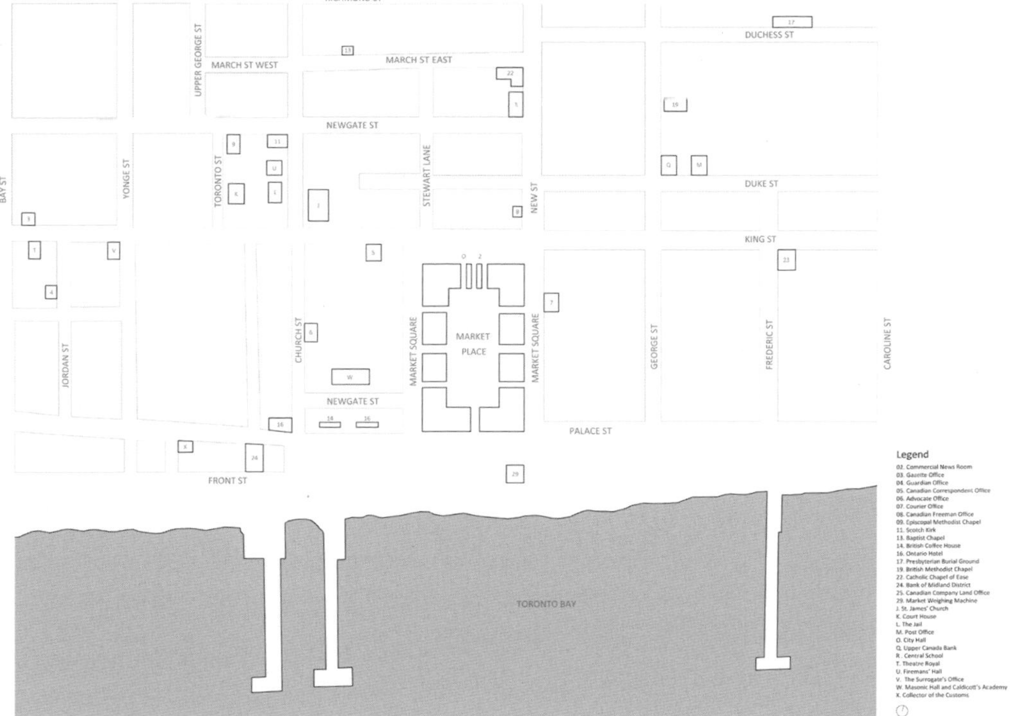

Figure 6.1. Detail of the *Plan of the City of Toronto, Capital of Upper Canada* showing the context of the New Market House and Place, Toronto, 1834. By Alpheus Todd. Redrawn by Stephanie Vo, Nicole Li (research assistants) and author.
The ground floor of the market is represented and the legend is based on the original plan which does not contain a scale. On this view, the West Market Place Street is named Market Square and it is located to its west; and Nelson Street is called Market Square and is to its east.

goods into the Market Place. The market, which the 1834 Public Market Act mentions would be open daily save for Sundays, was accessible through gates that opened before sunrise and closed at 4 p.m., with the exception of Saturdays, when activities could extend until 9 p.m.[14] On market days, some farmers and other vendors sold their products from the carriages parked in the courtyard. It was by all accounts a vibrant and messy site—and sight—bustling with life, noise and activity. In *Reminiscences of a Canadian Pioneer for the Last Fifty Years: An Autobiography*, published in 1884, Samuel Thompson, an editor and politician, describes it as being "rarely free of cabbage leaves, bones, and skins."[15] Still, despite the apparent chaos, similar goods were grouped in their own areas. Dairy products and eggs were concentrated on the southern part of the site along the square; and farmers sold their produce in the vicinity of the northern façade.[16] Thirty-six butchers' stalls lined the two longitudinal façades facing the courtyard, which was surrounded by a wooden gallery on the second floor.[17] Butchers would attach hooks to the posts and cross-beams supporting this elevated walkway to display their products.[18] The elevations facing the other two streets, described in 1833 as "dead walls," were mainly solid and were open by the entranceways; there were also high, narrow apertures that helped ventilate the butcher stalls.[19] These east and west street-facing façades thus contrasted with the more porous north and south ones, enabling patrons to enter stores directly from the street.

Public health concerns marked the life of the market from early on, in part because of the risks inherent in displaying raw meat and the fear of diseases. The aforementioned Market Act included many details about the work of butchers, given their concentration in the market. It specified that if the products they sold were not wholesome, they could face penalties, from paying a fee, to being convicted, or having their permit suspended. More specifically, the act stated that

> Any Butcher, or other Person selling or exposing for sale in market, or in any other part of this City, any unwholesome, stale, emaciated, blown, stuffed, tainted, putrid, or measly pork, meat, poultry, or other provision, shall forfeit ten shillings, for each offence; and the meat, pork, poultry, and provisions so exposed, shall without delay upon view of the Mayor, or an Alderman, or upon complaint under oath before them, or any of them, be seized, and destroyed by the Clerk of the Market.[20]

In addition to the efforts to control the quality of the meats and byproducts on display, the regulations also sought to protect the health of both sellers and buyers by addressing the cleanliness of spaces—surfaces and furniture within stalls, the area where meat was kept, and the public spaces in front of the stands.[21] This extended to the cellars beneath the complex. These dark and humid spaces were used for storage and were not immune to flooding. Regulations indicated that the ones leased by butchers needed to remain clean and accessible for potential inspection.[22]

Moreover, besides the perils invited by the food supply activities it hosted, the Market House's inadequate construction also contributed to public health concerns. As early as April 1834, less than a year after the market's completion and a month before the Public Market Act was enacted, James McMillan reported to the mayor on the lack of ventilation, unfinished floors in the cellars, flooding, and stagnant waters.[23] Concerns about market activities added urgency to finding solutions, amidst varied perceptions of disease transmission and differing opinions on the need for public health requirements. The city's regulations of 1834, Logan Atkinson writes, were partly influenced by the fear of the spread of cholera amid a series of outbreaks, initially identified in the Town of York in 1832.[24] In the broader debate about the nature of contagion, two perspectives dominated. The contagionist side, he explains, hypothesized that "disease was passed from person to person through more or less direct contact," the solution being to quarantine people and to restrict access to spaces already afflicted.[25] According to the anti-contagionist view, meanwhile, "disease was simply 'in the air,'" the remedy being to eliminate "the conditions thought most conducive to the generation of miasma ... by removing garbage, eliminating standing water, and thoroughly cleaning the streets and basements of the cities to prevent the fumes of rotting animal and vegetable matter from contaminating the air."[26] The Market Committee made recommendations to address some of these issues.[27] In 1835 it proposed, among other things, that "cellar windows [...] be made on the outside, to admit of free circulation of air, as in their present state, the cellars are [useless] and unwholesome." The apprehension articulated in these records about the dampness and humidity of the cellars is an indication of the anti-contagionist view. Guarding against diseases was further justification for inspecting cellars for standing waters, cleaning spaces and surfaces, and removing rotting material.

However, despite the recommendations and regulations intended to keep the market clean, both the underground spaces and their infrastructure remained hidden, obscuring ongoing sanitary problems from the public. In 2015, archeological excavations of the site prior to the North St. Lawrence Market Redevelopment shed some light on the drainage system integrated to remove standing water and outflows from butchers' activities. They revealed that secondary brick drains flowed into a central conduit made of stone and enclosed by an irregular arch, earning it the nickname "porcupine."[28] According to Robertson, this infrastructure was similar to the one built for the hospital; that this usage appears in more than one place, preceding the more widespread development of drains and sewers in the city, indicates the importance of collecting effluents from the market site and moving them beyond it.[29]

In the market's early years, public health considerations were taken into account by way of inspecting the products displayed and sold, regulating the areas where these transactions occurred, controlling the conditions of spaces, like cellars, and integrating new infrastructure. But the market was about more than just supplying food. The additional uses provided by its spatial organization allowed the gathering of large groups which sometimes turned into unruly mobs.

Political unrest characterized the city in the years immediately following the New Market House's construction,[30] and the public also converged there to express their views, but the coexistence of politics and market was not an ideal situation in this context. For example, in late July of 1834, Toronto's first mayor, William Lyon Mackenzie, called a public meeting to discuss how city taxes should be assessed. The event turned into a riot, during which someone assaulted him. When it reconvened the next day, a fight broke out. Amid the commotion, the gallery on the second floor collapsed under the crowd's weight. Beneath it hung butchers' hooks, and some people fell onto them. Three people died, many were injured, and this tragedy shocked the population.[31]

The 1830s were, therefore, a tumultuous period in the city's history, both in terms of health, given the 1832 cholera outbreak, its subsequent waves, and the related city regulations, and in terms of politics. But the 1840s also proved eventful: a new mixed-use city hall opened in 1845, south of the market on the other side of Front Street. Initially, it also included a police station, a jail and additional market spaces.[32] In 1849, a fire devastated an area of the city including the northern side of the Market House. While there was interest in preserving part of what remained of the market, ultimately it was demolished to allow for a new complex.

1851 Market Building and Links

The fire that destroyed the northern portion of the market facing King Street freed up the site for the construction of the St. Lawrence Hall in 1850, while the demolition of the rest of the New Market House made way for what was initially called the St. Lawrence Arcade—also known as the St. Lawrence Market—which opened a year later. Hence, the 1851 market building came to stand between the newly completed City Hall and St. Lawrence Hall (figures 6.2 and 6.3) at the crossroad of civic and cultural loci.

This new complex had a different layout than its predecessor. Robertson writes it resembled the capital letter "I", with two crossbar ends.[33] The north crossbar was the St. Lawrence Hall, along King Street, while the south one, along Front Street (figure 6.4), stood across from the City Hall.[34] Both ends had entrances to the market and were linked by the vertical bar of the "I"—a covered butchers' arcade which ran perpendicularly to King and Front Streets. In plan, the latter appears to have mainly been built down the center of the previous market's courtyard, away from those earlier buildings, their foundations and cellars. This might have been done to provide butchers with new and more adequate spaces. It measured two hundred by twenty-nine feet, and it hosted their stalls on both sides of the central passage.[35] In addition to this principal covered area, the market also included open-air spaces: west and east market places, containing stalls for other vendors; the hay and grain markets, along Front Street; a vegetable and poultry market behind City Hall; and a fish market closer to the water's edge, as depicted in the Boulton map of 1858 and figure 6.3.[36]

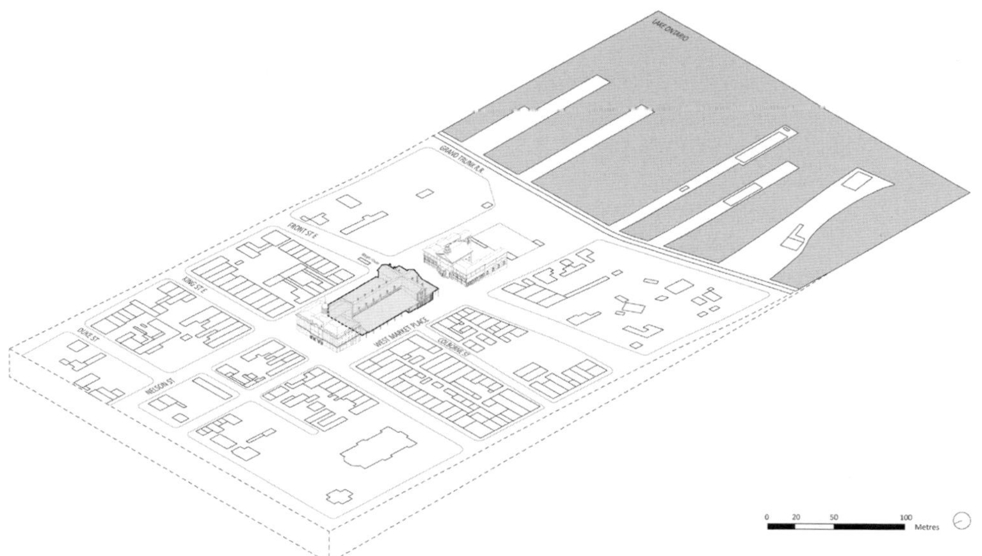

Figure 6.2. Contextual view of the St. Lawrence Market around 1858, Toronto. Based on William Sommerville Boulton, *Atlas of the City of Toronto and Vicinity*, XXVII. Toronto: J. Ellis, 1858. The City Hall and the St. Lawrence Hall are based on orthographic drawings from the City of Toronto Archives (Fonds 200, Series 2347 and Series 1465, File 351, Item 23). In addition, digital photos from the Toronto Reference Library also helped represent the St. Lawrence Market and the St. Lawrence Hall. Visualization by author with Stephanie Vo, Andrea Bickley and Nicole Li (research assistants). A light solid grey hatch identifies the market building. The City Hall hosted additional market-related activities. The blocks and footprints of nearby buildings are shown in plan; and all three, the St. Lawrence Hall, the St. Lawrence Market and the City Hall are represented. This visualization aims to provide insight into the evolving market and its relation to its context. It does not intend to address the exact topography, but to show that there was a slope, indicated by a dashed line.

The central arcade was emblematic of the market's role. It was situated at the crossroad of three types of networks: trade links between people and products, which supplied the stalls; family connections, which often extended into formal or informal partnerships; and, polluting practices, which spread beyond the market, impacting the city's environment and public health.

The networks of people and trade was key to the life of the market, as is evident in newspaper articles about it during the Christmas period. Indeed, the St. Lawrence Arcade was one of the Toronto's main attractions, especially during that festive season, when it was a popular destination for visitors to the

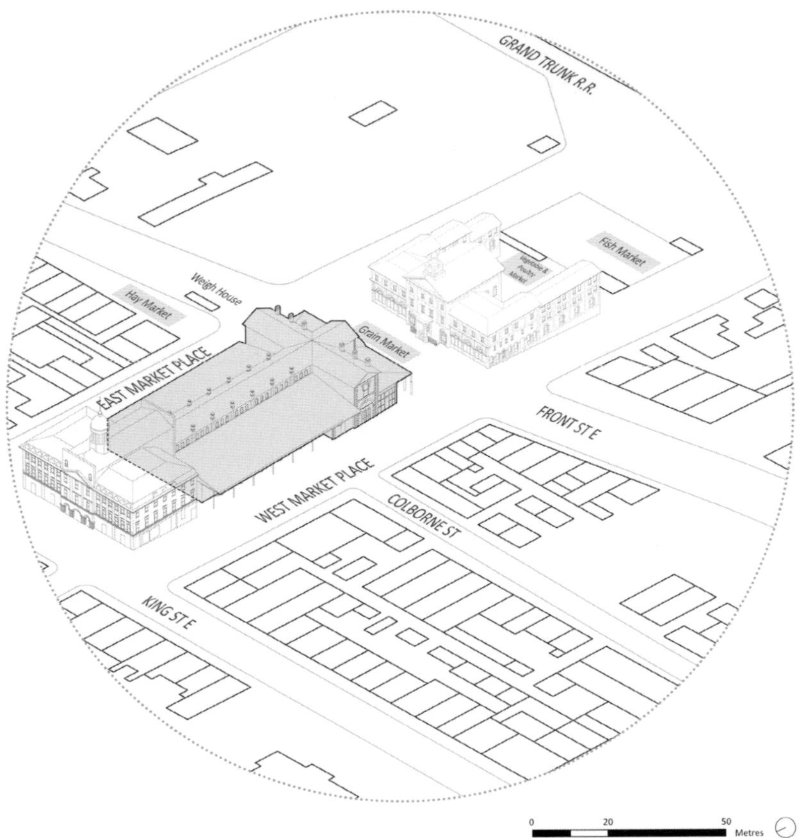

Figure 6.3. View of the St. Lawrence Market around 1858, with the St. Lawrence Hall (south of King Street) and the City Hall (south of Front Street). For sources, see figure 6.2. In this illustration, additional market activities are specified with the use of a light grey hatch.

city as well as residents and their children.[37] In the daily *Globe,* an article published on December 24, 1855, meticulously lists thirty-two vendors in the meat trade and itemizes the products displayed and their provenance, providing insights into local, regional and broader North American links.[38] The butchers John Wickson and Philip Armstrong,[39] for example, leased stalls six and nine respectively, and the writer of the article saw fit to report the source of their products. Wickson displayed beef from Kentucky, Ohio, and the nearby community of Markham. His sheep were "fed by Mr. Palmer of Richmond Hill and Mr. A. Speers of Dundas Street."[40] Armstrong's beef cattle were "fed by Mr. Anderson, of Georgiana, 1 Devon steer, by W. Armstrong, of Markham,

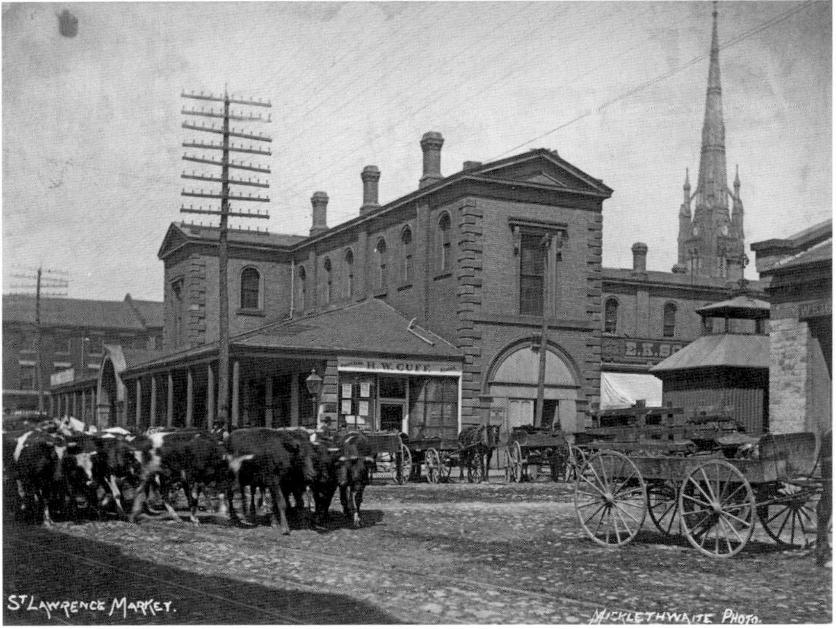

Figure 6.4. St. Lawrence Market, between 1885 and 1895. North Building. Photograph by F.W. Micklethwaite. Courtesy of the City of Toronto Archives, Fonds 1478, Item 21.

and one heifer by S. Morehead, of Scarboros'. There were also on sale at this stall, a lot of excellent sheep from [nearby] London."[41]

Not only were Wickson and Armstrong arcade neighbors, roughly across one another at its northern end, but they were also linked through family ties. In Jackson W. Armstrong's introduction to *Seven Eggs Today: The Diaries of Mary Armstrong, 1859 and 1869*, he writes that Mary, the author of the diaries, was the daughter of James Wickson and had married Philip Armstrong in 1837.[42] For the year 1859, Mary Armstrong describes her daily routine and regularly mentions going to the St. Lawrence Market on Saturdays, where she sold the output of her farming activities—calves, eggs, or butter—and items she crafted, such as aprons.[43] In addition to her father and husband being in the same métier, Mary was part of a wider network of butchers. Her brothers, Samuel, who entered into a partnership with her husband between 1859 and 1860, and John, who had a spot at the St. Lawrence Market, were also butchers, as was her stepdaughter's husband, Robert Pallett.[44] Even her son, Thomas, ended up working in the medical field only after first having partaken in the meat trade.[45] Although not all members of the family were in meat related businesses, these relationships reveal a network of kin and commercial links running through butchers' families. While such paths converged in the St. Lawrence Market, they also occurred north of a toll gate to the city. This is where Philip Armstrong and his family lived, owned and farmed additional lands, and where John Wickson and his spouse moved later.[46] The Armstrongs ran a slaughterhouse in the vicinity of Yonge Street, an important route linking the city to the countryside.[47] But as articulated in an 1851 bylaw, operating a slaughterhouse within city limits had the potential to be a source of disease:

> No person shall butcher or slaughter for sale, any Ox, Cow, Heifer, Steer, Hog, Calf, Sheep, or Lamb, within the city in any case, nor within the Liberties, unless his slaughter house shall be constructed in such a manner as shall prevent nuisances to the adjoining premises or neighborhood, and that no offal or impurity shall be allowed to remain in or near such slaughter house, and no Pigs shall be kept or fed by him at or near such slaughter houses under the penalties hereinafter provided; and that it shall be the duty of the City Inspector to visit all slaughter houses within the City and Liberties, at least once a week, and to report in writing thereon to the Standing Committee on Public Markets.[48]

William Davies, one of the other vendors described in the *Globe*'s Christmas market article of 1855, represents a case that illustrates the confluence of the market and food networks on an industrial scale. Davies was undoubtedly an ambitious individual. He emigrated from England to Canada in 1854 and began with a modest stand at the St. Lawrence Market in the mid-1850s, where he sold bacon, pork, lard, butter, and eggs.[49] In his letters, he writes about making sausage and the challenge of acquiring sheep guts and skin. As a result of these difficulties, he explored the possibility of importing materials from England toward such an endeavor.[50] While his business in the market was productive, he sold his stall lease at a profit and in the summer of 1856 he moved to the countryside to establish a farm.[51] Later, he went into wholesale meat production and eventually started to export large quantities of his goods, becoming a leading figure in the Toronto meat industry. He operated a meatpacking building located on Front and Frederick Streets, close to the St. Lawrence Market in the 1860s and 1870s.[52] In the late 1870s, he relocated his activities to a larger site east of the city—at the nexus between Front Street, the Don River, which flowed into Lake Ontario, and the train tracks (figure 6.5)—where proximity to the rail infrastructure enabled the speedy supply of his company and the transport of his products.[53] There, he developed one of the largest facilities of its kind in the British Empire, where hogs were slaughtered and their products and by-products processed, packed and shipped to places as far away as England.[54] From thirty thousand hogs in the mid-1870s, by the

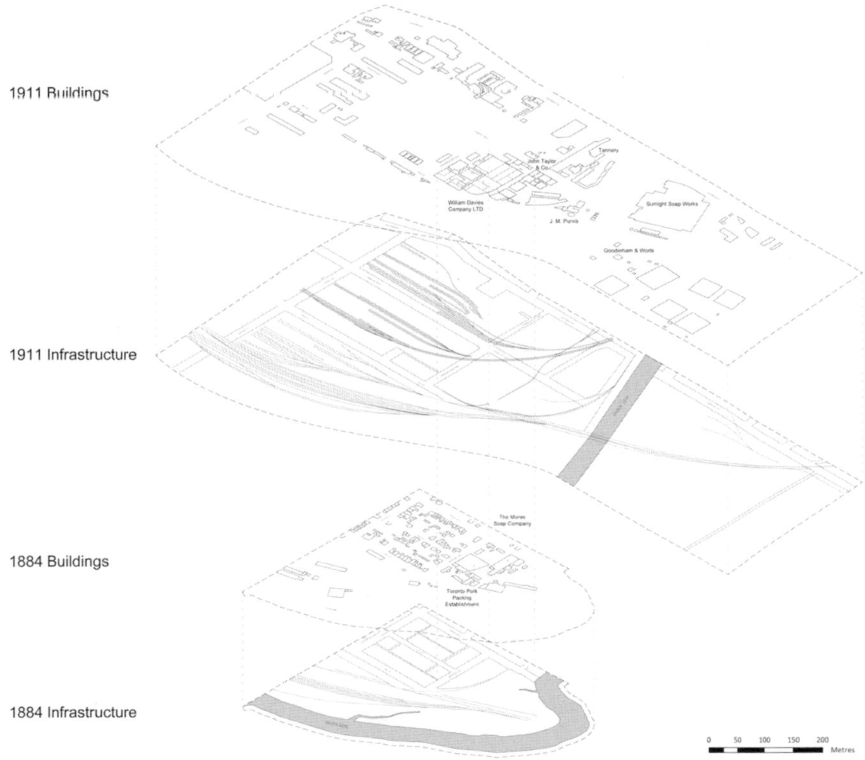

Figure 6.5. Exploded view of the context in which the William Davies Company was located along the Don River, based on the 1884 and 1911 Toronto Fire Insurance maps. Visualization by author with Stephanie Vo and Nicole Li (research assistants). In 1884, the facility was called the Toronto Pork Packing Establishment, and the 1911 plan identifies it as the William Davies Company LTD.

turn of the twentieth century, the company's shipments increased to close to five hundred thousand a year.[55] An examination of a detailed fire insurance plan from 1911 depicts the William Davies Company's main facility and provides some indication of the interior layout of the plant. It identifies a variety of spaces such as: hog pens, hog house, large ice house, refrigerating plant, packing, chill room, cutting and hanging areas, canning and sausage room, a fertilizing plant, and a pickle and jam factory. Other nearby industries likely relied on their neighbors' byproducts. For example, the Morse Soap Company, which also produced candles and lard oil, initially stood on the northeast side of the block;[56] the Sunlight Soap Works, across the Don River; and the Wickett & Craig tannery, north of Front Street (figure 6.5).

While these facilities took advantage of resources produced in their vicinity, at the same time the effluent they generated had a deleterious impact on the environment, and eventually on the health of the city's inhabitants. In *Reclaiming the Don: An Environmental History of Toronto's Don River Valley*, Jennifer Bonnell writes:

> For most industrial operations along the Don, the river offered a convenient disposal site for industrial wastes. Animal carcasses, lime from tanning operations, corrosive lye from soapworks, and industrial byproducts such as gasoline all found their way into the river. Organic wastes such as animal offal and manure put heavy stress on the river's supply of dissolved oxygen, a vital ingredient for the maintenance of aquatic life and the decomposition of wastes. In limited quantities, organic wastes will be broken down by microorganisms present in river water. As tanneries, breweries, and other industries multiplied along the lower river in the latter half of the nineteenth century, however, the river's ability to assimilate these wastes would have been seriously compromised.[57]

Indeed, the population of Toronto grew very rapidly, from just over 30,000 in 1851 to more than 180,000 in 1890,[58] and it would not be until the first decade of the following century that the city would become equipped with a wastewater treatment plant.[59] Prior to that, the city built drains and sewers incrementally in hopes of reducing the spread of disease.[60] Developing this infrastructure was complex, lengthy, and costly for residents, and it did not take place without political tension. In the meantime, effluent and waste ended up in rivers and the Toronto Bay, raising concerns about water quality.[61] In the nineteenth century, typhoid claimed the lives of many Toronto residents.[62] In her extensive examination of public health in Toronto from 1850 to 1900, Heather MacDougall notes that sanitation emerged as a public health priority for both those who espoused the "zymotic" theory—a nineteenth-century postulation of how contagious disease spread—and for contingent-contagionists who followed the "sanitary idea."[63] She also writes that some visitors to the market perceived its stench as a health threat and communicated their concerns to the medical officer.[64] Overall, while participating to the supply of the city at various scales, some food processing activities ended up contributing to pollution, which was a concern around the sites where goods were transformed and where they were sold.

Finally, it should be noted that during the early stage of this period, the St. Lawrence Market was also connected to social change. For example, soon after the St. Lawrence Hall doors opened, anti-slavery events were organized there, and in September 1851, it housed the North American Convention of Colored

Freemen. The latter meeting was a major abolitionist event, the goal of which was to help slaves escape to Canada. In addition, during the hall's early years of operation, it frequently hosted a diverse array of cultural and entertainment events, including fundraising concerts for orphans.[65]

Expansion

By the turn of the twentieth century, sanitation efforts, aided by scientific discoveries and public policies, gradually began to yield results. The St. Lawrence Market also evolved, especially after 1899, when the City Hall moved to another location on Queen Street, freeing its premises and providing an opportunity for the market to grow.

In 1898, members of the Market Commission toured a number of markets across North America and provided a report recommending strategies on how to improve and expand the St. Lawrence Market.[66] Cleanliness was considered the responsibility of both the market commissioner, in charge of swiftly removing "all the dirt and the filth in or about" it, and the dealers.[67] The latter had to "clean their stalls inside and outside, and the pavement thereof, daily, before leaving them, and [...] keep them at all times in a neat and creditable condition, and subject to inspection by the officials; no article in an unwholesome or offensive condition shall be kept, offered, or sold in or about the market."[68]

In this Market Commission's short but informative report, a large section is also dedicated to the topic of cold storage, which epitomized modernization. In their "opinion no modern market building can be considered complete without proper facilities are provided for controlling the greater and lesser supplies of perishable products [... among them] fish, fruit, eggs, butter, poultry, game, and meats of every kind."[69] Therefore, to facilitate the stocking of the main ground floor, they recommended the inclusion of cold storage underground, close to elevators. Notably, prior to their integration in the market, butchers used in their cellars ice harvested from rivers and waterways to keep meats. As waters were polluted and ice could contaminate food, public health measures had to be developed to differentiate the use of ice for food preservation from its use for other purposes.[70]

In both the North and South Markets, the roofs and their openings were also important considerations in combating disease. The report recommended the integration of skylights to bring daylight and to help provide ventilation.[71] Moreover, heating considerations further contributed to the future vision; and the Market Commission envisioned relatively homogeneous stalls, with the ones dedicated to fish to be serviced with "proper water facilities, sinks, etc." so that they could be easily kept clean.

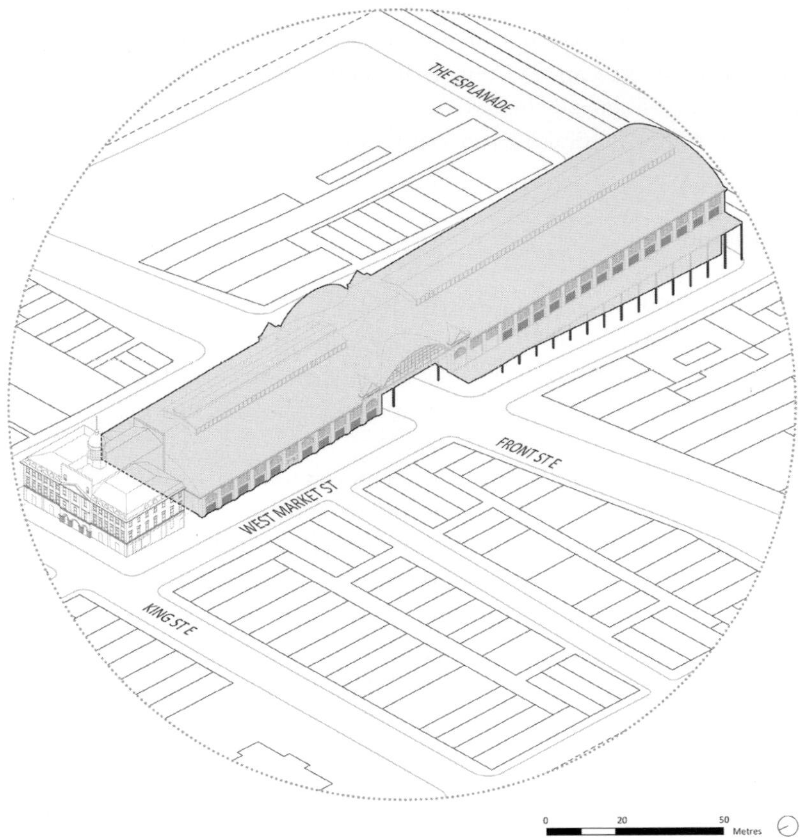

Figure 6.6. Virtual model of the St. Lawrence Market in the early 20th century. Based on data from the City of Toronto Archives, Fonds 200, Series 544, File 23; the *Atlas of the City of Toronto* by the Chas. E. Goad Company, Insurance Plan, 1910; and photographs from the Toronto Public Library Digital Archive, 1 -1211. Visualization by author with Andrea Bickley and Nicole Li (research assistants).

By 1904, the new market complex was complete. It comprised two buildings linked by a canopy (figures 6.6 and 6.7). The larger wholesale market replaced the 1851 building (figure 6.8), and parts of the old City Hall were integrated into the new South St. Lawrence Market.[72]

Yet when the butchers moved to the newly opened market, they found it lacking. In some ways, the new building was viewed as inferior to the previous one, with potential implications for sanitation. According to an article published in the *Globe*, the butchers did not have access to either cold storage or

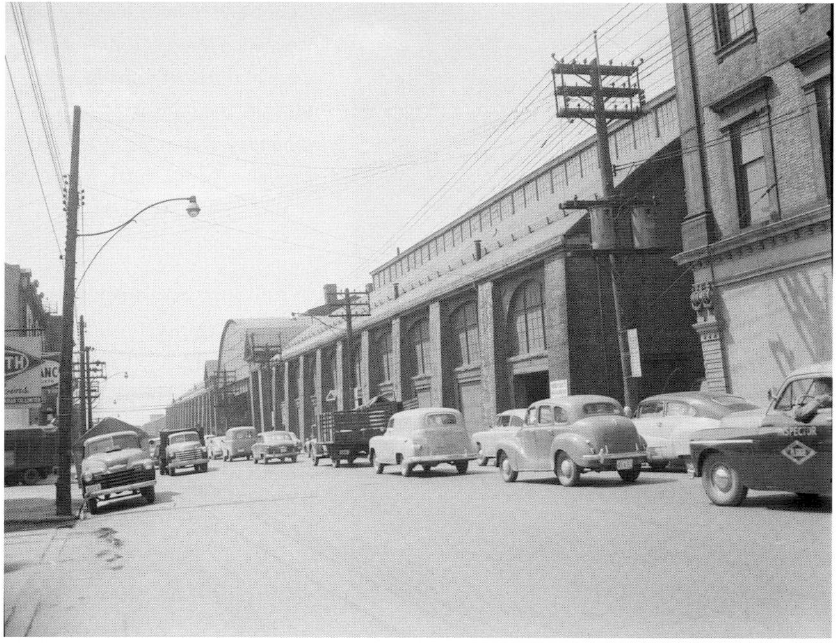

Figure 6.7. St. Lawrence Market [1950?], view of the North and South Markets, as well as the canopy. Courtesy of the City of Toronto Archives, Fonds 1128, Series 380, Item 132.

covered stalls, and they expressed their discontent. One of John Mallon & Co.'s vendors asked:

> Where is the cold storage with which the building was to be equipped? An efficient cold storage system would be a decided acquisition to the market, and a proper system would be far preferable to the use of ice, besides being more economical in space. Of course, an expensive system is out of the question, but if we can get it at the same cost as ice it will pay butchers to use it. Another grievance which we have is the absence of a covering to our stalls; our goods are entirely without protection, and the place is becoming filled with sparrows. These constitute a great nuisance, which will be multiplied many times when they commence building their nests in a month or two. The butchers have suffered considerable loss owing to the impossibility of regulating the temperature satisfactorily. In the old market we could keep our meat from Christmas to Easter in good condition, but we cannot do so here, exposed, as it is, to the varying temperature.[73]

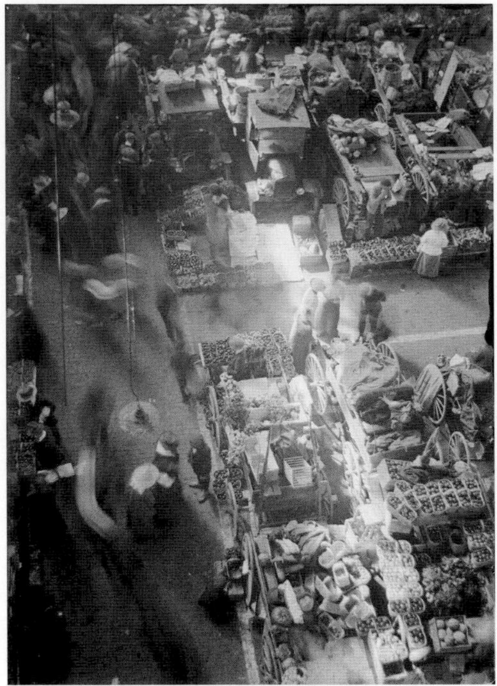

Figure 6.8. Market day, St. Lawrence Market (interior). View of the North St. Lawrence Market. September 13, 1919. Courtesy of the City of Toronto Archives, Fonds 1231, Item 612.

While not in support of a cold storage system, another butcher, Mr. W. Brown, also complained about the heating in the building, which led to financial losses. The superintendent of the market addressed the cold storage concern by bringing a report to the committee. In addition, he suggested that the sparrow issue could be resolved by temporarily obtaining owls from the zoo.[74]

By 1905, most of these issues appear to have been resolved. According to Robertson, the South St. Lawrence Market hosted fifty-eight vendors and was equipped with four cold storage spaces and sixteen storage rooms below the main floor. It also had a restaurant, washrooms, elevators, and a printing office—the latter being located in spaces of the previous City Hall which, by then, had become part of the market complex. Opposite, in the north building, the wholesale market typically hosted farmers, hucksters, wholesale butchers, and loads of hay.[75]

The twentieth century had arrived in the St. Lawrence Market. Still, some echoes of its past remained. For example, one of the stalls in the new South Market was operated by the William Davies' Company. In a photograph from 1911, it appears well stocked, signaling the company's status (figure 6.9).[76] The abundance displayed in this record contrasted with the description of Davies's stall in the Christmas market half a century earlier.[77] By then, the business had expanded further, with the creation of a retail chain of over thirty additional stores in Toronto,[78] the intensification of the meatpacking industrial activities along the Don River (illustrated on the top of figure 6.5), and an involvement with the Harris Abattoir.[79]

The first part of the twentieth century witnessed multiple transformations and shocks for the city. In October 1918, during the worst month of the Spanish Influenza, half of Torontonians fell sick and thirteen hundred died

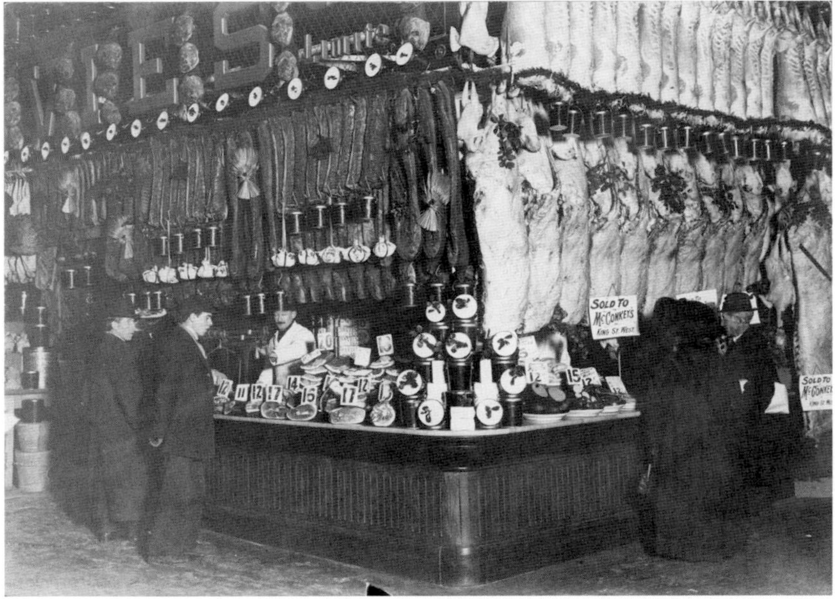

Figure 6.9. William Davies stall, St. Lawrence Market. [ca. 1911]. Photoprint (12x17). Courtesy of City of Toronto Archives, Fonds 1244, Item 338B.

from it; the Great Depression in the 1930s triggered a middle-class flight to the suburbs; and the early post-WWII boom dramatically increased housing and services.[80] During this period, Toronto's population rose sharply, from 208,040 in 1901 to 675,754 in 1951.[81] The city's sanitation and related rules improved—e.g., milk pasteurization became compulsory in 1914, a municipal abattoir was constructed in 1913,[82] downtown slums were inspected, and infrastructure, including planned sewerage, expanded. However, the spatial growth that accompanied the demographic one inevitably meant that the St. Lawrence Market began to fade from the spotlight. Grocery stores and chains sprang up across Toronto; nonetheless, the building and its retail activities carried on.[83]

Decline and Revitalization

By the 1950s, it was evident that the aging St. Lawrence Market needed repairs. In addition, in 1954 the canopy connecting the north and south buildings was removed, but more importantly, that same year, the Ontario Food Terminal opened roughly ten kilometers to its west.[84] Considering this momentous development for wholesale trade and the provisioning of the city, discussions began

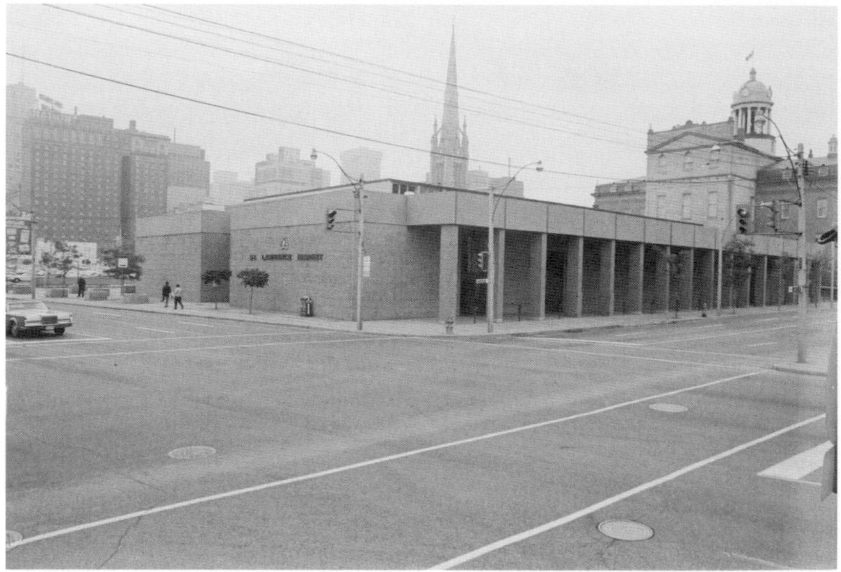

Figure 6.10. St. Lawrence Market, 1972. View of the 1968 North Market building from the corner of Jarvis St. and Front Street, looking north-west. Courtesy of the City of Toronto Archives, Fonds 2032, Series 841, File 2, Item 12.

about the market's fate. In tune with the era's trend, proposals emerged that rethought its use, prioritizing cars over pedestrians. In the early 1960s, two schemes focused on increasing revenue by addressing the parking issue created by the increase of vehicles in the area. Both projects proposed integrating parking inside the market, either with the help of ramps on its perimeter—including the St. Lawrence Hall—or, by alternating functions with parking on weekdays and holding the market on Saturdays. Besides issues with access and structural load that the proposals did not fully address, the lack of "proper exhaust equipment" was also identified as a concern. These considerations seem to have deterred the city from moving forward with these alternatives.[85]

The market's future remained precarious nonetheless. Ultimately, its north building was demolished in 1967 and replaced by a modest structure that stood on the site until 2016 (figure 6.10). However, when the South Market building was also set for demolition in the early 1970s, a line appears to have been crossed in the collective consciousness of concerned citizens, many of whom joined forces to save the market because it was a piece of their city's history.[86] Mobilization efforts included the advocacy work of the Time and Place group, some members of which were associated with the Friends of Old City Hall and had prior experience with preserving the 1899 edifice.[87] With

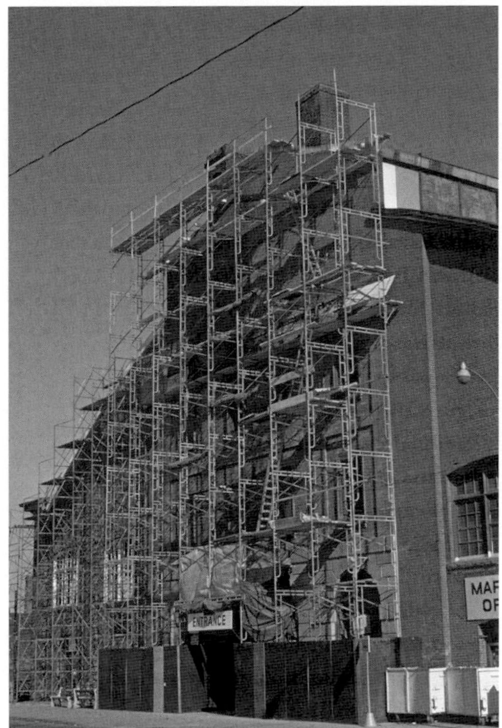

Figure 6.11. View of scaffolding on St. Lawrence Market. May 13, 1975. Courtesy of the City of Toronto Archives, Fonds 1520, File 16, Item 8.

the publication and dissemination of a pamphlet titled *A Sense of Time and Place*, they raised awareness and motivated citizens and associations to preserve Toronto's heritage.[88] Their activities included creating a flyer, organizing tours of the South Market, and responding to local authorities who were gearing up to tear it down on the grounds of structural unsoundness.[89] As a result, they were successful in overturning the city's original decision, and the building was saved. Instead of being demolished, it was renovated in the mid-to-late 1970s (figure 6.11), with the addition of more retail space below grade and a new gallery space.

The most recent phase in the market's timeline is the North St. Lawrence Market Redevelopment. In 2009, the City of Toronto launched a competition to intensify the use of the site by replacing the North Market building of 1968 with a multilevel one and diversifying the activities present on the site. According to the accompanying brief, the new mixed-used proposal had to carry on both a farmers' market and an antiques' market and include a courthouse, administrative offices, and an underground parking garage.[90] Moreover, the development also aimed to provide a vision for the market's future, one that intertwined "design excellence," sustainability and historic sensitivity.[91] In 2010, the design proposal of Rogers Stirk Harbour + Partners and Adamson Associates Architects was selected (figure 6.12). In anticipation of this construction, a temporary market opened in 2015 south of the historical St. Lawrence Market building to accommodate the farmers' and Sunday antique markets.[92] In 2019, a joint venture of Buttcon Limited and Atlas Corporation was granted the contract by the City Council to build the new North Market.[93] Given the disruptions caused by COVID-19, the work was delayed, with a

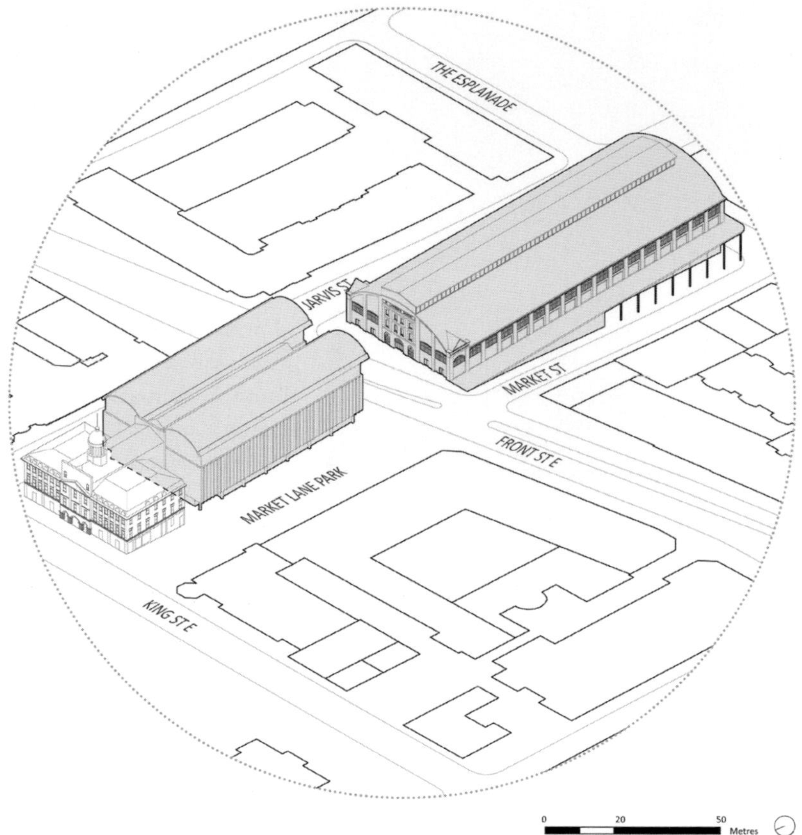

Figure 6.12. Massing of the North St. Lawrence Market Redevelopment. Based on City of Toronto 3D Massing Data 2019, Site Visits, North St. Lawrence Market and competition drawings and renderings by Adamson Associates Architects and Rogers Stirk Harbour + Partners. Visualization by author with Andrea Bickley and Nicole Li (research assistants).

revised completion date of mid-2023.[94] Attention has also been given to the public realm: Market Street has been revitalized and the regeneration of Market Lane Park is in progress.

It is worth mentioning that during the pandemic, the St. Lawrence Market adopted a number of public health measures and diversified its shopping options, illustrating yet another sign of resilience, adjusting to different eras and their challenges.[95] After more than two centuries of history, the St. Lawrence Market continues to endure.

Junctures

This chapter sought to explore how, since the 1830s, the St. Lawrence Market has been an important site where different aspects of the city's evolution converged, in urban transformations, in trades and commercial practices, and in public health and technological innovations.

The market's built form and the context in which it is located have been characterized by constant flux. Historically, both the north and south portions of the site saw notable changes. The north one witnessed a series of construction and demolition cycles—with the latest North St. Lawrence Market Redevelopment approaching completion. The south one also underwent transformations, from a fish market to a fruit and vegetable one—at the back of the former City Hall—to a covered market hall, which still stands today through community mobilization efforts. The program of the South Market diversified to include a Market Gallery and further extended its retail floor space, specifically below the main market area. Also, a temporary market has been erected to its south. In addition, significant land development incrementally occurred along the waterfront through infilling, enabling new infrastructure and faster transportation routes. Hence, while initially set close to the Toronto Bay, with time and land expansion into the lakefront, today, the market's distance from the shore has increased.

This work also underscored the importance of the market's spaces, both above and below grade. For example, subterranean areas like cellars, cold storage, and drains were essential to the operation of these buildings, and research shows that they were inspected, and if not maintained properly, they were considered a source of public health concern. Moreover, the outflows of some activities that supplied the market polluted sites and waterways beyond its physical limits. More broadly, the St. Lawrence Market was influenced by various perspectives on public health at a time when knowledge about diseases and their spread was rapidly evolving. Importantly, these views contributed to the regulation of its operation. Therefore, for a good part of its history, it has been interwoven with environmental and sanitary issues and solutions pursued by city officials.

Furthermore, the St. Lawrence Market has been related to civic and sociocultural spaces. In the 1830s, the New Market House hosted Toronto's first City Hall. Also, the second City Hall in the south part of the site was the place where political decisions were made from the mid-1840s to the late 1800s, until a newer one, known today as the Old City Hall, was built along Queen Street. Even then, fragments of the former building were themselves incorporated into the South St. Lawrence Market in the early twentieth century. In addition, historically, the St. Lawrence Hall located to its north, did not limit itself to cultural festivities; it hosted many philanthropic and advocacy events. Soon after it opened, the latter included anti-slavery meetings, as well as a major abolitionist event.[96]

Overall, in the span of over two centuries, the St. Lawrence Market has witnessed a wide range of changes: from a simple wooden structure to a contemporary complex—still under construction—equipped with innovative technologies; from the use of often unhealthy cellars to the introduction of new systems of preservation; from disorderly rioters, to inspired and activist citizenry. Its presence in the cityscape also varied, and it has intensified with the latest development. Its composition transformed too, evolving from a courtyard layout, to an I-shaped building, to linked, or separate covered market halls. So has its role: while historically, it played an important part in supplying the city, today it is a colorful place with a variety of specialized products and diverse experiences.

At the same time, despite all these transformations, the St. Lawrence Market has also persisted as a fixture for Torontonians. Although no longer the main destination for inhabitants' food provision, it continues to serve as a year-round attraction for residents, foodies and visitors alike, featuring many vendors. Its early link to civic space through the first City Hall survives via the soon-to-open provincial courtrooms and the revitalization of the public realm. Finally, it has remained anchored in the neighborhood and keeps contributing to its character.

In conclusion, the St. Lawrence Market has emerged not only as an iconic landmark in the city's ever-changing urban landscape but also as an important juncture in Toronto's social, political, and public health history.

Acknowledgments

This research was supported by the Department of Architectural Science, the Faculty of Engineering and Architectural Science, including a 2018 and a 2021 Dean's Research Funds, and the Toronto Metropolitan University. I thank Andrea Bickley, Stephanie Vo and Nicole Li who contributed to the visualizations. I also acknowledge the assistance of the librarians at the Toronto Metropolitan University, and I thank the City of Toronto Archives team, the Market Gallery staff members and Tony Masucci at the City of Toronto for providing me with copies of historical bylaws. I am grateful to Samantha L. Martin and to Lenore Hietkamp for their constructive comments on an early draft.

Notes

1. From "Land Acknowledgement," City of Toronto, accessed June 2021, https://www.toronto.ca/city-government/accessibility-human-rights/indigenous-affairs-office/land-acknowledgement/. The land acknowledgement also mentions: "Toronto is covered by Treaty 13 with the Mississaugas of the Credit." For more information on Treaty 13, see "The Toronto Purchase Treaty No. 13 (1805)," Mississaugas of the Credit First Nation, May 28, 2017, https://mncfn.ca/the-toronto-purchase-treaty-no-13-1805/. See also "The Indigenous History of Tkaronto," University of Toronto Libraries, last modified September 28, 2022, https://guides.library.utoronto.ca/c.php?g=251707&p=1675204.
2. Peter Hunter, *Upper Canada Gazette*, November 5, 1803; Graeme Mercer Adam, *Toronto, Old and New: A Memorial Volume, Historical, Descriptive and Pictorial, Designed to Mark the Hundredth Anniversary of the Passing of the Constitutional Act of 1791, Which Set Apart the Province of Upper Canada and Gave Birth to York (Now Toronto) to Which Is Added a Narrative of the Rise and Progress of the Professions, and of the Growth and Development of the City's Industries and Commerce, with Some Sketches of the Men Who Have Made or Are Making the Provincial Capital* (Toronto: The Mail Printing Company, 1891), 16.
3. Today, New Street is Jarvis Street and Market Street is Front Street. Hunter, *Upper Canada Gazette*.
4. Hunter, *Upper Canada Gazette*.
5. John Ross Robertson, *Robertson's Landmarks of Toronto: A Collection of Historical Sketches of the Old Town of York, from 1792 until 1833, and of Toronto from 1834 to 1893*, 1 (Toronto: J. Ross Robertson, 1894), 61.
6. Simon Washburn, "New Market House," *Patriot and Farmer's Monitor* (York, Upper Canada) December 21, 1832, 7.
7. Henry Scadding, *Toronto of Old: Collections and Recollections* (Toronto: Adam, Stevenson & Co., 1873), 42.
8. James Maurice Stockford Careless, "Toronto," in *The Canadian Encyclopedia*. Historica Canada, last modified March 11, 2022, https://www.thecanadianencyclopedia.ca/en/article/toronto.
9. Nelson Street replaced New Street.
10. For a detailed description of this market, see Stephen Otto, "The Creation of Toronto's First City Hall and Market Buildings," Spacing Magazine, March 4, 2016, http://spacing.ca/toronto/2016/03/04/the-creation-of-torontos-first-city-hall-and-market-buildings/. A physical model of an interpretation of the New Market House was built in 1985 for an exhibition titled "Meeting Places: Toronto's City Halls" which was curated by Steve Otto and Douglas Richardson. The model was made by students enrolled in the Department of Architectural Science/Landscape Architecture of Ryerson Polytechnical Institute (currently

Toronto Metropolitan University) and it is part of the Market Gallery collection. Photos of it can be consulted at the City of Toronto Archives.

11. Otto, "The Creation of Toronto's First City Hall and Market Buildings."
12. Otto, "The Creation of Toronto's First City Hall and Market Buildings."
13. Samuel Thompson, *Reminiscences of a Canadian Pioneer for the Last Fifty Years. An Autobiography* (Toronto: Hunter, Rose & Co., 1884), 265-266. In his publication, he refers to this market as the Old Market House.
14. According to the 1834 Public Market Act, the market was open between 5 a.m. and 4 p.m. from May 1 to November 1 and between 7 a.m. and 4 p.m. the rest of the year, except for Saturdays when it closed at 9 p.m. William Lyon Mackenzie, "By-Law 2. Public Market Act" (Toronto, May 27, 1834), Section V, item 3, 8–9.
15. Thompson, *Reminiscences*, 266.
16. George Walton, *York Commercial Directory, Street Guide, and Register, 1833–4: With Almanack and Calendar for 1834* (York: Thomas Dalton, 1833), 47. See also Otto, "The Creation of Toronto's First City Hall and Market Buildings."
17. Jamie Bradburn, "Revisiting the Past Lives of St. Lawrence Market. An Archaeological Assessment Reveals Earlier Incarnations of the North Market," *Torontoist*, September 15, 2015, https://torontoist.com/2015/09/revisiting-the-past-lives-of-st-lawrence-market/; Scadding, *Toronto of Old: Collections and Recollections*, 43.
18. Thompson, *Reminiscences*, 266.
19. Isaac Fidler, *Observations on Professions, Literature, Manners and Emigration, in the United States and Canada: Made during a Residence There in 1832* (London: Whittaker, Treacher, 1833), 263. Cited in Peter Popkin, *Stage 2–3 Archeological Assessment. 92 Front Street East, Saint Lawrence Market North, Part of the Market Block, Town of York Plan, City of Toronto* (Toronto: Golder Associates, 2015), 3. Report kindly shared with me by the Market Gallery.
20. Mackenzie, "By-Law 2. Public Market Act," Section I, Item 4, 3.
21. Mackenzie, "By-Law 2. Public Market Act," Section I, Item 10, 6.
22. Mackenzie, "By-Law 2. Public Market Act," Section I, Item 9, 5.
23. Council Papers, James McMillan to William Lyon Mackenzie, Mayor, April 14, 1834. City of Toronto Archives, Fonds 200, Series 1081, Items 1–8. Also cited in Popkin, *Stage 2–3 Archeological Assessment*, 4-5.
24. Logan Atkinson, "The Impact of Cholera on the Design and Implementation of Toronto's First Municipal By-laws, 1834," Urban History Review 30, no. 2 (2002): 4. See also Elam Stimson, *The Cholera Beacon, Being a Treatise on the Epidemic Cholera: As It Appeared in Upper Canada, in 1832–4: With a Plain and Practical Description of the First Grade, or Premonitory Symptoms, and the Various Forms of Attack, by which the Disease May be Detected in Its Curable Stage: Together with Directions for Successful Treatment. Designed for Popular Instruction*, 63184 (Dundas: G. H. Hackstaff, 1835); and Fidler, *Observations on Professions*, book 2, chapter 3, 274–306.

25. Proponents of this view were "in favor of quarantine, the encirclement of towns, the isolation of the sick, and other standard regulatory measures that had been employed in an ad hoc way in the great cities of Europe for some centuries." Atkinson, "The Impact of Cholera," 4.
26. Atkinson, "The Impact of Cholera," 4–5. An important proponent of miasma theory was Edwin Chadwick. See Stephen Halliday, in "Death and Miasma in Victorian London: an Obstinate Belief," *British Medical Journal Publishing Group* 323, no. 7327 (2011). Additionally, background on anticontagionism can be found in Erwin Ackerknecht, "Anticontagionism between 1821 and 1867: The Fielding H. Garrison Lecture," *International Journal of Epidemiology* 38, no. 1 (2009). I am indebted to Samantha L. Martin for this reference.
27. Council Papers, Report no. 4 of the Market Committee, June 13, 1835. Cited in Popkin, *Stage 2–3 Archeological Assessment*, 5.
28. John Rieti, "Displaying St. Lawrence Market's 1831 Drain Could Cost City $2M," *CBC News* (Toronto) 2017, https://www.cbc.ca/news/canada/toronto/st-lawrence-market-costs-1.4298986.
29. This underground infrastructure was an important finding that delayed the new development and generated debate about preserving and displaying the drainage system to the public. It was estimated that this endeavor would add 1.6 to 2 million Canadian dollars to the redevelopment project. John Lorinc, "North St. Lawrence Market Dig Delves Deep into Toronto's Foodie History," January 8, 2017, https://www.thestar.com/news/gta/2017/01/08/north-st-lawrence-market-dig-delves-deep-into-torontos-foodie-history.html; Catherine Brace, "Public Works in the Canadian City: The Provision of Sewers in Toronto 1870–1913," *Urban History Review / Revue d'histoire urbaine* 23, no. 2 (March 1995): 41.
30. That decade witnessed a growing call for political reform and included the Lower and Upper Canada rebellions of 1837–38.
31. For more information on this tragedy, see Robertson, *Robertson's Landmarks of Toronto* (1894), 62; Otto, "The Creation of Toronto's First City Hall and Market Buildings;" and "Awful Event," *Patriot and Farmer's Monitor* August 1, 1834, 4.
32. For a detailed research on this City Hall and associated market spaces, see Stephen Otto, "Second City Hall (1845-99)," in City of Toronto Archives, Fonds 92, Item 342. It was also referred to as the New Market House.
33. Robertson, *Robertson's Landmarks of Toronto* (1894), 64.
34. It is interesting to note that for a period of time, the Board of Heath Office was located in the City Hall. See W. R. Brown, *Brown's Toronto General Directory* (Toronto: Maclear & Co., 1856), 36.
35. Robertson, *Robertson's Landmarks of Toronto* (1894), 64–65.
36. William Sommerville Boulton, *Atlas of the City of Toronto and Vicinity* (Toronto: J. Ellis, 1858), map XXVII.

37. John Ross Robertson, *Robertson's Landmarks of Toronto: A Collection of Historical Sketches of the Old Town of York, from 1792 until 1837, and of Toronto from 1834 to 1908* (Toronto: J. Ross Robertson, 1908), 148.
38. "The St. Lawrence Market," *Globe* (Toronto, ON) December 24, 1855, 2.
39. P. Armstrong had been listed as a butcher in the New Market House building, see Walton, *York Commercial Directory, Street Guide, and Register*, 48.
40. "The St. Lawrence Market."
41. "The St. Lawrence Market."
42. Armstrong, *Seven Eggs Today*, 4.
43. Armstrong, *Seven Eggs Today*, 104-133.
44. Armstrong, *Seven Eggs Today*, 1–14.
45. Armstrong, *Seven Eggs Today*, 52.
46. J. Armstrong (ed), *Rowsell's City of Toronto and County of York Directory for the 1850–51* (Toronto: Henry Rowsell, 1850), 4.
47. Armstrong, *Seven Eggs Today*, 53.
48. John George Bowes, "By-law Number 173. An Act to Amend the Law Relating to the Public Markets of the City of Toronto" (Toronto, September 12, 1851), 4.
49. William Davies, *Letters of William Davies, Toronto 1854–1861*, ed. William Sherwood Fox (Toronto: University of Toronto Press, 1945), 40 (Letter 5, March 25, 1855).
50. Davies, *Letters*, 67 (Letter 27, Good Friday 1856).
51. A year later, in a letter to his brother, he admitted regretting this decision after having heard about how one of his fellow butchers was doing in the market. Davies, *Letters*, 90 (Letter 45, August 17th 1857).
52. Information about this meatpacking building is available on the "Davies/Taylor Site," Lost Rivers, accessed June 20, 2020, http://lostrivers.ca/content/points/daviestaylor.html, as well as the "Don Valley Historical Mapping Project," accessed June 20, 2020, https://maps.library.utoronto.ca/dvhmp/davies.html.
53. "Davies/Taylor Site," Lost Rivers. For additional information on William Davies & Co., see John Douglas Sutherland Campbell, *Industries Of Canada: Historical and Commercial Sketches of Toronto and Environs, Its Prominent Places and People, Representative Merchants and Manufacturers, Its Improvements, Progress and Enterprise* (Toronto: M.G. Bixby, 1886), 86.
54. Campbell, *Industries of Canada*, 86.
55. Bliss, Michael. "Davies, William." In *Dictionary of Canadian Biography*, vol. 15. University of Toronto/Université Laval, 2003, accessed June 10, 2020, http://www.biographi.ca/en/bio/davies_william_15E.html. According to one version, it was Toronto's prolific production of pig-related meats that led to its nickname "Hogtown."
56. For a record of a product it produced, see Geo. D. Morse & Co., "Jas. L. Morrison, John Taylor, Geo. D. Morse & Co., manufacturers of Soap, Candles & Lard Oil. Printed ephemera from the Metropolitan Toronto Library"

Toronto, [187–?], https://www.canadiana.ca/view/oocihm.38717/1?r=0&s=6. It was later replaced by the John Taylor and Co Ltd.

57. Jennifer Bonnell, *Reclaiming the Don: an Environmental History of Toronto's Don River Valley* (Toronto: University of Toronto Press, 2014), 35; 37.
58. Risa Barkin and Ian Gentles, "Death in Victorian Toronto, 1850–1899," *Urban History Review / Revue d'histoire urbaine* 19, no. 1/2 (1990): 16 (table 3).
59. Brace, "Public Works in the Canadian City," 41.
60. Heather A. MacDougall, Robert Roddy, and Arthur R. Boswell, "The Genesis of Public Health Reform in Toronto, 1869–1890," *Urban History Review / Revue d'histoire urbaine* 10, no. 3 (February 1982): 1–9.
61. Brace, "Public Works in the Canadian City," 33–43.
62. Barkin and Gentles, "Death in Victorian Toronto," 23.
63. Heather MacDougall, "Public Health in Toronto's Municipal Politics: The Canniff Years, 1883–1890," *Bulletin of the History of Medicine* 55, no. 2 (Summer 1981): 186; Heather Anne MacDougall, *Activists and Advocates: Toronto's Health Department, 1883–1983* (Toronto: Dundurn Press, 1990). See also MacDougall, Roddy, and Boswell, "The Genesis of Public Health Reform in Toronto," 2; Heather MacDougall, "Public Health and the 'Sanitary Idea'" in *Essays in the History of Canadian Medicine*, ed. Wendy Mitchinson and Janice Dickin McGinnis (Toronto: McClelland and Stewart, 1988); Christopher Hamlin, "What Becomes of Pollution? Adversary Science and the Controversy on the Self-Purification of Rivers in Britain, 1859–1900" (PhD diss., University of Wisconsin-Madison, 1987); Margaret Pelling, *Cholera, Fever and English Medicine, 1825–1865* (Oxford: Oxford University Press, 1978); and Brace, "Public Works in the Canadian City," 33–43.
64. MacDougall, *Activists and Advocates*, 57.
65. Robertson, *Robertson's Landmarks of Toronto* (1898), 325.
66. They visited markets in Montreal, Boston, New York, Philadelphia, Baltimore, Washington, Cleveland, and Buffalo, according to the report. *Report of Market Commission* (Toronto: Market Commission, 1898), 1.
67. *Report of Market Commission*, 3.
68. *Report of Market Commission*, 4.
69. *Report of Market Commission*, 5.
70. "An Infectious Idea: Clean and Nutritious Food," City of Toronto Archives, accessed June 20, 2020, http://bit.ly/3ThHS3b.
71. *Report of Market Commission*, 7.
72. In addition, the St. Lawrence Hall was less frequented, so there were plans and discussions on how to revitalize it. One of the proposals included a technical school. Robertson, *Robertson's Landmarks of Toronto* (1908), 149.
73. "The Butchers Are Protesting," *Globe* (Toronto, ON), February 12, 1903, 10.
74. "The Butchers Are Protesting."

75. Robertson, *Robertson's Landmarks of Toronto* (1908), 149.
76. By then, Davies had already retired from the lucrative company he had established. See Bliss, "Davies, William."
77. "The St. Lawrence Market."
78. *The Toronto City Directory 1911,* vol. 36 (Toronto: Might Directories Limited, 1911), 548.
79. Ian MacLachlan, *Kill and Chill: Restructuring Canada's Beef Commodity Chain* (Toronto: University of Toronto Press, 2001), 146.
80. "The First Half of the 20th Century, 1901–51," Toronto History Museums, City of Toronto, accessed June 20, 2020, https://www.toronto.ca/explore-enjoy/history-art-culture/museums/virtual-exhibits/history-of-toronto/the-first-half-of-the-20th-century-1901-51/.
81. Toronto's History: Popular Topics, City of Toronto, accessed July 2022, http://bit.ly/3AaJgxO
82. MacLachlan, *Kill and Chill*, 25; and "An Infectious Idea: Clean and Nutritious Food."
83. "The First Half of the 20th Century."
84. For a comprehensive study of the establishment of wholesale terminal markets in other cities in North America, see Helen Tangires, *Movable Markets: Food Wholesaling in the 20th Century City* (Baltimore: John Hopkins University Press, 2019).
85. "Two Plans Considered: City May Convert Market to Parking Garage," *Globe and Mail* (Toronto, ON), March 29, 1960; "The Past Has a Future," *Globe and Mail* (Toronto, ON), September 7, 1960.
86. "Citizens' Committee is Formed to Preserve Old Market Building," *Globe and Mail* (Toronto, ON) September 15, 1971.
87. Howard V. Walker, "New Life for Old Toronto Market," *Globe and Mail* (Toronto, ON) July 29, 1975.
    The City of Toronto Archives contain photos illustrating the decaying conditions of the building prior to renovations. See City of Toronto Archives, Fonds 200, Series 1465, File 755.
88. John Sewell, *A Sense of Time and Place* (Toronto: City Pamphlets, 1971).
89. See City of Toronto Archives, Fonds 1493, File 3 (South St. Lawrence Market).
90. "St. Lawrence Market North Building," Canadian Competitions Catalogue, University of Montreal, accessed June 10, 2020, https://www.ccc.umontreal.ca/fiche_concours.php?lang=en&cId=163.
91. Competition Brief, North St. Lawrence Market Redevelopment, City of Toronto, accessed June 10, 2020, https://www.toronto.ca/services-payments/venues-facilities-bookings/booking-city-facilities/st-lawrence-market/north-st-lawrence-market-redevelopment/.

92. In the course of the year 2022, the Sunday antique market hosted in the Temporary North Market closed and moved to another location.
93. "North Saint Lawrence Market Redevelopment. Progress Update," City of Toronto, accessed June 22, 2021, https://www.toronto.ca/services-payments/venues-facilities-bookings/booking-city-facilities/st-lawrence-market/north-st-lawrence-market-redevelopment/progress-update/.
94. "North Saint Lawrence Market Redevelopment."
95. For example, in order to help support vendors and facilitate the supply of shoppers, in February 2021, it partnered with a delivery service through the online Inabuggy app. See "St. Lawrence Market Online Ordering and Home Delivery Launches with Inabuggy," City of Toronto, February 4, 2021, https://www.toronto.ca/news/st-lawrence-market-online-ordering-and-home-delivery-launches-with-inabuggy/.
96. "Looking back at Toronto's historic anti-slavery convention of 1851," *TVO*, February 13, 2020, https://www.tvo.org/article/looking-back-at-torontos-historic-anti-slavery-convention-of-1851; Robertson, *Robertson's Landmarks of Toronto* (1898), 325.

Archival sources

The City of Toronto Archives. (Fonds 92, Item 342).
———. (Fonds 124, File 2, Item 63).
———. (Fonds 200, Series 1081, Items 1-8).
———. (Fonds 200, Series 1092, Item 6, September 11, 1841).
———. (Fonds 200, Series 1465, File 351, Item 23 and File 755).
———. (Fonds 200, Series 2347).
———. (Fonds 1128, Series 380, Item 132).
———. (Fonds 1231, Item 612).
———. (Fonds 1244, Item 338B).
———. (Fonds 1478, Item 21).
———. (Fonds 1493, File 3).
———. (Fonds 1526, File 16, Item 8).
———. (Fonds 2032, Series 841, File 2, Item 12).

Bibliography

Ackerknecht, Erwin. "Anticontagionism between 1821 and 1867: The Fielding H. Garrison Lecture." *International Journal of Epidemiology* 38, no. 1 (2009): 7–21.

Adam, Graeme Mercer. *Toronto, Old and New: A Memorial Volume, Historical, Descriptive and Pictorial, Designed to Mark the Hundredth Anniversary of the Passing of the Constitutional Act of 1791, Which Set Apart the Province of Upper Canada and Gave Birth to York (Now Toronto) to Which Is Added a Narrative of the Rise and Progress of the Professions, and of the Growth and Development of the City's Industries and Commerce, with Some Sketches of the Men Who Have Made or Are Making the Provincial Capital.* Toronto: Mail Printing Company, 1891.

Armstrong, Frederick Henry. *A City in the Making: Progress, People & Perils in Victorian Toronto*. Toronto: Dundurn Press, 1988.

Armstrong, Mary, and Jackson W. Armstrong. *Seven Eggs Today: The Diaries of Mary Armstrong, 1859 and 1869*. Life Writing Series. Waterloo, ON: Wilfrid Laurier University Press, 2004.

Atkinson, Logan. "The Impact of Cholera on the Design and Implementation of Toronto's First Municipal By-Laws, 1834." *Urban History Review* 30, no. 2 (2002): 3–15.

"Awful Event." *Patriot and Farmer's Monitor*, August 1, 1834, 4.

Barkin, Risa, and Ian Gentles. "Death in Victorian Toronto, 1850–1899." *Urban History Review / Revue d'histoire urbaine* 19, no. 1/2 (1990): 14–29.

Bliss, Michael. "Davies, William." In *Dictionary of Canadian Biography*. University of Toronto/Université Laval, 2003. Accessed June 10, 2020, http://www.biographi.ca/en/bio/davies_william_15E.html.

Bonnell, Jennifer. *Reclaiming the Don: An Environmental History of Toronto's Don River Valley*. Toronto: University of Toronto Press, 2014.

Boulton, William Sommerville. *Atlas of the City of Toronto and Vicinity*. Map. Toronto: J. Ellis, 1858.

Bowes, John George. "By-Law Number 173. An Act to Amend the Law Relating to the Public Markets of the City of Toronto." September 12, 1851.

Brace, Catherine. "Public Works in the Canadian City; the Provision of Sewers in Toronto 1870–1913." *Urban History Review / Revue d'histoire urbaine* 23, no. 2 (March 1995): 33–43.

Bradburn, Jamie. "Looking Back at Toronto's Historic Anti-Slavery Convention of 1851." *TVO*, February 13, 2020. https://www.tvo.org/article/looking-back-at-torontos-historic-anti-slavery-convention-of-1851.

———. "Revisiting the Past Lives of St. Lawrence Market. An Archaeological Assessment Reveals Earlier Incarnations of the North Market." *Torontoist*, September 15, 2015. https://torontoist.com/2015/09/revisiting-the-past-lives-of-st-lawrence-market/.

Brown, W. R. *Brown's Toronto General Directory*. Toronto: Maclear & Co., 1856.

Campbell, John Douglas Sutherland. *Industries of Canada: Historical and Commercial Sketches of Toronto and Environs, Its Prominent Places and People, Representative Merchants and Manufacturers, Its Improvements, Progress and Enterprise*. Toronto: M. G. Bixby, 1886.

Cane, James. *Topographical Plan of the City and Liberties of Toronto*. Map. Toronto: Cane, James, 1842.

Careless, James Maurice Stockford. "Toronto." In *The Canadian Encyclopedia*. Historica Canada. https://www.thecanadianencyclopedia.ca/en/article/toronto.

"Citizens' Committee Is Formed to Preserve Old Market Building." *Globe and Mail* (Toronto, ON), September 15, 1971, 5.

City of Toronto. "Land Acknowledgement." Accessed June 20, 2021. https://www.toronto.ca/city-government/accessibility-human-rights/indigenous-affairs-office/land-acknowledgement/.

———. "North Saint Lawrence Market Redevelopment. Progress Update." Accessed July 22, 2021. https://www.toronto.ca/services-payments/venues-facilities-bookings/booking-city-facilities/st-lawrence-market/north-st-lawrence-market-redevelopment/progress-update/.

———. "St. Lawrence Market Online Ordering and Home Delivery Launches with Inabuggy." February 4, 2021. https://www.toronto.ca/news/st-lawrence-market-online-ordering-and-home-delivery-launches-with-inabuggy.

———. Toronto History Museums. "The First Half of the 20th Century, 1901–51." Accessed June 20, 2020. https://www.toronto.ca/explore-enjoy/history-art-culture/museums/virtual-exhibits/history-of-toronto/the-first-half-of-the-20th-century-1901-51/.

City of Toronto Archives. "An Infectious Idea: Clean and Nutritious Food." Accessed June 20, 2020. http://bit.ly/3ThHS3b

———. "Toronto's History: Popular Topics." Accessed July 2022. http://bit.ly/3AaJgxO

Davies, William. *Letters of William Davies, Toronto 1854–1861*. Edited by William Sherwood Fox. Toronto: University of Toronto Press, 1945.

Don Valley Historical Mapping Project. "Don Valley Historical Mapping Project." Accessed June 20, 2020. https://maps.library.utoronto.ca/dvhmp/davies.html.

Fidler, Isaac. *Observations on Professions, Literature, Manners and Emigration, in the United States and Canada: Made During a Residence There in 1832*. London: Whittaker, Treacher, 1833.

Goad, Chas. E. *Atlas of the City of Toronto and Vicinity From Special Survey Founded on Registered Plans and Showing All Buildings and Lot Numbers*. Map. Toronto, 1884, 118-119.

Halliday, Stephen. "Death and Miasma in Victorian London: An Obstinate Belief." *British Medical Journal Publishing Group* 323, no. 7327 (2011): 1469–71.

Hamlin, Christopher. "What Becomes of Pollution? Adversary Science and the Controversy on the Self-Purification of Rivers in Britain, 1850–1900." PhD diss., University of Wisconsin-Madison, 1987.

Hunter, Peter. *Upper Canada Gazette*, November 5, 1803.

Lorinc, John. "North St. Lawrence Market Dig Delves Deep into Toronto's Foodie History." January 8, 2017. https://www.thestar.com/news/gta/2017/01/08/north-st-lawrence-market-dig-delves-deep-into-torontos-foodie-history.html.

Lost Rivers. "Davies/Taylor Site." Accessed June 20, 2020. http://lostrivers.ca/content/points/daviestaylor.html.

MacDougall, Heather. "Public Health and the 'Sanitary Idea.'" In *Essays in the History of Canadian Medicine*, edited by Wendy Mitchinson and Janice Dickin McGinnis. Toronto: McClelland and Stewart, 1988.

———. "Public Health in Toronto's Municipal Politics: The Canniff Years, 1883–1890." *Bulletin of the History of Medicine* 55, no. 2 (Summer 1981): 17.

———. *Activists and Advocates: Toronto's Health Department, 1883–1983*. Toronto: Dundurn Press, 1990.

MacDougall, Heather A., Robert Roddy, and Arthur R. Boswell. "The Genesis of Public Health Reform in Toronto, 1869–1890." *Urban History Review / Revue d'histoire urbaine* 10, no. 3 (February 1982): 1–9.

Mackenzie, William Lyon. "By-Law 2. Public Market Act." Toronto, May 27, 1834.

MacLachlan, Ian. *Kill and Chill: Restructuring Canada's Beef Commodity Chain*. Toronto: University of Toronto Press, 2001.

Mississauguas of the Credit First Nation. "The Toronto Purchase Treaty no. 13 (1805)." May 28, 2017. https://mncfn.ca/the-toronto-purchase-treaty-no-13-1805/.

Morse, Geo. D. & Co. *Jas. L. Morrison, John Taylor, Geo. D. Morse & Co., Manufacturers of Soap, Candles & Lard Oil*. Printed Ephemera from the Metropolitan Toronto Library. Toronto, [187–?]. https://www.canadiana.ca/view/oocihm.38717/1?r=0&s=6.

Otto, Stephen. "The Creation of Toronto's First City Hall and Market Buildings." *Spacing Magazine*, March 4, 2016. http://spacing.ca/toronto/2016/03/04/the-creation-of-torontos-first-city-hall-and-market-buildings/.

P., John. "Remembering the Abolition of the Toll Gates of York County: December 31: Snapshots in History." Toronto Public Library, Local History & Genealogy blog. December 31, 2016. https://torontopubliclibrary.typepad.com/local-history-genealogy/2016/12/remembering-the-abolition-of-the-toll-gates-of-york-county-december-31-snapshots-in-history.html.

Pelling, Margaret. *Cholera, Fever and English Medicine, 1825–1865*. Oxford: Oxford University Press, 1978.

Popkin, Peter. *Stage 2-3 Archeological Assessment. 92 Front Street East, Saint Lawrence Market North, Part of the Market Block, Town of York Plan, City of Toronto*. Toronto: Golder Associates, 2015.

Report of Market Commission. Toronto: Market Commission, 1898.

Rieti, John. "Displaying St. Lawrence Market's 1831 Drain Could Cost City $2m." *CBC News* (Toronto), 2017. https://www.cbc.ca/news/canada/toronto/st-lawrence-market-costs-1.4298986.

Robertson, John Ross. *Robertson's Landmarks of Toronto: A Collection of Historical Sketches of the Old Town of York, from 1792 until 1833, and of Toronto from 1834 to 1893*. Toronto: J. Ross Robertson, 1894.

———. *Robertson's Landmarks of Toronto: A Collection of Historical Sketches of the Old Town of York from 1792 until 1833, and of Toronto from 1834 to 1898: Also, Nearly Two Hundred Engravings of Old Houses, Familiar Faces and Historic Places, with Maps and Schedules Connected with the Local History of York and Toronto*. Toronto: J. R. Robertson, 1898.

———. *Robertson's Landmarks of Toronto: A Collection of Historical Sketches of the Old Town of York, from 1792 until 1837, and of Toronto from 1834 to 1908*. Toronto: J. Ross Robertson, 1908.

Rowsell's City of Toronto and County of York Directory for the 1850–51. Edited by J. Armstrong. Toronto: Henry Rowsell, 1850.

Scadding, Henry. *Toronto of Old: Collections and Recollections*. Toronto: Adam, Stevenson & Co., 1873.

Sewell, John. *A Sense of Time and Place*. Toronto: City Pamphlets, 1971.

Stimson, Elam. *The Cholera Beacon, Being a Treatise on the Epidemic Cholera: As It Appeared in Upper Canada, in 1832–4: With a Plain and Practical Description of the First Grade, or Premonitory Symptoms, and the Various Forms of Attack, by Which the Disease May Be Detected in Its Curable Stage: Together with Directions for Successful Treatment. Designed for Popular Instruction*. Dundas: G. H. Hackstaff, 1835.

Tangires, Helen. *Movable Markets. Food Wholesaling in the 20th Century City*. Baltimore: John Hopkins University Press, 2019.

"The Butchers Are Protesting: Claim the City Has Broken Faith with Them in Rental of Stalls. Also in Failure to Provide Car Accommodation. Serious Dissatisfaction among Tenants of St. Lawrence Market – Grivances for Which They Ask a Remedy." *Globe* (Toronto, ON), February 12, 1903, 10.

"The Past Has a Future." *Globe and Mail* (Toronto, ON), September 7, 1960, 6.

"The St. Lawrence Market." *Globe* (Toronto), December 24, 1855, 2.

The Toronto City Directory 1911. Embracing an Alphabetical List of All Business Firms and Private Citizens – a Classified Business Directory; a Miscellaneous Directory – Containing a Large Amount of Valuable Information and a Complete Street Guide, Also Suburban Directories of Bedford Park, Davisville, Earlscourt, Eglinton, Humber Bay, Mimico, Moore Park, New Toronto, North Toronto, Runnymede, Spadina Park, Swansea, Todmorden and Weston. Toronto: Might Directories Limited, 1911.

Thompson, Samuel. *Reminiscences of a Canadian Pioneer for the Fifty Years. An Autobiography*. Toronto: Hunter, Rose & Co., 1884.

Todd, Alpheus. *Plan of the City of Toronto, Capital of Upper Canada*. Map. Toronto: Toronto Public Library, 1834.

Toronto Fire Insurance Plan. Vol. 3. 1911. Toronto. University of Toronto Libraries, Map and Data Library. Accessed June 20, 2020. https://mdl.library.utoronto.ca/collections/geospatial-data/toronto-fire-insurance-plans-volume-3/index.

"Two Plans Considered: City May Convert Market to Parking Garage." *Globe and Mail* (Toronto, ON), March 29, 1960, 1.

University of Montreal. Canadian Competitions Catalogue. "St. Lawrence Market North Building." Accessed June 10, 2020. https://www.ccc.umontreal.ca/fiche_concours.php?lang=en&cId=163.

University of Toronto Libraries. "The Indigenous History of Tkaronto." Last modified September 28, 2022. https://guides.library.utoronto.ca/c.php?g=251707&p=1675204.

Walker, Howard V. "New Life for Old Toronto Market." *Globe and Mail* (Toronto, ON), July 29, 1975, 1.

Walton, George. *York Commercial Directory, Street Guide, and Register, 1833–4: With Almanack and Calendar for 1834*. York: Thomas Dalton, 1833.

Washburn, Simon. "New Market House." *Patriot and Farmer's Monitor* (York, Upper Canada), December 21, 1832, 7.

CHAPTER 7

BETWEEN A GOVERNMENT PROJECT AND A COMMERCIAL SPACE FOR ORDINARY CITIZENS

Dongan Market, 1903–1937

Xusheng Huang

Introduction

The emergence of the covered market hall was a symbol of modernity in the European city, which met the demands of the rising bourgeoisie in the new industrial urban world. However, the situation in Asia was different: the covered market hall came to be used in preindustrial Beijing, even though the city had only a small number of industrial workers in the first half of the twentieth century. As such, this chapter offers an alternative case study—that of Dongan Market (*Dongan Shichang* or Eastern Peace Market)—which looks beyond the linear model of modernization so often used in studies of architectural typologies. As a microcosm of political, social, and economic changes in Beijing, Dongan Market flourished during the twentieth century.[1] This chapter traces its formation in 1903 and transformation over the following decades, until 1937 when Beijing was invaded by the Japanese and then became embroiled in World War II.

Dongan Market was a landmark and one of the first and most famous permanent public markets built in Beijing. The special geopolitical location of the market and Wangfujing Street, illustrated in figure 7.1, was near Dongan Gate, one of the main entrances to the Imperial City, close to the Legation Quarter, from where foreign powers exercised significant political influence over the Chinese government. Therefore, from the time of its establishment, the market became a primary focus of the government's urban improvement plan. As a new public sphere in the early twentieth century, it was shaped by the clash between the local government's efforts to promote urban improvement and the daily needs of local people who claimed their right to urban commercial spaces.

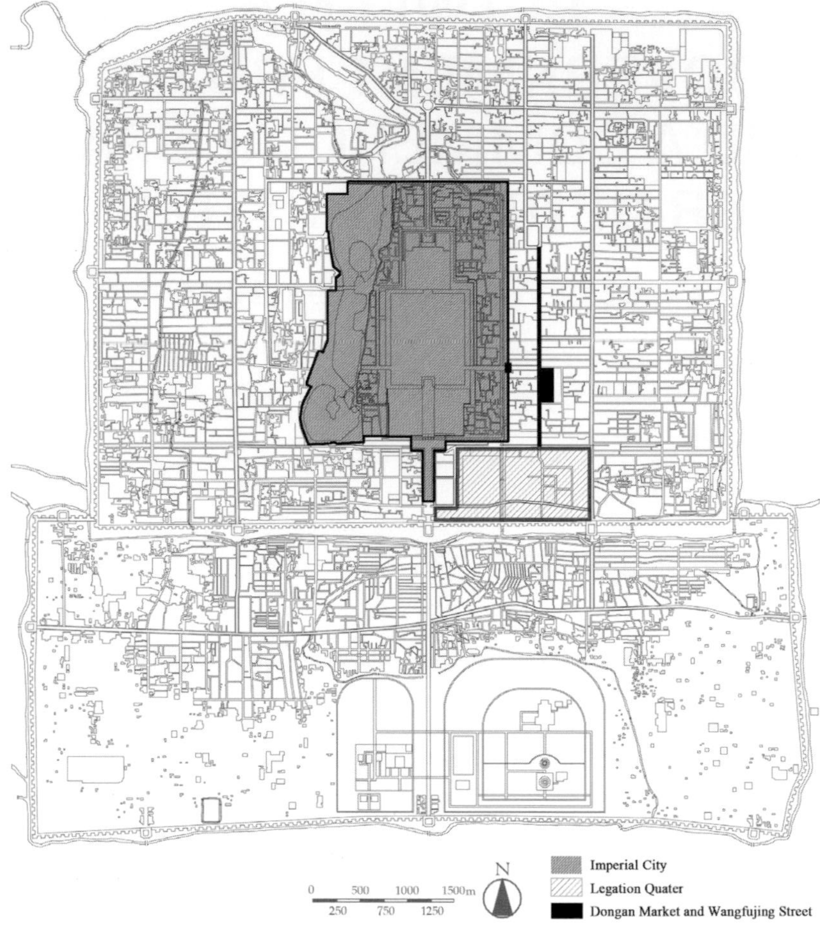

Figure 7.1. The location of Dongan Market and Wangfujing Street (black), in relation to the Imperial City (dense lines) and the Legation Quarter (sparse lines). Redrawn by the author based on 新测北京内外城全图 [The New Survey Map of the Inner and Outer City, Beijing], 1910s, 61.5 × 82.1 cm (Shanghai: Commercial Press, 1921).

There were three main types of traditional commercial space in Beijing in the late Qing period (1840–1912): the shopping street, the street market, and the temple market.[2] Qian Gate Street was a famous example for the first type, situated outside the Qian Gate of the Inner City wall and renowned for its many shops and restaurants (figure 7.2). The street market opened on certain days of the month, selling specific goods, such as rice, meat, fruit, flowers, birds, sugar, etc. Wandering through a bird market (figure 7.3) was not merely a commercial

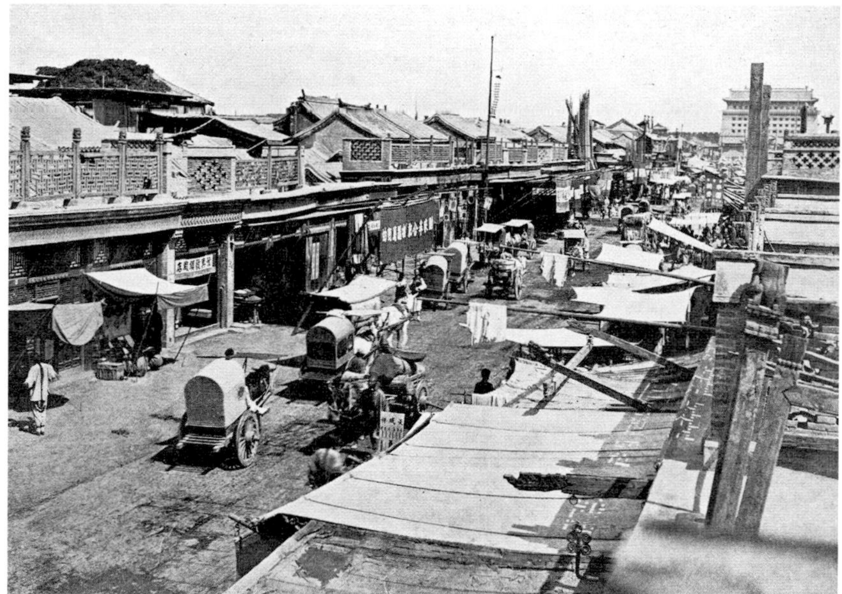

Figure 7.2. Qian Gate Street in the 1900s. Photograph by Sanshichiro Yamamoto. In *Peking* (Beijing: Yamamoto photography studio, 1906), fig 1.

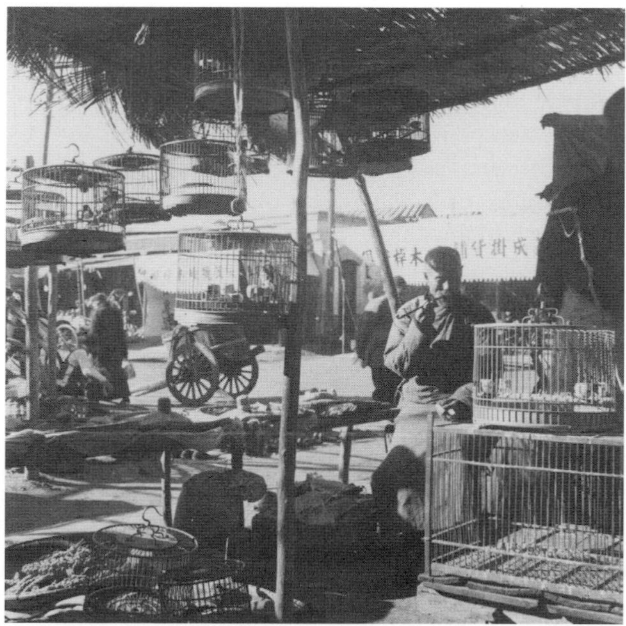

Figure 7.3. Bird market in Beijing. Photograph by Hedda Hammer, 1933–1946. The Hedda Hammer Morrison Photographs of China 1933–1946, Harvard-Yenching Library.

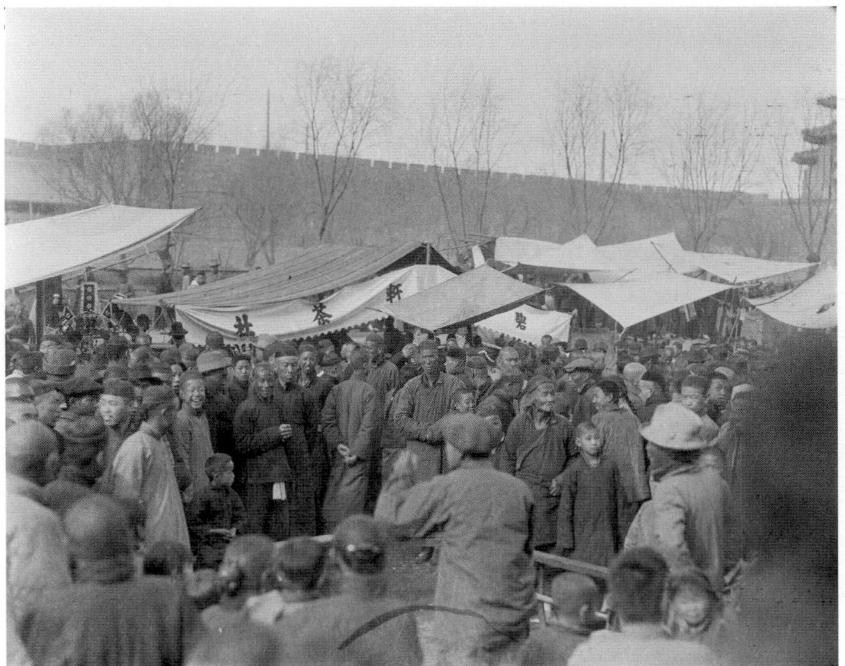

Figure 7.4. The Pantao Daoist Temple fair. Photograph by Sidney D. Gamble, 1924–1927. Sidney D. Gamble Photographs, David M. Rubenstein Rare Book & Manuscript Library, Duke University, gamble_397A_2281.

activity but also a recreational one—a gentleman's lifestyle in old Beijing, when "Chinese gentlemen carry around [birds] in their cages."[3] The temple market, also called temple fair or market fair, was typically located in the courtyard of a temple or in the surrounding streets "every ten or fifteen days and for not more than two days at a time."[4] For example, the Temple of Guarding the Country (Huguo Si) fair near Sixi was held three times a month and the Pantao Daoist Temple fair inside the Dongbian Gate took place once a year and featured performances by entertainers, storytellers, magicians, and singers (figure 7.4).

In the first half of the twentieth century, Beijing, like other Chinese cities, experienced dramatic change due to waves of political upheaval: the invasion of the Eight-Nation Alliance in 1900; the collapse of the Qing dynasty in 1911; the end of the Beiyang government in 1928, when Beijing lost its status as the capital;[5] and finally the occupation by the Japanese army in 1937.[6] On the heels of these political and social developments, a variety of new-style commercial spaces, named *Shangchang* or *Shichang*, emerged in Beijing specifically, including retail stores, combined shopping and leisure centers, and new types of urban markets.[7]

It is a challenge to categorize these new commercial spaces due to their considerable differences in scale, layout, and form. Yet beyond these factors, the emerging *Shangchang* or *Shichang* was a significant departure not only from traditional Chinese street or temple markets, but also from contemporary Western retail spaces.[8] Although influenced by Western department stores,[9] the commercial spaces that developed in early twentieth-century Beijing were more akin to a traditional market subsumed within one building complex or under covered roofs. Zehui Chi observed that the most notable feature of these new-style commercial spaces was their permanent and fixed location, a characteristic shared by neither the traditional temporary open markets nor the temple markets.[10] In *Social Life of the Chinese in Peking*, Jermyn Chi-hung Lynn opined that these new structures were "not exactly department stores like those in Europe and America;"[11] at the same time, he noted that they were different from Chinese temple markets and suggested calling them "bazaars."

Dongan Market demonstrated the emerging trend of new commercial constructions that resisted traditional classification systems. On the one hand, it was not restricted to being held on a certain day or to selling specific goods; rather, it was a permanent market with all kinds of stores. On the other hand, unlike traditional shopping streets and street markets that took place in the city streets or temple markets in temple courtyards, which depended on other spaces to be able to operate, Dongan Market was the first independently organized urban structure for commercial use in Beijing. It was thus the city's most notable new commercial space. According to a 1933 article, the Store of Industrial Promotion and the Qingyun Pavilion were as prosperous as Dongan Market, but less magnificent, while the Xisi and Dongsi department stores were in a state of disrepair compared to Dongan Market and were frequented by few middle- and upper-class people.[12] Lynn described Dongan Market as "certainly a place which no visitor to Peking can afford to miss. … The oldest as well as the largest bazaar in this city."[13] Sociologist Sidney Gamble stated that the spaces of Dongan Market "are more like big covered streets than buildings."[14] He went on to describe a typical scene in the market:

> Shops selling almost every imaginable article, toys, jewelry, furs, clothing, books, pictures, candies, cakes, are on each side of the big passageways, while in the center are tables or stalls on which are spread out brassware, notions, tongue scrapers, combs, chopsticks, fruit, candies. All of the tables are cleared every night, the unsold goods being packed up and carried away in big baskets.[15]

Dongan Market was characterized by its several commercial streets, which seen together formed "a city itself,"[16] with several large, separate markets, theaters, and stores inside the huge structure.[17] This was in contrast to Western bazaars, which were typically characterized by "a series of courtyards and rooms with skylights, light wells, and multileveled, continuous galleries."[18] To a great extent, Dongan Market was a commercial urban hub that remained closely related to traditional market spaces but offered Beijing the new sight of brick buildings with arched windows and covered walkways with skylights. These were built with modern materials—steel, glass, and iron—which were all still novel at the time of construction. The market was able to provide a wide range of food, shopping, and leisure activities to satisfy local citizens' everyday needs, the upper classes' expectation of luxury, and tourists' curiosity.

Ultimately, this chapter argues that the characteristics of Dongan Market did not merely represent but were also involved in shaping and contributing to Beijing's modernization, and that the market was a social and political arena of interaction between the government, officials, elites, merchants, consumers, and vendors. It looks closely at how Western ideas of sanitation, hygiene, and circulation, specifically in the context of market buildings, were quickly adopted in Beijing. The ways that these ideas were accepted, interpreted, and used differently by the competing forces mentioned above provide important insight into how public health and architecture intersected in early twentieth-century China.[19]

The Formation and Development of Dongan Market

The site of Dongan Market was originally a military training ground, but it had been abandoned since the mid-Qing dynasty (1736–1820). In 1903, street vendors were forced by the Inner City Administration of Public Works and Patrol to move to the vacant lot along Wangfujing Street because of roadworks on Dongan Gate Avenue.[20] These vendors occupied that area with temporary sheds, which later became the location of Dongan Market (figure 7.1). Initially, conditions at the market were rudimentary: there were no permanent buildings, only booths that were simply set up to sell food, toys, basic necessities, etc.[21]

In 1905, the Metropolitan Police Board of the Inner City decided that a permanent market should be built through a partnership between the government department that owned the land and a private investor who leased it and subsequently constructed, rented, and ran it. The Inner City Administration of Public Works and Patrol intended to provide financial support of more than five thousand taels of silver to the investor and contractor, Qingtai Ren. But Ren rejected the funding in order to avoid government intervention in and political influence over the project. It was eventually agreed that Ren would receive a two-year contract. He himself would raise the funds to construct the buildings and internal streets, thereby enabling him to retain the property

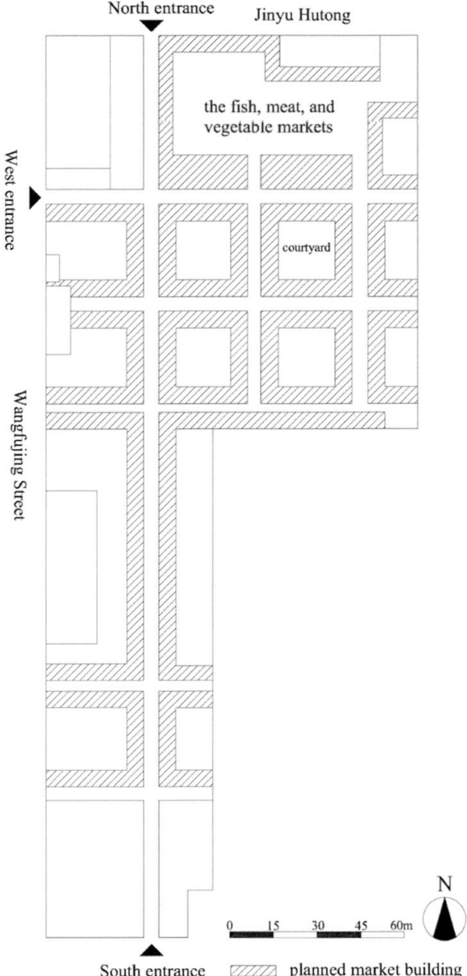

Figure 7.5. Plan of Dongan Market, 1906. Hatches show planned market buildings. Open spaces between buildings represent streets that were not covered yet. A garden to the south planned as an extension was not there yet. Redrawn by the author, based on The First Historical Archives of China, Archives of Police Department; Xiaochuan Yu and Hiroshi Katano, "The Evolution of the Public Market in the Modern China: The Case Study of Dongan Market in Beijing," *Journal of Architecture and Planning (Transactions of AIJ)* 67, no. 559 (2002): 120, fig. 2.

rights and manage the market. The Inner City Administration of Public Works and Patrol would be responsible for collecting taxes, maintaining public facilities, and regulating how the market would be run. Later, the Metropolitan Police Board of the Inner City published a series of rules that governed all aspects of the market's operations: building construction, renting, marketing, reporting, and so on.[22]

By June 1906, the market had begun to take shape. Fifty-four of the planned eighty-eight stores had been constructed, and twenty-four were open for business.[23] Figure 7.5 illustrates the grid plan with streets lined with single-story shops, which occupied around 2.4 hectares—around 310 meters from north to south, 59 meters from east to west on the south side, and 127 meters from east to west on the north side.[24] But the two-year contract was not renewed by the Metropolitan Police Board of the Inner City, which then paid Ren more than ten thousand taels of silver to take it over. This situation reflected the complex

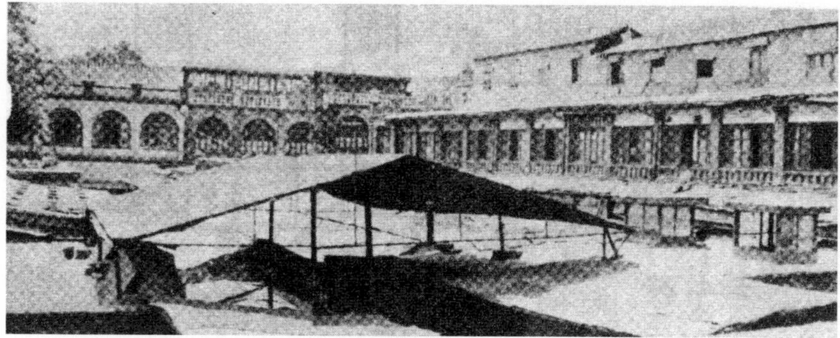

Figure 7.6. The roof covering was built after the 1912 fire. Photographer unknown. In Shaozhou Wang, 中国近代建筑图录 [Photo Archives of Early Modern Chinese Architecture] (Shanghai: Shanghai Scientific & Technical Publishers, 1989), 101.

relationship between the government and private investors. For instance, the presence of unstable authorities and the unilateral change in market regulation meant that return on investment and custom could not be guaranteed. According to the statement by Ren in the newspaper *Impartial Daily (Tianjin)*, "a lot of obstacles" greatly reduced the rental and occupancy rates. The fundamental underlying factor had to do with conflicting interests: the government tried to regulate the market as a representative case of urban reform, but it neglected its commercial interests, while Ren saw developing the market as his "lifelong honor," a case of "business promotion under new policies."[25]

The architectural history of Dongan Market has been shaped by catastrophic fires. The first great loss was due to the Renzi mutiny in 1912, when the market was pillaged and burned down by soldiers, although it was soon reconstructed. After the founding of the new Republic, the Metropolitan Police Board of the Inner City was combined with Metropolitan Police Board of the Outer City to establish the Capital Police Board in 1913, which managed Dongan Market.[26] The same year, the Public Chamber of Commerce of Dongan Market was created, and in 1915, the Chamber, together with the Capital Police Board, started to build roofs to cover the market streets and open spaces where temporary stalls were set up (figure 7.6). As the number of permanent commercial establishments increased, the market extended significantly southward: by 1917, there were two additional entrances to Dongan Market along Wangfujing Street.[27]

As shown in figure 7.7-1, the market's flourishing was interrupted by a second fire in 1920, when buildings were largely destroyed. The Municipal Council and Capital Police Board encouraged the merchants to rebuild the market and published detailed regulations on construction, design, fire safety, and lighting.[28] The planned passages between the storefronts and the streets,

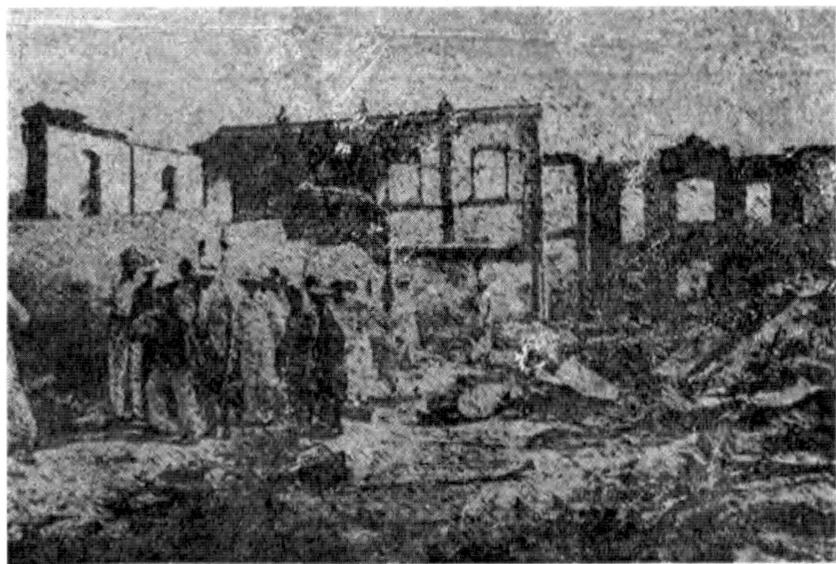

Figure 7.7-1 Dongan Market after the fires in 1920. Photographer unknown. In 时报图画周刊 [Weekly Illustrated Supplement to The Eastern Times], 3, 1920.

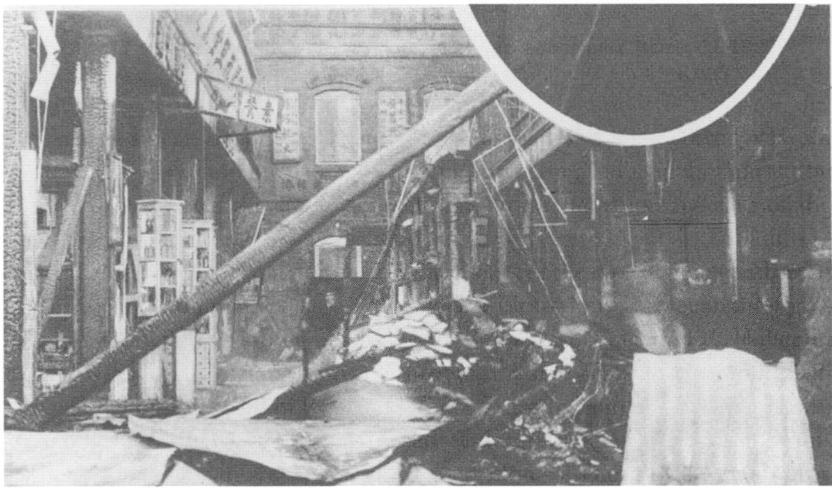

Figure 7.7-2 Dongan Market after the fires in 1926. Photographer unknown. In 东方杂志 [East Miscellany], 23, no. 8, 1926.

conceived before the fire, were no longer allowed, and a decision was made to widen the market's streets.[29] Unfortunately, even these regulations did not prevent another fire from occurring in 1926 (figure 7.7-2).

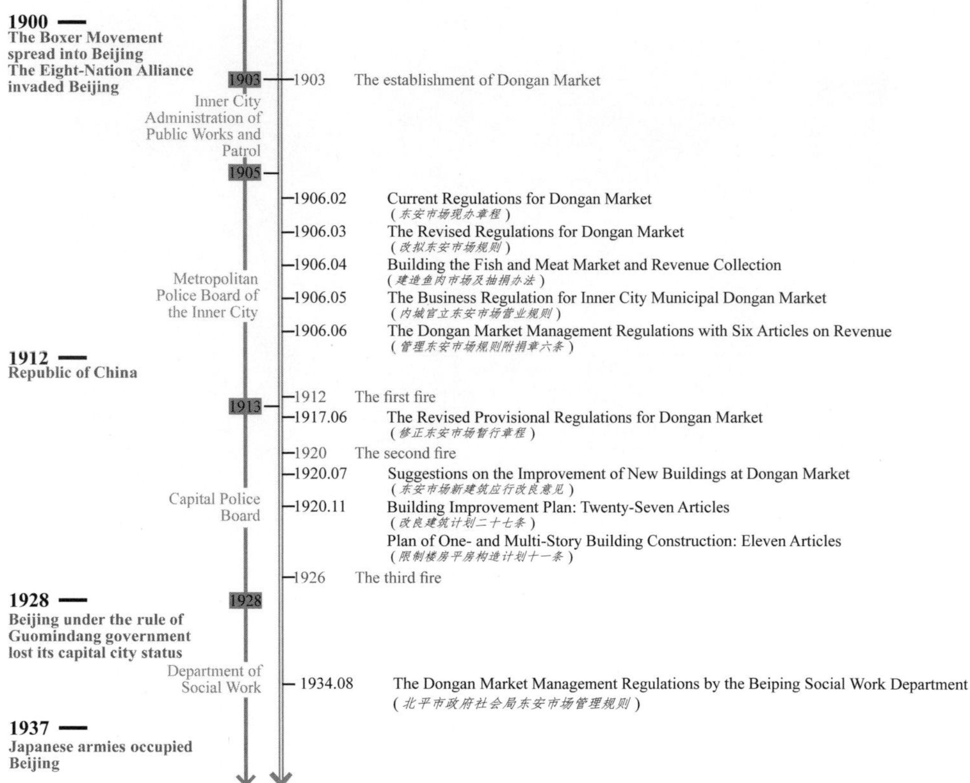

Figure 7.8. The transformation of Dongan Market: political background, key points, administrative offices and regulations. Drawn by the author.

When Beijing lost its capital city status in 1928, the municipal government was reorganized into five departments: Public Safety, Finance, Public Works, Sanitation, and Social Work. The latter replaced the Capital Police Board and ended up taking charge of Dongan Market.[30] Despite the repeated and numerous changes in the government agencies with which it was affiliated, the market was always under the direct management of the Dongan Market Administrative Office.[31] Figure 7.8 summarizes and clarifies the transformation of the market in terms of the changing political background, administrative offices, and regulations.

Before 1928, Dongan Market was not a typical market that developed in phases, but an example of repeated post-disaster reconstruction. It maintained nearly the same perimeter and area, except for an extension southward after 1915 into an area that was previously unused and undeveloped. The market's

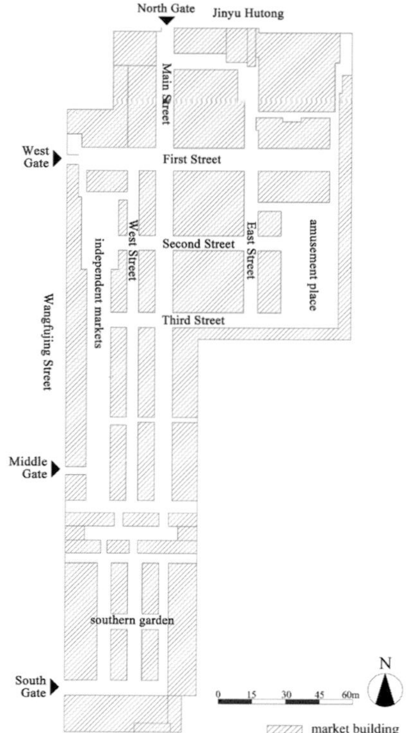

Figure 7.9-1. Street and open space in Dongan Market, 1930s. The amusement place on this plan was later gradually occupied by commercial buildings. Redrawn by the author. Based on Hongwen Liu, cartographer, in Shanyuan Dong, 阛阓纪胜——东风市场八十年 [Note of Market: Dongfeng Market over Eighty Years] (Beijing: Worker Press, 1985), 181; Xiaochuan Yu and Hiroshi Katano, "The Evolution of the Public Market in the Modern China: The Case Study of Dongan Market in Beijing," *Journal of Architecture and Planning (Transactions of AIJ)* 67, no. 559 (2002): 120, fig 4.

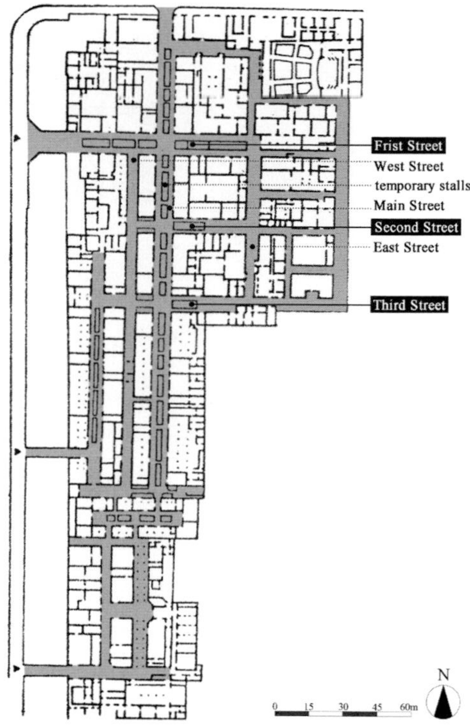

Figure 7.9-2. Plan of Dongan Market in 1948. The temporary stalls and sheds on Main Street and First Street were also shown in this plan. Shaozhou Wang, 中国近代建筑图录 [Photo Archives of Early Modern Chinese Architecture] (Shanghai: Shanghai Scientific & Technical Publishers, 1989), 101.

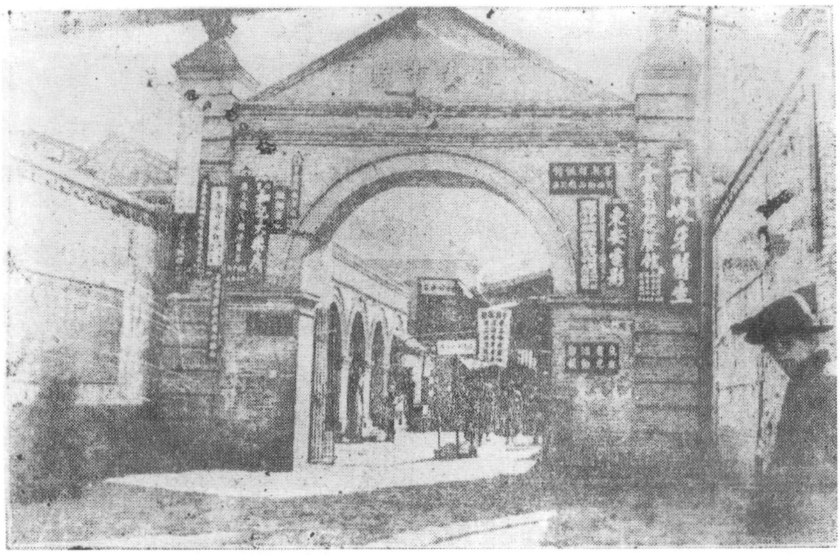

Figure 7.10. Entrance of Dongan Market in 1910s. Photographer unknown. In Editorial Office of Library of China, 北京指南 [Guide to Peking] (Shanghai: Library of China, 1916).

streets were initially covered in 1915, and when the whole market was rebuilt after the second fire, the roofs were rebuilt as well.[32]

Because the market experienced damage from fire and subsequent reconstructions on several occasions, the available plans, newspaper articles, archival information, and personal memoirs are important sources to piece together a general picture of the space. Figures 7.9–7.11 illustrate the plan, the building, and the interior of Dongan Market. It was designed in the 1930s as a grid with four entrances (the North Gate, West Gate, Middle Gate, and South Gate), three avenues from north to south (East Street, Main Street, and West Street), and another three from east to west (First Street, Second Street, and Third Street). An open area for entertainment surrounded by two-story buildings stood in the eastern portion of the site, and a garden originally located in the southern part was eventually replaced by stores. Main Street and First, Second, and Third Streets were lined with two-story buildings, sheltered by an iron roof, and paved with bricks. The brick façades on the street side had arched or square shop windows on the ground and first floors, the design of which was expected to remain consistent by the government after the post-fire reconstruction.[33]

The indoor covered market was still a rare sight in Beijing, and it attracted visitors and window shoppers who especially liked "modern" and "Western" goods and fashions. As such, it was described as exuding an "implicit foreign bourgeois atmosphere, or rather, aristocratic taste."[34] Nevertheless, temporary

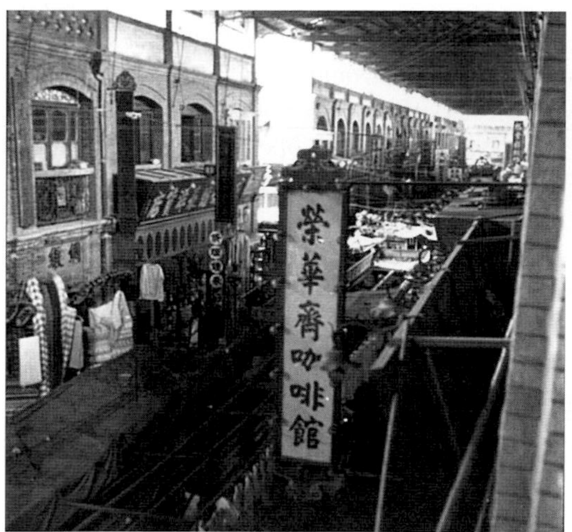

Figure 7.11-1. The covered street of Dongan Market, after 1920. Photographer unknown. In Heng Zhao and Changwei Li, "旧时北京的商业中心 [Commercial Centers in Old Beijing]," 南方都市报 [Southern Metropolis News], April 4, 2015.

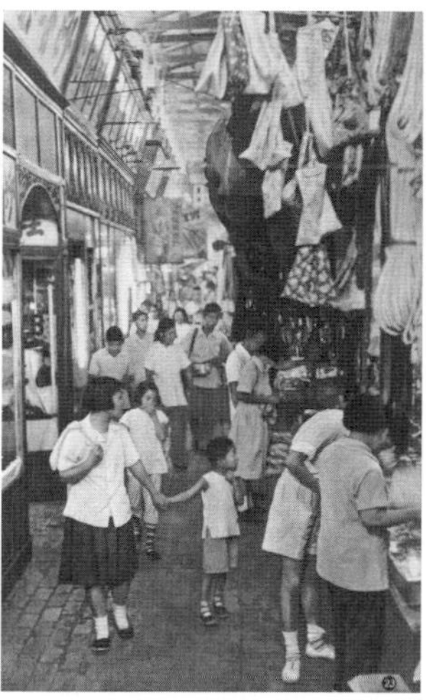

Figure 7.11-2. The covered street of Dongan Market in the 1950s. Photograph by A. Hoffman. In "东安市场 [Dongan Market]," 人民画报 [People's Pictorial], 11, 1956.

tables or stalls selling a variety of humble goods were also to be found down the middle of the market's streets. In 1933, the Report of the Chamber of Commerce of Dongan Market listed 925 businesses; 267 were permanent stores (selling silk, books, foods, drugs, antiques, jewelry, and other goods) while the other 658 were booths in open spaces.[35] The market also housed tea houses, theaters, clinics, photographic shops, and small factories, as well as open-air performance spaces.[36] Such scenes were noted by Jermyn Chi-hung Lynn:

> Near this theater is the big compound which has become the amusement resort of poor people in Peking. … In front of these small and dirty houses there are many stalls where hot dogs and other eatables can be had for a few coppers. … But it is the boxers and magicians who hold their exhibitions in the open air that have made this place very famous.[37]

The development of the market was the result of both government promotion and private participation. Especially after the first and second fires, most shops were reconstructed by the merchants themselves.[38] However, the site's development was led by and took place under the strict control of the government. Regardless of whether or not the merchants built the stores, the lease had to be paid. In addition, merchants were not allowed to sublet or sell their buildings to others themselves and could only do so through the government.[39] Most importantly, the Administrative Office, market police officers, and related government departments played the main role in the operation of the market. The market thus ultimately generated significant profit for the government.[40]

The Market as a Government Project: Architectural, Hygienic and Social Control

From the late Qing period, modern urban reform in China was a continuous process that bore witness to the emergence and development of municipal institutions.[41] Market reform in late Qing and Republican Beijing was part of a revolution in urban improvement. The Chinese intellectual elite were deeply aware of the importance of learning from the West. Key elements included modern building technology, urban administration, transportation facilities, and an understanding of sanitation. As government projects, urban markets aimed to emphasize urban sanitation, beauty, and improved transportation:

> There are three necessities of urban administration: sanitation, beauty, and convenience [for traffic]. … It is the market that can play roles in all these three. … When establishing the municipal market, the goods for sale can be well selected and easily regulated, owing to them being placed together. The [risk of] disease and infection will naturally be reduced. Accordingly, the goal of sanitation is achieved. … Since ancient times, our country has had a long history of trading in open spaces. When animal carcasses are exposed in the street, and the booths are nearly in the middle of the street, it destroys [urban] beauty and is inconvenient [for traffic].[42]

Construction and sanitation were two significant factors in the local government's attempt to cast markets in Beijing as demonstrable and tangible symbols of urban improvement. The evolution of construction regulations is a case in point. The first regulations governing Dongan Market, proposed in February 1906, only mentioned that the general contractor was responsible for construction. The Revised Provisional Regulations for Dongan Market in 1917, however, introduced strict requirements: structures should "comply with the regulations for construction, should comply with the property line along the road, and ensure that there is not a ragged [road line]."[43] After the second fire, the regulations published in 1920 further elaborated on construction methods, materials, and tectonics with plans and other drawings, and included articles on fire safety.[44] These regulations were generally in line with similar ones in foreign countries at that time. Most officials and advisors of the

Municipal Council participating in the preparatory meeting on rebuilding the market were professionals with degrees, and some had graduated from overseas universities.[45]

However, the market was still believed to have a lot of problems and shortcomings.[46] At the beginning of the project to build the market, the plan was to model it upon Les Halles in Paris, especially the use of a steel roof for fire safety,[47] although this did not ultimately happen. Later, in 1920, an article in the official government bulletin investigated food market precedents in the West, including Les Halles, as well as the Cattle Market in Glasgow, Quincy Market in Boston, and markets in Berlin, England, New York, New Orleans, etc. The study examined their scope, architecture, and especially their property and operational rights, and concluded that municipal markets were the predominant type, with other types as special cases, and thus, that Dongan Market should be built as a municipal one. It further examined the markets' investment and profit, and argued that the advantage of this revenue for the government would be that "all the incidental and setting-up expenses could be gradually recovered; after repaying the construction cost, [the market] could be a new source of municipal finance."[48] Thus, the municipal market model was seen to be in line with modern global trends; moreover, it was believed that the Beijing government should learn from foreign precedents.

As Qiqian Zhu, the founder of the Beijing Municipal Council and its first director, stated in an article, Dongan Market was not on par with its modern Western counterparts. In the 1930s, he proposed a plan to rebuild it:

> The government could firstly provide funding to acquire several acres of the empty area to the south of the market, and, modeled on the new market in Paris, to build a steel covering with pillars on the ground, which could delineate the spaces for several stores. The pathways could also be incorporated under this roof for people wandering [through the market]. Stores will prepare their own displays to attract customers and to encourage purchasing. This is the first kind of shop fitting. The second is for food, cultural goods, and other booths that don't need independent space. Similar goods should be grouped together in wooden and glass cabinets. For the area encompassing the Western food restaurant, hot pot restaurant, theater, and playing field, this should have separate access and probably should be rebuilt in another place, rather than under the covered roof, to avoid congestion at the entrance.[49]

Importantly, the transformation of the building's layout was also closely related to sanitation. As early as 1906, the market regulations proposed a covered open space for the sale of vegetables, fish, and meat, where the ability to drain dirty water was the primary consideration.[50] Furthermore, a special regulation focused on establishing a separate area for the fish, meat, and vegetable markets at the northeastern end of Dongan Market. It is worth quoting this regulation in full as it demonstrates the ambition and thoroughness of the plans:

> From an investigation of the ways in which fish, meat, and vegetable markets are built in the West, they should not be linked to residential areas. Using [the market] for [both] eating and accommodation is not allowed. The hygiene conditions should be improved, because exposure to filth easily causes illness. Today, as there are rows upon rows of stores in Dongan Market swarming with visitors, it would not be appropriate to build the fish, meat, and vegetable markets inside Dongan Market. However, because it has already been planned and it is difficult to find another site, [we have decided to] partition off an area for selling fish, meat, and vegetables on the northeastern side, and to build a high wall on the boundary in order to prevent contact with other stores. On the top of the wall, a triangular wooden structure covered with iron should be built. The roof should be higher than the wall for the sake of ventilation, while the eaves should be lower to withstand wind and snow. The floor should be paved with cement from Tangshang so it can be flushed with water. Sewers should also be built in accordance with the relevant regulation.[51]

The hygiene requirements applied not only to the food market but to all areas of Dongan Market. The market installed public garbage bins, which were emptied daily, while individual storekeepers were asked to do their own cleaning every morning. Punitive sanctions were outlined to prevent storekeepers from "discarding dirty water at will and harming public interests."[52]

In Republican Beijing, the Municipal Council stated that hygiene could be understood in two ways: individual and public. The article in the Municipal Bulletin stated that "the administration for sanitation is personal to some extent, but public to a greater extent, so public hygiene has priority."[53] Therefore, it was an important factor in building an indoor municipal market. Since food sanitation was closely related to public health, the public market was promoted as a means of preventing unsafe food from being sold. The gradual eradication of outdoor trading and informal markets in Beijing was understood as a sign of great progress for the modern, hygiene-aware administration.[54]

Alongside the improvement in sanitation in the market, the government also placed an emphasis on individual hygiene, as part of the image of a "civilized citizen." For example, in the 1906 market regulations, indecent performances, promiscuous songs, pornography, aphrodisiacs, abortions, and spells were prohibited in order to promote an "enlightened culture."[55] Market management regulations also emphasized the importance of customers' own cleanliness for the market.[56] It was noted that without personal hygiene, public hygiene would be meaningless, and vice versa.[57] For the government, the interaction between the two became a chance to connect individuals with the state. By promoting the hygiene of the individual, the state claimed that it was "protecting our nation and strengthening our people," thereby fostering the country's prosperity and preserving its honor in the face of the colonial crisis.[58]

This increased emphasis on hygiene, traffic flow, fire safety, and building regulations shows how the twin ideas of science and modern civilization were deeply embedded in the Chinese city and society. Modern Western medical science, based in particular on an understanding of bacteria and body circulation, was quite different from Chinese traditional hygiene and medicine, which was grounded in the idea of "guarding life" by preserving the system of vitalities through breathing, movement, massage, sexual economy, appropriate ingestion regimes, etc., to ensure the proper flow of *qi* within the body and balance *yin* and *yang*.[59] However, as with the significant impact of modern medicine and treatment of disease on Western cities in the eighteenth century,[60] this correlation of biology and physiology with urban reform was increasingly accepted and adopted by the Chinese elites and government as a "modern" and "scientific" way of reshaping Beijing's urban space during the first half of the twentieth century. For instance, the indoor market as a clean public space under new spatial regulations was proposed as a replacement for the unclean traditional street market.[61]

Furthermore, Dongan Market embodied the Beijing government's intensified efforts to use markets as a means of increasing its social control over the daily life of its citizens. The Business Regulations for the Inner City Municipal Dongan Market stipulated that "the police at the market guard the market and patrol on day and night shifts. Both buyers and sellers who break the police regulations will be punished accordingly."[62] Figure 7.12, from a popular Beijing pictorial, depicts a scene where a police officer intervenes in daily disputes to maintain the market order. Through the operation, management, and maintenance of the market by the Administrative Office and the police, the government's authority expanded into the social lives of urban residents. With goods and activities increasingly subject to political censorship, traditional activities, such as astrology and midwifery, as well as some "indecent" opera performances, were forbidden because of their "insalubrity" and "immorality." Through changing its citizens' customs, ethos, and social life, the government's goal was not merely to create a "civilized" national image but also to exercise a "modern" form of discipline over the everyday lives of both sellers and buyers through the municipal market space, thereby establishing control over and surveillance of them by the state.

Control over disease in urban environments is regarded by Foucault as an implicit metaphor for the emergence of a disciplinary society, wherein public

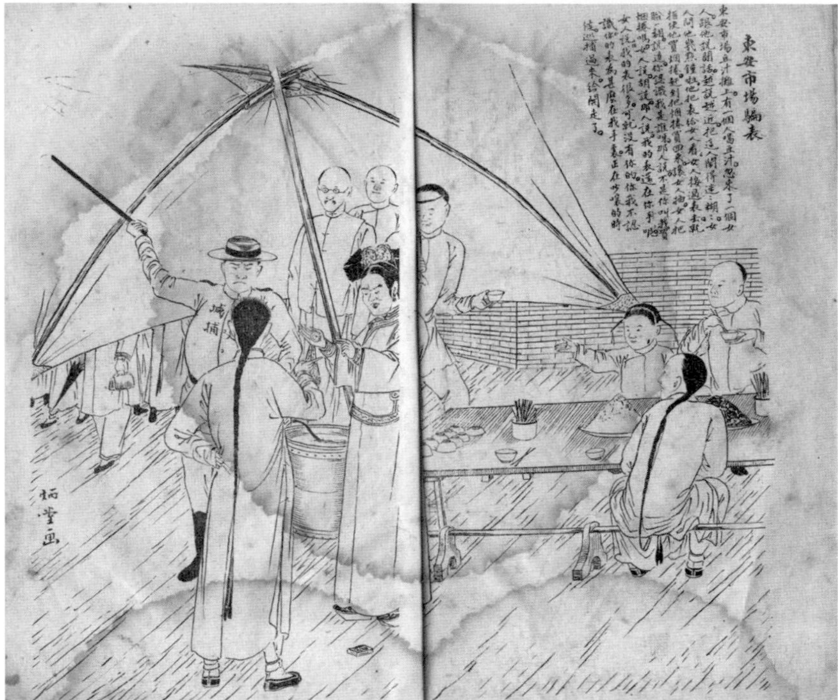

Figure 7.12. A man defrauded of a watch by a woman, but driven out by a policeman at a bean soup booth. Bingtang Liu, cartographer. In "东安市场骗表 [Defrauding of a Watch in Dongan Market]," 北京画报 [Beijing Pictorial], 1, May 23, 1906.

health became a means of social control.[63] Concomitant with the building renovations in Dongan Market, there were gradually improved regulations through which modern principles of sanitation and administration were constantly imposed on citizens' daily lives via the continual surveillance of the state. At the same time, however, the local culture and customs regularly resisted such state control and national unification.[64] The transformation of Dongan Market in Beijing revealed this common theme of the process of modernization. Despite the government's aim of urban improvement, citizens were unwilling to change their traditional lives to cooperate with this government project.

Society: Resistance from Ordinary Citizens

In Beijing, the government's urban improvement efforts were often met with open resistance and unenthusiastic responses. In Dongan Market, various regulations issued by the government imposed strict restrictions on certain aspects of the daily activities of buyers and sellers. For the merchants, these regulations limited their profits, as they were forced to use expensive fireproof materials and to comply with property boundaries, thereby preventing them from encroaching on public areas for their stores. Therefore, to reduce their financial losses, they sometimes refused to comply with the government's orders in an attempt to retain their existing customs and ways of operating.

After the 1920 fire, the Municipal Council asked all merchants to follow the new construction regulations, including putting up brick walls, concrete stairs, and tiled roofs. However, violations were already evident during construction: seven irregular buildings were noted.[65] The use of low-quality wood even caused a building to collapse, which drew considerable public attention.[66] The Capital Police Board attributed responsibility to the Municipal Council for having carried out an inadequate inspection and believed "there must be more irregularities that have not been detected."[67] But the Municipal Council rejected this explanation and argued that the failure to build a government-owned market was the fundamental cause.[68] The Capital Police Board and Municipal Council finally decided to inspect the construction process used at the market and developed a regulation governing inspections. Nevertheless, the merchants still reported experiencing financial difficulties and reduced profits as a way of fighting against the government's plans for this regulation.[69] One outcome of this struggle was that the regulation stipulated only that wood could not be used for the building envelope. However, fraud and corner-cutting remained very common:[70] many merchants "still use wood, which can catch fire easily."[71] Indeed, the market again suffered heavy losses in a fire in 1926. This proved that the government's intended improvements would not necessarily succeed, despite their beneficial nature.

Another government order had been met with resistance in March 1906, when the Metropolitan Police Board of the Inner City asked all entertainment businesses to move out of Dongan Market. Their performances were believed to be indecent, thereby threatening the "civilized" urban image of Beijing. Until that point, the commercial spaces of Beijing had in general maintained a traditional market environment that incorporated recreational activities. Sidney Gamble observed that "organized recreation was highly commercialized."[72] It was believed that it was difficult to conduct commerce without any form of recreational activity alongside it, such as traditional storytelling and entertainment by female singers, or new-style facilities like pool or billiards, cinemas, and peep boxes, etc.[73]

As a result, the merchants of Dongan Market directly challenged the concept of "civilized" urban space and claimed that their own interests should be respected. They wrote petitions to the Ministry of Civil Affairs, noting the decline of the market and their losses from the prohibition on entertainment.

They even borrowed the government's idea of a "national tax and livelihood" to defend their right to run entertainment businesses.[74] The Metropolitan Police Board of the Inner City finally provided clarification in October 1906, informing the public that entertainment was permitted in the market, except for those forms that were considered "immoral."[75] Following this, recreational business grew rapidly. In December of the same year, the Jixiang Tea Garden was opened within the bounds of Dongan Market. It was the first theater in the Inner City, breaking the ban on them by the Qing government. Because of the success of the Tea Garden, Dongan Market received wide media coverage and soon flourished.[76]

The chambers of commerce of Dongan Market played a significant role in the merchants' struggle with the government. The merchants established the Commerce Board of Dongan Market in 1906 and the Public Chamber of Commerce of Dongan Market in 1913.[77] Both dealt with commercial and public affairs and attempted to participate in administrative decisions. During the two post-fire reconstructions, the Public Chamber of Commerce of Dongan Market represented the merchants in negotiations with government agencies about the retention of property and rental rights.[78] Meanwhile, it also cooperated with the government, for example by providing assistance and inspections regarding the day-to-day management of the market and the quality of buildings.[79] Much like a traditional guild, the chambers of commerce acted as intermediaries between the ruler and the ruled and protected the commercial interests of their members by working with the government more than by fighting it.[80]

It is noteworthy from these events that beneath this placid surface of everyday commercial activities, Beijing was experiencing political unrest in the first half of the twentieth century. For geopolitical and economic reasons, Wangfujing Street, on which Dongan Market was located, was frequently chosen as a place for demonstrations or public speeches, for example during the eruption of the May Fourth Movement, which involved student protests and worker demonstrations and became a significant force in the social, political, and urban transformation of Beijing.[81] As shown in figure 7.13, during the June Third Movement in 1921, Peking University students spoke to the public near Dongan Market.

In this volatile political environment, the late Qing, Beiyang, and Guomindang governments were continually concerned about how the use of the market might lead to unrest. Reflecting these concerns, the 1934 Dongan Market regulation declared that "it is prohibited for anyone to use this market to hold a secret gathering."[82] Yet in contrast to its strict control of crowds in temple markets throughout history, the government had become aware of the importance of popular movements. Therefore, the Beijing municipal government held three Health Campaign Assemblies between 1934 and 1936 to

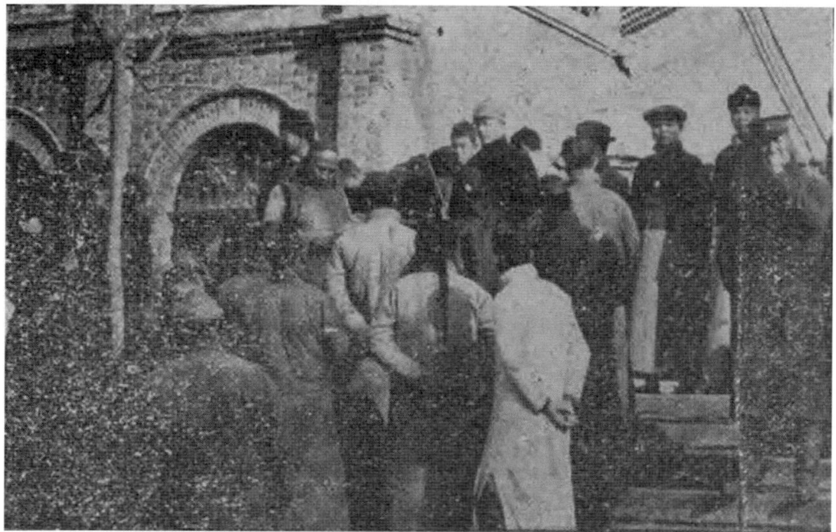

Figure 7.13. The Peking University speech team near Dongan Market during the June Third Movement on June 3, 1921. Photographer unknown. In 北大生活 [Life at Peking University], December 1921, 39.

promote health. However, the participants were mostly government officials or from the upper classes, which shows that the national mobilization efforts were still insufficient to reach the grassroots. Even so, the campaigns still led to great progress in sanitation measures. As Gamble argued, "health lectures and demonstrations produce distinct improvements, and in a district where such a campaign has been carried on it is not at all unusual to find the stores covering and protecting from flies food that is offered for sale."[83]

The elites in Beijing achieved a consensus with the government on urban and social control, believing that the market could be a place for enlightening and educating the general population. The Capital Library, the first official library of Beijing, was opened within Dongan Market in 1907 as a way to increase the citizens' knowledge and to enlighten the public.[84] The elites endorsed policies aimed at changing the city's "backward" image and improving public and personal hygiene, both of which were believed to be strongly related to the fate of the nation under the shadow of the colonial crisis. A government leaflet for the Cleaning Movement Procession of 1928 stated that "only healthy and strong people can form a healthy and strong society, which can then constitute a healthy and strong country."[85] The elites' support of the government's reforms on hygiene, construction, and planning contributed to the emphasis placed on knowledge and public opinion in expanding the power of the authorities.

Dongan Market ultimately remained prosperous during the period of political turmoil, partly because buyers wanted to retain access to this stable and luxurious environment. The elites, however, were constantly critical of and disappointed by those who enjoyed the peaceful and thriving shopping and recreational facilities: they regarded this as a demonstration of indifference to and lack of concern about the ongoing conflicts between warlords and the national crisis in Beijing. They also lamented the role that the market played as the dumping ground for foreign goods and criticized the citizens for ignoring the threats to the country from outside forces and instead hypocritically indulging in and enjoying such goods. However, the fact was that, as Yue Dong's study has shown, only the elites could normally afford the prices and services at the market and enjoy the convenience of international trade.[86] They were at the top of the social hierarchy, benefiting from luxurious lifestyles and continuing to take advantage of what Dongan Market offered.[87]

On the other hand, Dongan Market remained prosperous during the period of political instability because the merchants found ways to fight for their rights other than by starting riots. As mentioned above, the market's chambers of commerce were the medium through which merchants wrote petitions to and negotiated with the government to protect their property rights after the 1912 and 1920 fires. The Dongan Market Administrative Office also acted as an intermediary between the city government and the merchants.[88] Moreover, the merchants successfully asked for corruption to be punished in the 1921 scandal about reorganizing the location of stalls.[89] However, for the most part, the government's proposed improvements were usually faced with passive resistance from the merchants, rather than open objection. Hence, the struggle and compromises between the government, merchants, and customers, as well as the combination of traditional customs and modern characteristics at the market, functioned as the safety valve against a more radical revolution. Still, behind this compromise, radical changes to political and social life had begun to emerge.

Conclusion

In Beijing, in the first half of the twentieth century, a pervasive "urban improvement movement," based on modern knowledge and the incorporation of Western standards, endeavored to promote state-led social reforms, recreate national identity, and rescue the country from national crisis.[90] At the same time, as Di Wang states, the local culture and customs constantly resisted state control and national unification.[91] The transformation of Dongan Market in Beijing reveals this common theme of the process of modernization. Over the years, the state made various efforts—including adding roofs to, reforming, and regulating the market—aimed at regularizing the merchants and consumers. Still, ordinary citizens were generally unwilling to change their normal way of life to cooperate with the "government project" of urban improvement. Caught between the government and the citizenry, the elites played a complex role. They criticized the underdeveloped and disordered market environment, hoped to promote social reform by reregulating it, and, therefore, instead of representing the voice and interests of the public, were in favor of further increasing government control over the citizens. They enjoyed the services and convenience provided by these new markets, which distanced them further from the needs and way of life of ordinary people.

The development of Dongan Market, however, was not in line with what the government, the elites, the merchants or the customers wanted; nor was it in line with Western or traditional Chinese models. It offers a specific example of modernization arising from its particular economic, political, and social circumstances. In Republican Beijing, Dongan Market represented the struggle between different social actors claiming their right to urban space, especially through construction, spatial use, and sanitation. Generally, the development of Dongan Market, especially the post-fire reconstructions, was led by the local government. Little room was left for merchants to be involved in establishing the rules and making the plans. But merchants and their customers could choose to cooperate with, resist, or be indifferent to these regulations. The market was thus not only a showcase of a "modern" government project but also a place where merchants earned a living and where people congregated and participated in recreational activities. Hence, the market became a new public sphere shaped by the processes of conflict and negotiation, involving strategies by the government and counterstrategies by the people. Correspondingly, despite the presence of multiple traditional factors still preserved in its buildings, Dongan Market, like its predecessor, the department store in the West in the eighteenth and nineteenth centuries, represented the transition away from a traditional society and heralded the beginning of modern society.

Acknowledgments

This work is supported by the National Natural Science Foundation of China [Grant number 51708102].

Notes

1. Anne-Marie Broudehoux, *The Making and Selling of Post-Mao Beijing* (New York: Routledge, 2004), 102–43.
2. Besides these three commercial spaces, Beijing was also famous for casual hawkers selling everyday items.
3. Sidney David Gamble, *Peking: A Social Survey* (New York: George H. Doran, 1921), 213.
4. Gamble, *Peking*, 213. For more information on the temple market (庙市) and market fair (庙会) in Beijing, see Susan Naquin, *Peking: Temples and City Life, 1400–1900* (Berkeley: University of California Press, 2000), 626–38.
5. When the capital moved to Nanjing, Beijing was renamed Beiping in 1928. In 1937, the local puppet government under the Japanese regime revived its former name, Beijing. In this paper I use Beijing for consistency.
6. Beijing was named Beiping from 1928 to 1937; see previous note.
7. *Shangchang*: 商场; *Shichang*: 市场. Retail stores included the Store of Industrial Promotion (劝业场), Qingyun Pavilion (青云阁), Xisi Department Store (西四商场), Dongsi Department Store (东四商场), and No. 1 Department Store (第一楼) in the Dashilan area outside the Qian Gate. The New World Entertainment Center at Tianqiao was a combined shopping and leisure center. Dongan Market, the subject of this chapter, was a typical example of a new type of urban market.
8. Traditional markets in the West can broadly be classified as open-air markets, street markets, and traditional market houses. During the modernization period, there were a variety of transitional types, including the *magasin de nouveauté*, the bazaar, the large covered market hall, the exhibition hall, and the arcade, before the appearance of the department store. For further details on the transformation of commercial space in the West, see Johann Friedrich Geist, *Arcades: The History of a Building Type*, trans. Jane O. Newman and John H. Smith (Cambridge, MA: MIT Press, 1985); James Schmiechen and Kenneth Carls, *The British Market Hall: A Social and Architectural History* (New Haven: Yale University Press, 1999); Donatella Calabi, *The Market and the City: Squares, Streets and Buildings in Early Modern Europe*, trans. Marlene Klein (Aldershot: Ashgate, 2003); Helen Tangires, *Public Markets and Civic Culture in Nineteenth-century America* (Baltimore: Johns Hopkins University Press, 2002); Helen Tangires, *Public Markets* (New York: W. W. Norton, 2008).
9. See Fuhe Zhang, 北京近代建筑史 [The Modern Architectural History of Beijing from the End of the 19th Century to 1930s] (Beijing: Tsinghua University Press, 2004), 175–95. Some officials of the Municipal Council and experts were involved in building all these new commercial stores; for example, Ma Rong participated in both the reconstruction of the Store of Industrial Promotion and

in establishing the rules for rebuilding Dongan Market after the fire in 1920; see "重建市场计划 [A Plan to Rebuild the Market]," 爱国白话报 [Patriotic Vernacular News], June 14, 1920; 京都市政公所第二、三处关于召开筹建东安市场会议的通知及东安市场改良意见大纲等 [A Notice from the Second and Third Office of the Municipal Council about Convening a Meeting on Building Dongan Market, and an Outline of the Comment on Improving Dongan Market, etc.] (July 1, 1920–July 31, 1920), 北京市档案馆 [Beijing Municipal Archives] J017-001-00133.

10. Zehui Chi, Xuexi Lou, and Wenxian Chen (ed), 北平市工商业概况 [A Survey of Industry and Commerce of the City of Peiping] (Beijing: Department of Social Work, Beiping, 1932), 684.
11. Jermyn Chi-hung Lynn, *Social Life of the Chinese in Peking* (Beijing & Tianjin: China Booksellers, 1928), 83.
12. "东安市场 [Dongan Market]," 申报月刊 [Shenbao Monthly] 2, no. 10 (1933): 87–88.
13. Lynn, *Social Life of the Chinese in Peking*, 83.
14. Gamble, *Peking*, 213.
15. Gamble, *Peking*, 213.
16. Lynn, *Social Life of the Chinese in Peking*, 83.
17. According to Lynn, there were four bazaars and three large buildings inside Dongan Market. Lynn, *Social Life of the Chinese in Peking*, 83.
18. Geist, *Arcades*, 49.
19. Dongan Market as a representation of Republican Beijing has attracted the attention of many scholars. For example, Madeleine Yue Dong studies how the permanent indoor markets for the upper class in Beijing shaped the new social hierarchy that was based on consumption. Xiaochuan Yu summarizes the development of Dongan Market in the light of policies and rules. Jianwei Wang focuses on the social life and urban image of the market in order to understand Republican Beijing from a bottom-up point of view. See Madeleine Yue Dong, *Republican Beijing: The City and Its Histories* (Berkeley: University of California Press, 2003); Xiaochuan Yu, "从法令规制中看东安市场的形成及演变特征——近代北京商业空间的形成与变容过程的研究 [Review of Evolution of the Dongan Market in the Light of Policies and Rules: Research on the Evolution of Modern Commercial Spaces in Beijing]," in 建筑史论文集 [Collection of Papers on Architectural History], ed. Fuhe Zhang (Beijing: Tsinghua University Press, 2001); Jianwei Wang, "王府井与天桥：民国北京的双面叙事 [Wangfujing Street and Sky Bridge: An Pluralistic Narrative of Republican Beijing]," 学术月刊 [Academic Monthly] 48, no. 12 (2016).
20. Inner City Administration of Public Works and Patrol (内城工巡局), later renamed the Metropolitan Police Board of the Inner City (内城巡警总厅) in 1905. It was initially accountable to the Ministry of Police (巡警部) and later to

the Ministry of Civil Affairs (民政部). The Ministry of Police was reorganized and replaced by the Ministry of Civil Affairs in 1906.

21. The First Historical Archives of China, "光绪三十二年创办东安市场史料 [Archives Relating to the Creation of Dongan Market in 1906]," 历史档案 [Historical Archives], no. 1 (2000): 42; Quanchao Zong, "东安市场的过去和现在 [Dongan Market in Past and Present]," in文史资料选编 [Selections from Cultural History Materials], vol. 12, ed. Cultural History Materials Committee of Beijing Municipal Committee of CPPCC (Beijing: Beijing Press, 1982), 181–83.
22. The First Historical Archives of China, "光绪三十二年创办东安市场史料," 42–49.
23. The First Historical Archives of China, "光绪三十二年创办东安市场史料," 48.
24. The First Historical Archives of China, "光绪三十二年创办东安市场史料," 42.
25. The First Historical Archives of China, "光绪三十二年创办东安市场史料," 42, 46; Qingtai Ren, "东安市场声明归官 [A Statement About Dongan Market Taken Over by the Government]," 大公报(天津) [*Impartial Daily* (Tianjin)] April 8, 1907.
26. Together with the Municipal Council, founded in 1914, the Capital Police Board (京师警察厅) took over responsibility as the city government until 1928. The two bodies had clear individual responsibilities, but cooperated on matters of urban governance and they both reported to the Interior Ministry (内务部).
27. Xiaochuan Yu, "从法令规制中看东安市场的形成及演变特征——近代北京商业空间的形成与变容过程的研究," 156.
28. 京师警察厅关于函送修建东安市场计划、建筑表与京都市政公所的来往函及市政公所的布告等 [Letters between the Capital Police Board and Municipal Council about the Plan and List of Buildings of Dongan Market, and Announcements by the Municipal Council, etc.] (August 1, 1920–July 31, 1922), 北京市档案馆 [Beijing Municipal Archives] J017-001-00119.
29. 京师警察厅关于函送修建东安市场计划、建筑表与京都市政公所的来往函及市政公所的布告等.
30. For the changing urban administration, see Rui Ding, "北洋政府时期京师警察厅研究 [A Study on the Capital Police Board in the Era of the Beiyang Government]" (PhD diss., Graduate School of Chinese Academy of Social Sciences, 2011), 31–58; Mingzheng Shi, "Beijing Transforms: Urban Infrastructure, Public Works, and Social Change in the Chinese Capital, 1900–1928" (PhD diss. Columbia University, 1993), 26–35; Gamble, *Peking*, 70–80.
31. The members of the Dongan Market Administrative Office (东安市场管理处) were not always the same. According to the Municipal Archive of 1929, the office consisted of a manager, who had been appointed by the Capital Police Board in 1924, two staff members, a secretary, and twelve employees, including street

cleaners, garbage collectors, servants, and custodians. Cooperating with the Administrative Office, a police director, a manager, and several officers were appointed to be in charge of market safety and order. See 社会局对东安市场管理员的任免令、东安市场职员履历表及员司、夫役、巡官、长警花名册 [Remove and Appoint Order on Dongan Market by Department of Social Work, the Curricula Vitae of Officers of Dongan Market, and Rosters of Employees, Laborers, Police Directors, Managers, and Officers] (August 1, 1929–September 30, 1920), 北京市档案馆 [Beijing Municipal Archives] J002-001-00009; "内城官立东安市场营业规则 [The Business Regulation at Inner city Municipal Dongan Market]," in 清末北京城市管理法规 [Late Qing Beijing Urban Administrative Codes], ed. Tao Tian and Chengwei Guo (Beijing: Beijing Yanshan Press, 1996), 197–98.

32. It seems most streets were covered, but there is no conclusive evidence yet. Nevertheless, it is clear that the main street was covered.
33. 京师警察厅关于函送修建东安市场计划、建筑表与京都市政公所的来往函及市政公所的布告等.
34. Lao She, "离婚 [Divorce]," in 老舍小说全集 [Complete Collections of Lao She's Fictions], vol. 3, ed. Ji Shu and Yi Shu (Wuhan: Changjiang Wenyi Press, 2004), 349.
35. Zong, "东安市场的过去和现在," 186.
36. The coexistence of commerce with spectacle represents a fundamental characteristic of the idea of the market, both in China and the West, just as the Greek agoras and Roman fora in history served as sites for trade and commerce in tandem with entertainment and spectacle.
37. Lynn, *Social Life of the Chinese in Peking*, 87.
38. The Capital Police Board and Municipal Council stated that they "planned to take it over as a government-run market, to expand the scale, and thus to solve the problem once and for all." However, because of the war-time environment in Beijing and its surroundings, the plan was postponed. Merchants could not wait for the market to reopen; they were "very much looking forward to financing and constructing it by themselves." Ultimately, the government only claimed the land rights and maintained the merchants' private property rights. See 京师警察厅关于函送修建东安市场计划、建筑表与京都市政公所的来往函及市政公所的布告等.
39. According to the Revised Provisional Regulations for Dongan Market in 1917, in a situation of insolvency and nonpayment of rent, the government could lease the shop to others or, in the worst case, repossess it. Even in the case of privately owned properties, the owner could only collect the material back after building demolition, or opt for a small compensation.
40. 社会局对东安市场管理员的任免令、东安市场职员履历表及员司、夫役、巡官、长警花名册.

41. For the transformation of Beijing's municipal institutions, see Xusheng Huang, "Building Modern Beijing: Government-led Urban Reconstruction, 1900–1937," in *Proceedings of the 10th International Symposium on Architectural Interchanges in Asia*, ed. the Architectural Society of China (Beijing: China City Press, 2014), 975–79
42. "论市设市场 [Review of the Municipal Market]," 市政通告 [Municipal Bulletin], no. 24 (October 1919): section 论说 [Review]: 7.
43. 京师警察厅行政处关于送修正东安市场暂行章程的函 [Letter from the Administration Office of the Capital Police Board about Sending the Revised Provisional Regulations for Dongan Market] (from June 1, 1917), 北京市档案馆 [Beijing Municipal Archive] J181-018-07668; "改定东安市场暂行章程 [The Revised Provisional Regulations for Dongan Market]," in 京师警察法令汇纂 [Compilation of Laws and Decrees of Capital Police], ed. Capital Police Board (Beijing: Xiehua Press, 1916), 155–59.
44. Including "东安市场新建筑应行改良意见 [Suggestions on the Improvement of New Buildings at Dongan Market]" (July 1920); "改良建筑计划二十七条 [Building Improvement Plan: Twenty-Seven Articles]" (November 1920); "限制楼房平房构造计划十一条 [Plan of Single- and Multi-Story Building Construction: Eleven Articles]" (November 1920); see 京都市政公所第二、三处关于召开筹建东安市场会议的通知及东安市场改良意见大纲等.
45. 京都市政公所第二、三处关于召开筹建东安市场会议的通知及东安市场改良意见大纲等.
46. Qiqian Zhu, "王府井大街之今昔(附东安市场) [Wangfujing Street in the Past and Present (including Dongan Market)]," in文史资料选编, vol. 12, 213.
47. Zhu, "王府井大街之今昔," 214.
48. "食物之供给与卫生 [Food Supply and Hygiene]," 市政通告, no. 27 (April 1920): section 论说 [Review], 5–6.
49. Zhu, "王府井大街之今昔," 214.
50. The First Historical Archives of China, "光绪三十二年创办东安市场史料," 43.
51. Annex: no accommodation inside; no recreation activities to avoid people gathering; opening only in the morning; hiring two people to wash the floor after the market opens, for cleaning. See The First Historical Archives of China, "光绪三十二年创办东安市场史料," 47.
52. The First Historical Archives of China, "光绪三十二年创办东安市场史料," 47.
53. "食物之供给与卫生," section 论说 [Review], 1.
54. "食物之供给与卫生," section 论说 [Review], 1.
55. The First Historical Archives of China, "光绪三十二年创办东安市场史料," 49.
56. A report by Beiping Social Work Department in 1943 stated that "stores and customers should keep clean and observe order. … Stores shouldn't sell unhygienic food and medicine hazardous to health." 东安市场管理处关于修正管理规则、接收职业介绍所的呈文(附：管理规则) [Report from Dongan Market Administration Office about Revising Management Regulation and

Taking Over the Employment Agency (Annex: Management Regulation)] (January 1, 1943–December 31, 1943), 北京市档案馆 [Beijing Municipal Archive] J002-004-00192.

57. He Yu, "个人卫生和公众卫生(续) [Individual Hygiene and Public Hygiene (Continuation)]," 通俗医事月刊 [Popular Medical Monthly] 2, no. 3 (1920): 23.

58. Shiqing Zhao, "公众卫生之重要 [The Importance of Public Hygiene]," 晨报六周年纪念增刊 [The Sixth Anniversary of the Morning Post Commemorative Supplement] (December 1924): 116. From the beginning of the twentieth century, the Chinese government and social elites profoundly reevaluated their defeat from the Opium War in 1840 to the Eight-Nation Alliance's aggression in 1900 and worried the country was gradually being colonized by foreign powers. In this context, building a "modern" Beijing was regarded as a way to demonstrate that the capital of China should be recognized as the same kind of great, independent, and civilized capital city as those in the West. It did not deserve to be seen as "backward" or to be colonized. See Xusheng Huang, "Reforming Beijing in the Shadow of Colonial Crisis: Urban Construction for Competing with the Foreign Powers, 1900–1928" In *The International Planning History Society Proceedings, 17th IPHS Conference, History-Urbanism-Resilience*, ed. Carola Hein (Netherlands: TU Delft, 2016), 83–93.

59. See Ruth Rogaski, *Hygienic Modernity: Meanings of Health and Disease in Treaty-Port China* (Berkeley: University of California Press, 2004), 22-47.

60. Richard Sennett, *Flesh and Stone: The Body and the City in Western Civilization* (New York: W. W. Norton 1996), 256.

61. For instance, see "说食品卫生 [Remarks on Food Sanitation]," 市政通告, no. 50 (1914): section 论说 [Review], 2–3.

62. The First Historical Archives of China, "光绪三十二年创办东安市场史料," 49.

63. Foucault claims that the control of the plague implied the origin of disciplinary society. Michel Foucault, *Discipline and Punish: The Birth of the Prison*, trans. Alan Sheridan, 2nd ed. (New York: Vintage Books, 1995), 198.

64. See Di Wang, *The Teahouse: Small Business, Everyday Culture, and Public Politics in Chengdu, 1900–1950* (Stanford, CA.: Stanford University Press, 2008), 1–2.

65. 京师警察厅关于函送修建东安市场计划、建筑表与京都市政公所的来往函及市政公所的布告等.

66. "市场工程如是 [Example of Market Projects]," 爱国白话报, November 3, 1921; "市场塌房砸人 [Market Building Collapses and Injures People]," 爱国白话报, August 2, 1921; Lao Dan, "社会小言 [Comments on Society]," 群强报 [Masses' Strength Daily], August 2, 1921.

67. 京师警察厅关于函送修建东安市场计划、建筑表与京都市政公所的来往函及市政公所的布告等.

68. "After the fire of Dongan Market, the former President of the Municipal Council Wu planned to establish a new institution, to construct the solid buildings and to

rent them out to merchants. If merchants are allowed to build by themselves, no matter how the government supervises them, they always attempt to save money and choose basic materials." 京师警察厅关于函送修建东安市场计划、建筑表与京都市政公所的来往函及市政公所的布告等.

69. 京师警察厅关于函送修建东安市场计划、建筑表与京都市政公所的来往函及市政公所的布告等.
70. 京师警察厅关于函送修建东安市场计划、建筑表与京都市政公所的来往函及市政公所的布告等; "市场工程如是."
71. "大火后之东安市场 [Dongan Market after the Fire]," 晨报星期画报 [Morning Post Weekly Pictorial] 1, no. 32 (1926): 2.
72. Gamble, *Peking*, 223.
73. Gamble, *Peking*, 223.
74. The idea being that because business owners paid tax and contributed to the country's finances, the country should support business owners. Meanwhile, since the government claimed its objective was to build democracy and prosperity for people, it should support the merchants' needs for improving the bad living conditions. The First Historical Archives of China, "光绪三十二年创办东安市场史料," 48.
75. The First Historical Archives of China, "光绪三十二年创办东安市场史料," 50. For the negotiations, see The First Historical Archives of China, "光绪三十二年创办东安市场史料," 48–51.
76. Zong, "东安市场的过去和现在," 184. Ironically, however, after 1915, the performance area was gradually developed and occupied by permanent stores intensifying commercial uses. "试办商场 [Opening a Market for Trial]," 群强报, October 10, 1915.
77. Commerce Board of Dongan Market: 东安市场商民董事会; Public Chamber of Commerce of Dongan Market: 东安市场商民公益联合会. The Public Chamber of Commerce of Dongan Market, for example, was established after the second fire, and consisted of a president and four executive directors. Each row of shops elected a manager to attend meetings of the chamber.
78. Quanchao Zong, "历史上的东安市场 [Dongan Market in History]" in 纪念北京市社会科学院建立十周年历史研究所研究成果论文集 [Commemorative Proceedings of Research Results at the Institute of History for the 10th Anniversary of Beijing Academy of Social Science], ed. Editorial Committee of Yandu Chunqiu at Beijing Academy of Social Science (Beijing: Beijing Yanshan Press, 1988), 276; Shanyuan Dong, Bokang Chen, and Xiangyu Ma, "话说东安市场 [Tales of Dongan Market]," in 北京市东城区文史资料选编 [Selections from Beijing Dongcheng District Cultural History Materials], vol. 2, 142.
79. "市场工程如是"; "市场包工内幕 [The Inside Story of Contracting Market Buildings]," 爱国白话报, September 3, 1921.

80. For the traditional role of the guilds and an evaluation of it, see William Townsend Rowe, *Hankow: Commerce and Society in a Chinese City, 1796–1889* (Stanford, CA: Stanford University Press, 1984); William Townsend Rowe, *Hankow: Conflict and Community in a Chinese City, 1796–1895* (Stanford, CA: Stanford University Press, 1992).
81. "学生演讲被拘 [Students Arrested for Public Speech], " 爱国白话报, June 6, 1919. See Xusheng Huang, "Space, State, and Crowds: Urban Squares on Beijing's Central Axis in the 1910s," *Architectural Theory Review* 23, no. 2 (2019): 214–32.
82. The Dongan Market Management Regulations by the Beiping Social Work Department, see 东安市场管理处关于修正管理规则、接收职业介绍所的呈文(附：管理规则).
83. Gamble, *Peking*, 115.
84. The First Historical Archives of China, "光绪三十二年创办东安市场史料," 51–54.
85. "清洁运动大会纪录 [Record of the Cleaning Movement Meeting]," 卫生公报 [Government Bulletin on Hygiene], no. 1 (December 1928): 265.
86. Dong, *Republican Beijing*, 147–52.
87. Wuliao, "封存日货后之东安市场 [Dongan Market During the Prohibition of the sale of Japanese Goods]," 北洋画报 [Beiyang Pictorial], October 31, 1931. See also Yi Dong, 北平日记 [Beiping Diary] (Beijing: People's Publishing House, 2009), a diary of a college student from 1938 to 1943, which shows his daily life of shopping, eating, and recreational activity at Dongan Market.
88. "When the government agencies perform their duties on merchants, they would write to and handle the affairs jointly with the Market Administrative Office; merchants should report firstly to the Market Administrative Office, which will transmit their request to the agencies." See 北平市市长视察东安市场管理处及管理处业务概要 [An Overview of the Inspection of Dongan Market's Administrative Office by the Mayor of Beiping] (January 1, 1946–December 31, 1946), 北京市档案馆 [Beijing Municipal Archive] J001-002-00339.
89. "重建市场计划.", "对于东安市场此次风潮之意见 [A Comment on the Dongan Market Crisis]," 爱国白话报, November 19, 1921; "派员调查市场 [Dispatching the Inspector to the Market]," 爱国白话报, November 20, 1921; " 传讯市场商人 [Summoning the Market's Merchants]," 爱国白话报, November 22, 1921.
90. See Joseph Esherick, ed., *Remaking the Chinese City: Modernity and National Identity, 1900–1950* (Honolulu: University of Hawaii Press, 2002).
91. Wang, *The Teahouse*, 1–2.

Archival sources

北平市市长视察东安市场管理处及管理处业务概要 [An Overview of the Inspection of Dongan Market's Administrative Office by the Mayor of Beiping] (January 1, 1946–December 31, 1946). 北京市档案馆 [Beijing Municipal Archive] J001-002-00339.

东安市场管理处关于修正管理规则、接收职业介绍所的呈文(附：管理规则) [Report from Dongan Market's Administration Office about Revising Management Regulation and Taking Over the Employment Agency (Annex: Management Regulation)] (January 1, 1943–December 31, 1943). 北京市档案馆 [Beijing Municipal Archive] J002-004-00192.

京都市政公所第二、三处关于召开筹建东安市场会议的通知及东安市场改良意见大纲等 [A Notice from the Second and Third Office of the Municipal Council about Convening a Meeting on Building Dongan Market, and an Outline of the Comment on Improving Dongan Market, etc.] (July 1, 1920–July 31, 1920). 北京市档案馆 [Beijing Municipal Archives] J017-001-00133.

京师警察厅关于函送修建东安市场计划、建筑表与京都市政公所的来往函及市政公所的布告等 [Letters between the Capital Police Board and Municipal Council about the Plan and List of Buildings of Dongan Market, and Announcements by the Municipal Council, etc.] (August 1, 1920–July 31, 1922). 北京市档案馆 [Beijing Municipal Archives] J017-001-00119.

京师警察厅行政处关于送修正东安市场暂行章程的函 [Letter from the Administration Office of the Capital Police Board about Sending the Revised Provisional Regulations for Dongan Market] (from June 1, 1917). 北京市档案馆 [Beijing Municipal Archive] J181-018-07668.

社会局对东安市场管理员的任免令、东安市场职员履历表及员司、夫役、巡官、长警花名册 [Remove and Appoint Order on Dongan Market by the Department of Social Work, the Curricula Vitae of Officers of Dongan Market, and Rosters of Employees, Laborers, Police Directors, Managers and Officers] (August 1, 1929–September 30, 1920). 北京市档案馆 [Beijing Municipal Archives] J002-001-00009.

Bibliography

Broudehoux, Anne-Marie. *The Making and Selling of Post-Mao Beijing*. New York: Routledge, 2004.

Calabi, Donatella. *The Market and the City: Squares, Streets and Buildings in Early Modern Europe*. Translated by Marlene Klein. Aldershot: Ashgate, 2004.

Chi, Zehui, Xuexi Lou, and Wenxian Chen, eds. 北平市工商业概况 [A Survey of Industry and Commerce of the City of Peiping]. Beijing: Department of Social Work, Beiping, 1932.

Ding, Rui. "北洋政府时期京师警察厅研究 [A Study on Capital Police Board in the Era of Beiyang Government]." PhD diss., Graduate School of Chinese Academy of Social Sciences, 2011.

Dong, Madeleine Yue. *Republican Beijing: The City and its Histories*. Berkeley: University of California Press, 2003.

Dong, Shanyuan, Bokang Chen, and Xiangyu Ma. "话说东安市场 [Tales of Dongan Market]." In 北京市东城区文史资料选编 [Selections from Beijing Dongcheng District Cultural History Materials], edited by Cultural History Materials Committee of Beijing Dongcheng District Committee of CPPCC. Vol. 2, 139–59. Beijing: Beijing Press, 1982.

Dong, Yi. 北平日记 [Beiping Diary]. Beijing: People's Publishing House, 2009.

Esherick, Joseph, ed. *Remaking the Chinese City: Modernity and National Identity, 1900–1950*. Honolulu: University of Hawaii Press, 2002.

The First Historical Archives of China. "光绪三十二年创办东安市场史料 [Archives Relating to the Creation of Dongan Market in 1906]." 历史档案 [Historical Archives], no. 01 (2000): 42–54.

Foucault, Michel. *Discipline and Punish: The Birth of the Prison*. Translated by Alan Sheridan. New York: Vintage Books, 1995.

Gamble, Sidney David. *Peking: A Social Survey*. New York: George H. Doran, 1921.

Geist, Johann Friedrich. *Arcades: The History of a Building Type*. Translated by Jane O. Newman and John H. Smith. Cambridge, MA: MIT Press, 1985.

Huang, Xusheng. "Building Modern Beijing: Government-led Urban Reconstruction, 1900–1937." In *Proceedings of the 10th International Symposium on Architectural Interchanges in Asia*, edited by the Architectural Society of China. 975–79. Beijing: China City Press, 2014.

———. "Reforming Beijing in the Shadow of Colonial Crisis: Urban Construction for Competing with the Foreign Powers, 1900–1928." In *International Planning History Society Proceedings, 17th IPHS Conference, History-Urbanism-Resilience*, edited by Carola Hein. Vol. 1. 83–93. The Netherlands: TU Delft, 2016.

———. "Space, State, and Crowds: Urban Squares on Beijing's Central Axis in the 1910s." *Architectural Theory Review* 23, no. 2 (2019): 214–32.

Lao Dan. "社会小言 [Comments on Society]." 群强报 [Masses' Strength Daily], August 2, 1921.

Lao She. "离婚 [Divorce]." In 老舍小说全集 [Complete Collections of Lao She's Fictions], edited by Ji Shu and Yi Shu. Vol. 3. 171–402. Wuhan: Changjiang Wenyi Press, 2004.

Lynn, Jermyn Chi-hung. *Social Life of the Chinese in Peking*. Beijing: China Booksellers, 1928.

Naquin, Susan. *Peking: Temples and City Life, 1400–1900*. Berkeley: University of California Press, 2000.

Ren, Qingtai. "东安市场声明归官 [A Statement about Dongan Market Taken Over by the Government]." 大公报(天津) [Impartial Daily (Tianjin)], April 8, 1907.

Rogaski, Ruth. *Hygienic Modernity: Meanings of Health and Disease in Treaty-Port China*. Berkeley: University of California Press, 2004.

Rowe, William Townsend. *Hankow: Commerce and Society in a Chinese City, 1796–1889*. Stanford, CA: Stanford University Press, 1984.

———. *Hankow: Conflict and Community in a Chinese City, 1796–1895*. Stanford, CA: Stanford University Press, 1992.

Schmiechen, James, and Kenneth Carls. *The British Market Hall: A Social and Architectural History*. New Haven: Yale University Press, 1999.

Sennett, Richard. *Flesh and Stone: The Body and the City in Western Civilization*. New York: W. W. Norton, 1996.

Shi, Mingzheng. "Beijing Transforms: Urban Infrastructure, Public Works, and Social Change in the Chinese Capital, 1900–1928." PhD diss., Columbia University, 1993.

Tangires, Helen. *Public Markets*. New York: W. W. Norton, 2008.

———. *Public Markets and Civic Culture in Nineteenth-Century America*. Baltimore: Johns Hopkins University Press, 2002.

Wang, Di. *Street Culture in Chengdu: Public Space, Urban Commoners, and Local Politics, 1870–1930*. Stanford, CA: Stanford University Press, 2003.

———. *The Teahouse: Small Business, Everyday Culture, and Public Politics in Chengdu, 1900–1950*. Stanford, CA: Stanford University Press, 2008.

Wang, Jianwei. "王府井与天桥：民国北京的双面叙事 [Wangfujing Street and Sky Bridge: A Pluralistic Narrative of Republican Beijing]." 学术月刊 [Academic Monthly] 48, no. 12 (2016): 161–71.

Wuliao. "封存日货后之东安市场 [Dongan Market During the Prohibition of the Sale of Japanese Goods]." 北洋画报 [Beiyang Pictorial], October 31, 1931.

Yu, He. "个人卫生和公众卫生(续) [Individual Hygiene and Public Hygiene (Continuation)]." 通俗医事月刊 [Popular Medical Monthly] 2, no. 3 (1920): 23–25.

Yu, Xiaochuan. "从法令规制中看东安市场的形成及演变特征—近代北京商业空间的形成与变容过程的研究 [Review of Evolution of the Dongan Market in the Light of Policies and Rules: Research on the Evolution of Modern Commercial Spaces in Beijing]." In 建筑史论文集 [Collection of Papers on Architectural History], edited by Fuhe Zhang. Vol. 14, 155–63, 270. Beijing: Tsinghua University Press, 2001.

Yu, Xiaochuan, and Hiroshi Katano. "The Evolution of the Public Market in the Modern China: The Case Study of Dongan Market in Beijing." *Journal of Architecture and Planning (Transactions of AIJ)* 67, no. 559 (2002): 117–23.

Zhang, Fuhe. 北京近代建筑史 [The Modern Architectural History of Beijing from the End of the 19th Century to 1930s]. Beijing: Tsinghua University Press, 2004.

Zhao, Shiqing. "公众卫生之重要 [The Importance of Public Hygiene]." 晨报六周年纪念增刊 [The Sixth Anniversary of the Morning Post Commemorative Supplement] (December 1924): 116–22.

Zhu, Qiqian. "王府井大街之今昔(附东安市场) [Wangfujing Street in the Past and Present (including Dongan Market)]." In文史资料选编 [Selections from Cultural History Materials], edited by Cultural History Materials Committee of Beijing Municipal Committee of CPPCC. Vol. 12, 211–14. Beijing: Beijing Press, 1982.

Zong, Quanchao. "东安市场的过去和现在 [Dongan Market in the Past and Present]." In文史资料选编 [Selections from Cultural History Materials], edited by Cultural History Materials Committee of Beijing Municipal Committee of CPPCC. Vol. 12, 181–99. Beijing: Beijing Press, 1982.

———. "历史上的东安市场 [Dongan Market in History]." 纪念北京市社会科学院建立十周年历史研究所研究成果论文集 [Commemorative Proceedings of Research Results at the Institute of History for the 10th Anniversary of Beijing Academy of Social Science], edited by Editorial Committee of Yandu Chunqiu at Beijing Academy of Social Science. 271–92. Beijing: Beijing Yanshan Press, 1988.

"重建市场计划 [A Plan to Rebuild the Market]." 爱国白话报 [Patriotic Vernacular News], June 14, 1920.

"传讯市场商人 [Summoning the Market's Merchants]." 爱国白话报 [Patriotic Vernacular News], November 22, 1921.

"大火后之东安市场 [Dongan Market after the Fire]." 晨报星期画报 [Morning Post Weekly Pictorial] 1, no. 32 (1926).

"东安市场 [Dongan Market]." 申报月刊 [Shenbao Monthly] 2, no. 10 (1933): 87–88.

"对于东安市场此次风潮之意见 [A Comment on the Dongan Market Crisis]." 爱国白话报 [Patriotic Vernacular News], November 19, 1921.

"改定东安市场暂行章程 [The Revised Provisional Regulations for Dongan Market]." In 京师警察法令汇纂 [Compilation of Laws and Decrees of Capital Police], edited by Capital Police Board. 155–59. Beijing: Xiehua Press, 1916.

"论市设市场 [Review of the Municipal Market]." 市政通告 [Municipal Bulletin], no. 24 (October 1919): section 论说 [Review], 7–9.

"内城官立东安市场营业规则 [The Business Regulation at Inner City Municipal Dongan Market]." In 清末北京城市管理法规 [Late Qing Beijing Urban Administrative Codes], edited by Tao Tian and Chengwei Guo. 197–214. Beijing: Beijing Yanshan Press, 1996.

"派员调查市场 [Dispatching the Inspector to the Market]." 爱国白话报 [Patriotic Vernacular News], November 20, 1921.

"清洁运动大会纪录 [Record of the Cleaning Movement Meeting]." 卫生公报 [Government Bulletin on Hygiene], no. 1 (December 1928): 265–70.
"试办商场 [Opening a Market for Trial]." 群强报 [Masses' Strength Daily], October 10, 1915.
"市场包工内幕 [The Inside Story of Contracting Market Buildings]." 爱国白话报 [Patriotic Vernacular News], September 3, 1921.
"市场工程如是 [Example of Market Projects]." 爱国白话报 [Patriotic Vernacular News], November 3, 1921.
"市场塌房砸人 [Market Building Collapses and Injures People]." 爱国白话报 [Patriotic Vernacular News], August 2, 1921.
"食物之供给与卫生 [Food Supply and Hygiene]." 市政通告 [Municipal Bulletin], no. 27 (April 1920): section 论说 [Review], 1–6.
"说食品卫生 [Remarks on Food Sanitation]." 市政通告 [Municipal Bulletin], no. 50 (1914): section 论说 [Review], 2–3.
"学生演讲被拘 [Students Arrested for Public Speech]." 爱国白话报 [Patriotic Vernacular News], June 6, 1919.

CHAPTER 8

HYGIENE, URBANISM, AND FASCIST POLITICS AT ROME'S WHOLESALE MARKET

Ruth W. Lo

The opening of Rome's Wholesale Market in 1922 took place four months before the fascists seized power in the city. Although preliminary plans for a comprehensive food provisioning system had emerged shortly after Rome became Italy's capital in 1871, a wholesale market did not materialize until the first year of the Fascist Era. This turned out to be a propitious coincidence for a regime that saw agriculture as the key to improving Italy's economic situation, an engine for modernization, and a tool for eventually realizing imperial ambitions. Food was literally integral to nation building, in both an actual and ideological sense. As such, Mussolini's government promptly claimed the Wholesale Market as its own achievement, featuring it often in fascist propaganda as an exemplary building for the sanitary provisioning of food in the capital. The Wholesale Market was to be the central—and centralizing—structure within Rome's food distribution network, which would also include neighborhood market halls. While the official function of this system was to provide more hygienic conditions for food vending, its physical structures were locations from which the government exercised unprecedented biopolitical control of comestible resources. This chapter traces the development of Rome's Wholesale Market from its inception in the Liberal Era to its realization during the fascist period, with a coda dedicated to its current adaptive reuse. The analysis focuses, in particular, on the siting of the Wholesale Market in relation to the city, the integration of the transit system into the distribution hub, and the structure's architecture and function as reflections of fascist Italian political and economic realities.

The groundwork for a comprehensive food provisioning system before fascism was laid by Rome's mayor Ernesto Nathan, who assumed the office in November 1907. An influential figure, Nathan modernized Rome by municipalizing many of its public services, such as energy delivery and transit, to prevent their monopolization by private companies.[1] The new mayor also recognized that food was fundamental to the city's health and vitality, and

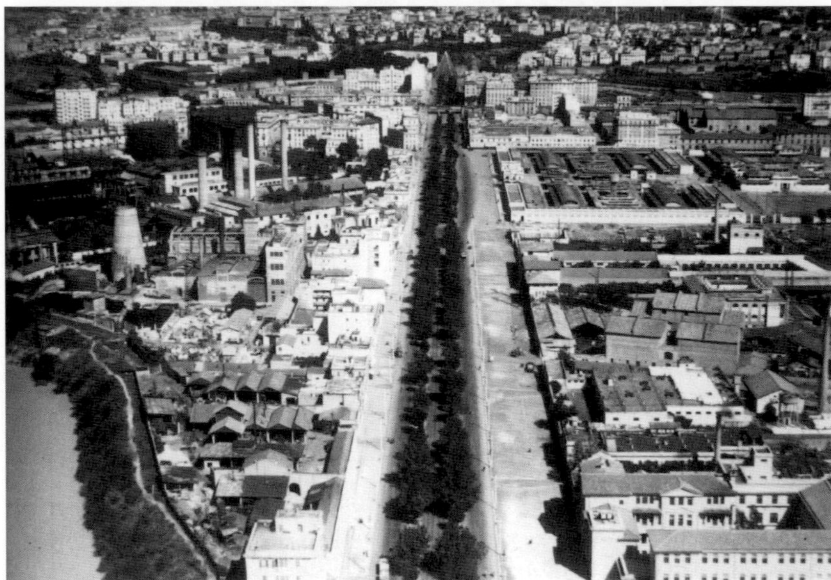

Figure 8.1. Perspectival view showing the Wholesale Market in the Ostiense industrial zone, ca. 1920s. Northwest of the market is Testaccio, where Rome's slaughterhouse was located. Courtesy of Archivio Storico Capitolino.

therefore that provisioning must be carefully planned as part of the design and development of Rome. Nathan was a proponent of centralizing responsibility within his administration, the Giunta Nathan, so the city could build more infrastructure for food vending and storage—that is, not just function as sanitation police—as well as establish more regulations to protect both producers and consumers. He was also in favor of constructing more neighborhood markets (*mercati rionali*) that would be integrated into the transit network to ensure that all citizens had easy access to fresh food. Nathan established the Food Commission, a municipal agency that oversaw food supply and determined the location of the Wholesale Market.[2]

The Food Commission picked an area in Ostiense, a neighborhood southeast of Rome's city center, opposite the slaughterhouse in Testaccio (figure 8.1). Two principal reasons drove this decision: hygiene and transit. For the former, the city wanted to establish an industrial zone downriver on the Tiber so food and manufacturing detritus would not flow through the city as it had in preceding centuries. For the latter, it had an ambitious plan for a new river port that would connect Rome to the sea at Ostia via a navigable canal.[3] Even though the canal project was never realized, it helped to intensify the industrial development of Ostiense, which was already home to the city's thermoelectric

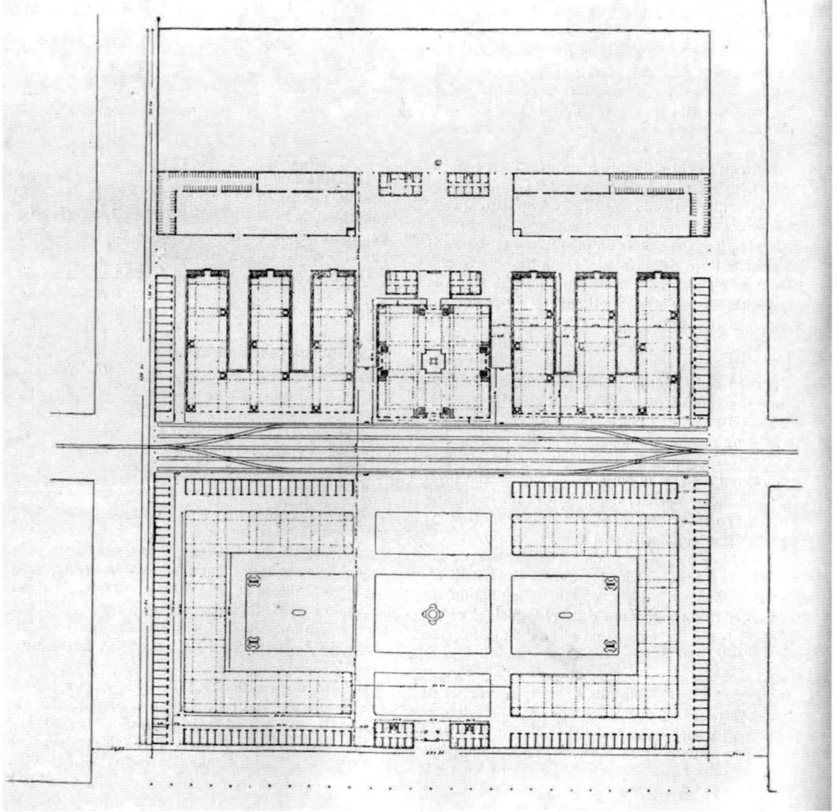

Figure 8.2. Plan of the Wholesale Market, Rome, 1922–27. Railroad tracks bisected the complex with the western side (bottom) for the vending of fruits and vegetables and the eastern side (top) for the selling of meats and seafood. Emilio Saffi, architect. Courtesy of *Rivista di Ingegneria Sanitaria e di Edilizia Moderna* 11, no. 9 (1915): 100.

plant, gas works, warehouses, and factories.[4] Furthermore, Ostiense was well connected both to existing railway lines that ran from Rome to the Castelli Romani and Pisa (two sources of agricultural goods for the capital) and the planned railway line to the seaport at Ostia.

The design of the Wholesale Market by Emilio Saffi, the Food Commission's appointed architect, was approved in 1910; it was a consummate reflection of the city's objective to integrate the transportation system in order to improve food provisioning. The area for the Wholesale Market, about seventy-five thousand square meters, was to comprise two sections, one dedicated to fruits and vegetables and the other to meats and seafood (figure 8.2). Bisecting the two areas were railroad tracks that connected the market directly with the existing

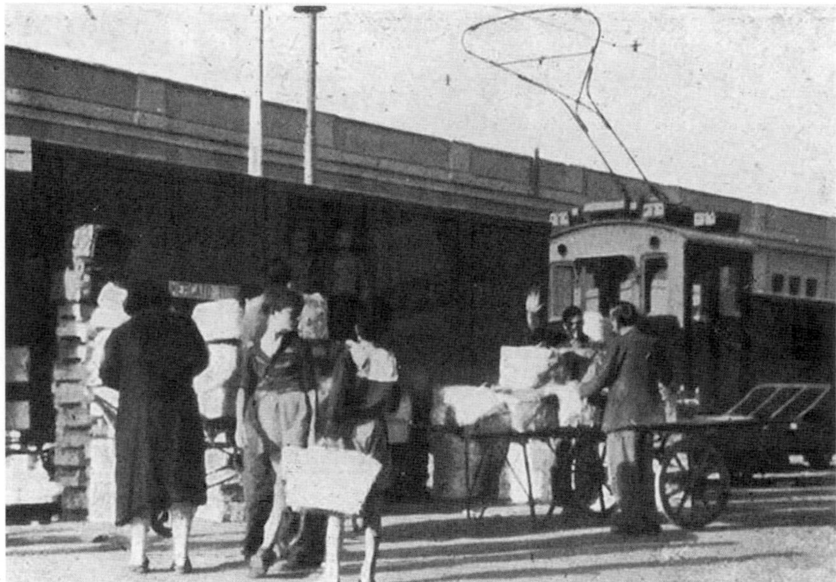

Figure 8.3. Tram with special cars for transporting alimentary goods at Via Negri by the Wholesale Market, Rome, ca. 1920s. Courtesy of Tramroma.

Rome-Pisa line and the future Rome-Ostia line.[5] This infrastructure was the literal lifeline that delivered sustenance from the countryside to nourish the city, as incoming goods to the Wholesale Market were then loaded onto trams and carts to be delivered to neighborhood markets for resale (figure 8.3).

Another key feature of Saffi's design was its planned centralization of the city's entire food supply in one location. This was an extraordinarily ambitious endeavor and rare even for larger cities in Europe and the United States at this time. An article in *Capitolium*, an urban planning journal created by the fascist regime, pointed out that no big city had concentrated all types of food wholesale in one place. Some of the most important markets, the author wrote, such as Covent Garden in London, the Grossmarkthalle in Munich, and the Lower Manhattan Market in New York, were wholesale markets for fruits and vegetables only.[6] The closest example to a comprehensive wholesale market was Les Halles in Paris, where all categories of food were offered within the glass and iron pavilions designed by Victor Baltard.[7] Rome's Wholesale Market was similarly organized by different food categories, but unlike Les Halles's repetitive, gridded system composed of pavilions and streets, the categories were contained within distinct zones and in separate buildings. The central railroad tracks served as the divider between two large areas: the fruit and vegetable market occupied the western side, while the meat and seafood markets were on

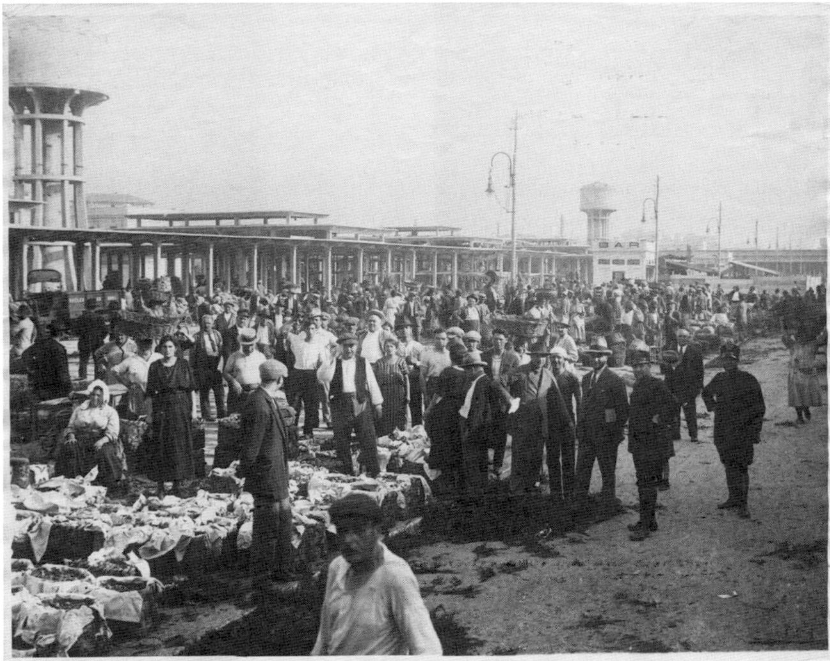

Figure 8.4. Inside the courtyard of the Wholesale Market complex, Rome, ca. 1925. Courtesy of Archivio Storico Capitolino.

the eastern side. The latter section was subdivided into a structure for lamb, poultry, and eggs, and another for seafood. Like other municipal markets, the architecture enabled the city to regulate sanitation and prices by centralizing the administrative and policing functions in one place.

Saffi's design of the pavilions was reminiscent of the typical nineteenth-century glass and iron markets across European cities. Many European metropolises modeled their central markets after Baltard's design for Les Halles in Paris, for example, Porta Palazzo in Turin and San Lorenzo in Florence.[8] Saffi also wanted his buildings in Rome to adhere to a simple architectural program by using modular design and exposed structural materials. Iron columns would support expansive buildings formed along a central hall flanked by aisles on each side with articulated bays. Curtain walls were to be composed of numerous fenestrations, and additional windows would rim the roof to provide abundant light into the interior.[9] However, at Rome's Wholesale Market, these pavilions were storage for foodstuff—rather than spaces for vending, as was typical in the markets of other major European cities.[10]

The commerce of fruits and vegetables would take place under the stalls (*capannoni*) and in the open-air, central courtyard (figure 8.4). Like the other

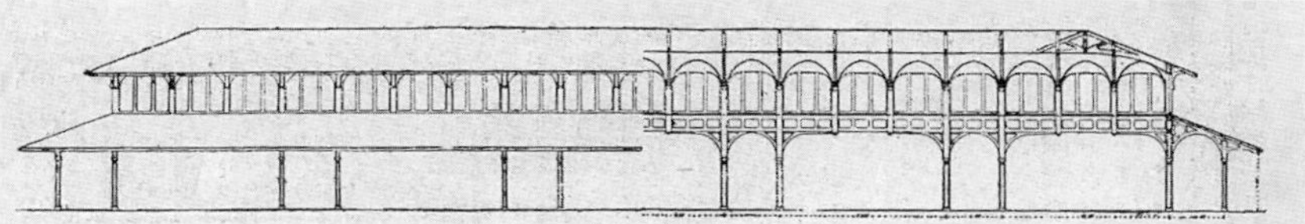

Figure 8.5. Elevation and longitudinal section of the fruit and vegetable market stalls at the Wholesale Market (unrealized design), Rome, 1922–27. Emilio Saffi, architect. Courtesy of *Rivista di Ingegneria Sanitaria e di Edilizia Moderna* 11, no. 9 (1915): 101.

structures in the complex, Saffi designed the stalls to be made of iron (figure 8.5); however, due to budgetary constraints, the stalls were ultimately built of reinforced concrete like the other structures at the Wholesale Market.[11] Underneath these continuous coverings, the wholesale and retail of extraprovincial produce would occur, while in the open courtyard, local producers—from Rome and its suburbs—offered their goods.[12] This clearly differentiated system allowed local farmers to have a more informal trading structure, giving them the opportunity to set up in the courtyard daily.

On the eastern side of the central railroad tracks were the seafood market, the lamb, poultry, and egg market (Ovipol), and the dry goods and flower market. Saffi designed these as independent pavilions to separate the storage, processing, and vending of the food categories. One of the main reasons was that the seafood and meat trades required different spatial configurations, equipment, and storage facilities.

The seafood market occupied the central lot between the two other identical pavilions. The city had intended this structure to replace the existing fish market on the Via di San Teodoro, which it considered outdated and inadequate for the growing capital after thirty years of usage.[13] Saffi's original drawings showed a symmetrical pavilion that had a square footprint and was constructed of iron and glass. Topped with iron cupolas, the structure would have continuous windows beneath the roof to allow plenty of light into the space. One of the most notable features of the seafood market was its incorporation of on-site mechanical refrigeration, a technological novelty for Italian markets, to prolong the life of the goods and promote a more sanitary trading environment. Refrigeration lockers and additional storage spaces were located directly beneath the market, and the industrial machinery that provided the cooling mechanism and ice was housed in a separate structure attached to the seafood market.[14]

The Ovipol market and the dry goods and flower market were identical structures on either side of the seafood market. The buildings assumed a tripartite organization, in the shape of the letter "E," presumably with each arm dedicated to the commerce of one type of goods (e.g., lamb, poultry, and egg; wine and oil; nuts and grains; and flowers). The Ovipol market at the Wholesale Market would replace the existing one located at Piazza Guglielmo Pepe by Termini railway station in the Esquilino neighborhood.[15] The butchering and commerce of cattle would continue at the slaughterhouse in nearby Testaccio, which would receive a technological upgrade in 1932 with the addition of refrigerated storage and ice-making machinery.[16] The city considered the incorporation of refrigeration at the Wholesale Market to be an exceptional achievement, as a municipal pamphlet proudly claimed that other major Italian cities would now be looking to Rome to improve their own food sanitation measures.[17]

In fact, the entire Wholesale Market complex integrated the modern utility systems that Nathan's administration municipalized. The market received its water via the ancient aqueducts of the Acqua Paola and the Acqua Marcia, and an extensive drainage system separated the collection of grey water from sewage.[18] Two water towers of reinforced concrete were erected in 1918 in the fruit and vegetable market, and a third was added later in 1926 to the meat market.[19] The gas plant across the Via Ostiense from the Wholesale Market provided the energy necessary for illuminations, since activities at the latter typically began long before sunrise.[20] Electricity came from the nearby Centrale Montemartini, the first municipal thermal-electric plant in Rome that Nathan instituted.[21] It was clear that Nathan's government intended the Wholesale Market to benefit from its proximity to the newly municipalized energy suppliers.[22]

When the Wholesale Market finally opened in June 1922, much of its architecture diverged from Saffi's original designs. The Giunta Nathan fell in 1913, bringing Rome's public works projects to a halt. Italy entered World War I in 1915, so building materials became scarce and manpower was limited in the city. Food availability across the country diminished, and the government instituted rations in order to prioritize the supply to troops on the frontline.[23] It was not until 1922 that the first section of the Wholesale Market (i.e., the fruit and vegetable market) entered into commerce; the seafood and meat markets remained under construction until 1926. Saffi's designs for the various pavilions were simplified, both in style and material, to accommodate postwar financial and resource realities. The original *stile Liberty* pavilions in iron and glass were ultimately made of reinforced concrete, a familiar construction method in Rome, and faced with brick. All of the roofs, including the fish market's iron cupolas, were changed to less complicated and more economical designs of sloping covers supported on concrete beams and columns. The stalls in the fruit and vegetable market also ended up in reinforced concrete, even though Saffi had intended them to be iron structures (figure 8.6).[24] Other Art Nouveau features, such as decorative ironwork and ornamental stucco, were eliminated. The biggest change in form, however, was to the Ovipol pavilion. The building's footprint changed from a letter "E" to a letter "C" shape, with

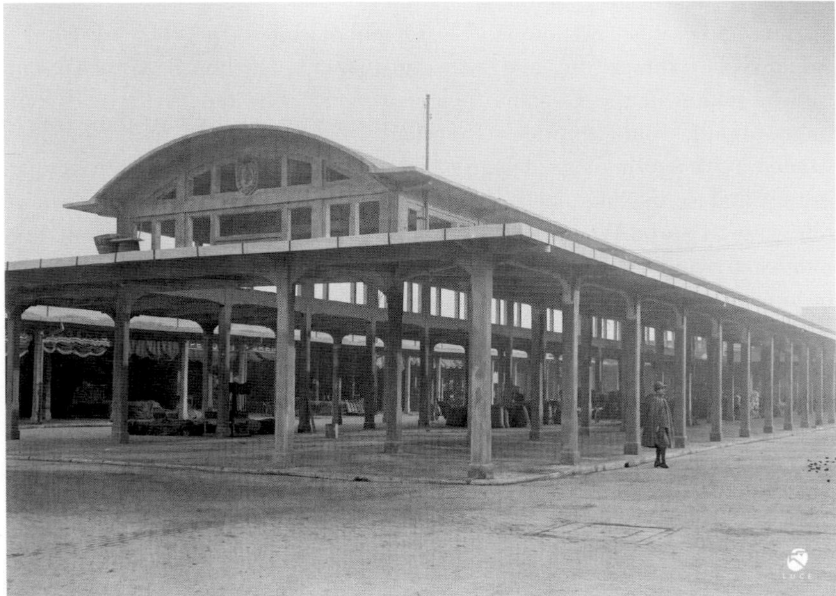

Figure 8.6. Reinforced concrete stalls at the Wholesale Market, Rome, 1926. Emilio Saffi, architect. Courtesy of Archivio Luce.

a water tower in the middle of the market's courtyard. The dry goods pavilion, on the other hand, was entirely eliminated.

Significant alterations in materials and the construction method notwithstanding, the pavilions retained their luminous interiors. Large expanses of windows abounded, puncturing the brick and stucco façades of the market buildings. While the pavilions did not have the glass enclosures that Saffi had intended, the realized versions found compromises through continuous ribbon windows under the rooflines (figure 8.7). In the seafood market, skylights covered atrium-like spaces and provided abundant light to the interior. This attention to natural illumination reflected the widespread belief that light and air, especially in food markets, were essential elements to regulating public health.

Under fascism, the government of Rome repeatedly attempted to rearrange the ways in which the city administered the Wholesale Market in order to control food supply, one of the most fundamental means of disciplining the citizens. Soon after the Wholesale Market opened, the city moved its jurisdiction from the Office of Food and Markets (established under the previous liberal government) to the Office of Urban Policing.[25] This was a reversal of the actions undertaken by previous administrations and signified the regime's attitude toward the role of food in Rome. In 1912 the Giunta Nathan merged the administration of food, previously the responsibility of the Office of

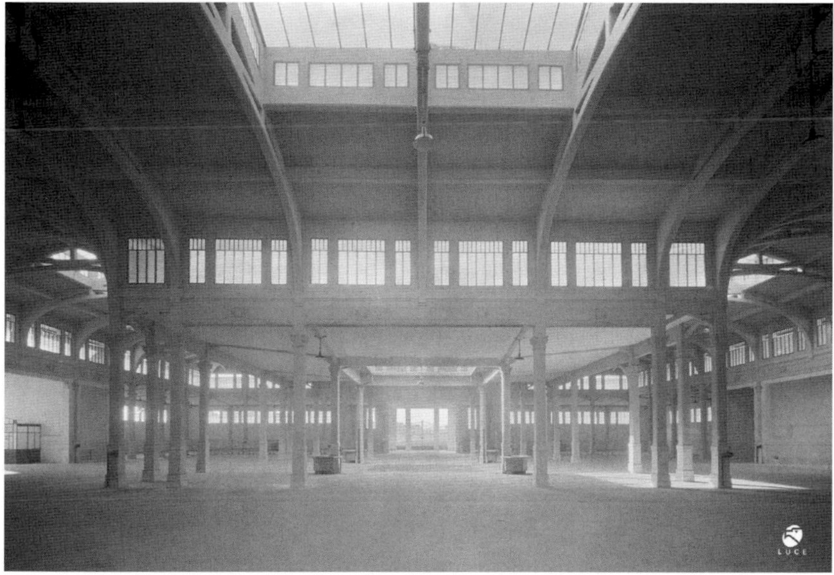

Figure 8.7. Internal view of the Seafood Pavilion at the Wholesale Market, Rome, 1926. Emilio, Saffi, architect. Image courtesy of Archivio Luce.

Urban Policing during the post-Risorgimento era, with the office that oversaw the development of the Roman countryside (*agro romano*).[26] The joining of the two functions was logical and in consonance with Nathan's plans to intensify agricultural production in the *agro romano* so it could increase the supply of food to Rome. In 1915, the city established the Office of Food and Markets as its own autonomous entity, which, as mentioned, was later absorbed back by the Office of Urban Policing in 1923, shortly after the fascists came to power.

This decision was an indication that the regime saw food provisioning as a matter of civic order. In other words, the administration was keenly aware that the improper management of food supply, or worse, a shortage of it, would lead to civil unrest. However, the city ultimately realized that the lack of a dedicated provisioning office was antithetical and counterproductive to national campaigns advocating the boosting of food production in Italy in order to achieve alimentary autarchy.[27] As such, in 1927, the city moved the administration of food in Rome from the Office of Urban Policing back to the Office of Food and Markets.[28] The newly restored agency became an important political tool for the fascist government of Rome, which was more than ready to utilize the Wholesale Market to meet the regime's ambitious goals concerning food in the capital as well as in Italy overall.

State-controlled newspapers and newsreels touted the efficiency and abundance of Rome's Wholesale Market. For example, a 1932 newsreel by Luce, the official state media company, emphasized the market's architecture and its integration into the city's transit network.[29] With the clamoring sounds of the markets in the background, the camera panned across the fruit and vegetable markets, showing the many pavilions and the water tower, before stopping at the monumental entrance. The camera then cut to a scene of the train tracks, where men loaded and unloaded abundant goods from rail cars and donkey-drawn carts. Under the reinforced concrete stalls laden with heaps of produce, merchants and buyers negotiated prices as market workers (e.g., weighers and porters) helped handle the goods. Toward the end of this two-minute newsreel, a brief scene showed foodstuff getting loaded onto trams that would travel through the city to the neighborhood markets. The film underscored the Wholesale Market as an orderly space of food commerce that served as a fascist biopolitical hub. Though its ostensible purpose was for local food provisioning, the structure became a national symbol that reinforced ideas of fascist agricultural success and autarchic goals in its mediated images.

Despite this and similar types of propaganda, historians and archival documents have pointed to the great failures of Rome's fascist government in managing food supply.[30] The city used the Wholesale Market to institute a system of price controls to prevent price surges and food shortage as a way of maintaining public order; that is, to avoid urban uprisings against the government. In the early 1920s, Rome's municipal government placed price caps on the "most essential" items, such as bread, pasta, lard, meat, and coal.[31] The list grew in 1927, due to the devaluation of the lira, to include olive oil, coffee, sugar, legumes, cheese, and sausages.[32] The price caps were centralized by the state after Italy's invasion of Ethiopia in 1935 and became even more rigorous as the nation experienced international sanctions.[33] These measures were disincentives for producers to bring their goods to the Wholesale Market, and instead, encouraged them to find more profitable ways to sell, for example, on the black market. The municipal overregulation contributed to the decline of the Wholesale Market during the later fascist years, and the city's new food infrastructure and architecture were ultimately unable to improve Rome's alimentary situation.[34] The regime's informants described general complaints about the high cost of living in the capital, but especially the price of food. One informant reported that citizens felt "food [was] the worst part of social and national well-being."[35]

The regime's attempts to use the Wholesale Market to comprehensively manage food in Rome ultimately failed, and the complex, along with other new structures in the city, was unable to counter the dire alimentary situation during fascism. The Wholesale Market continued to be operational after the

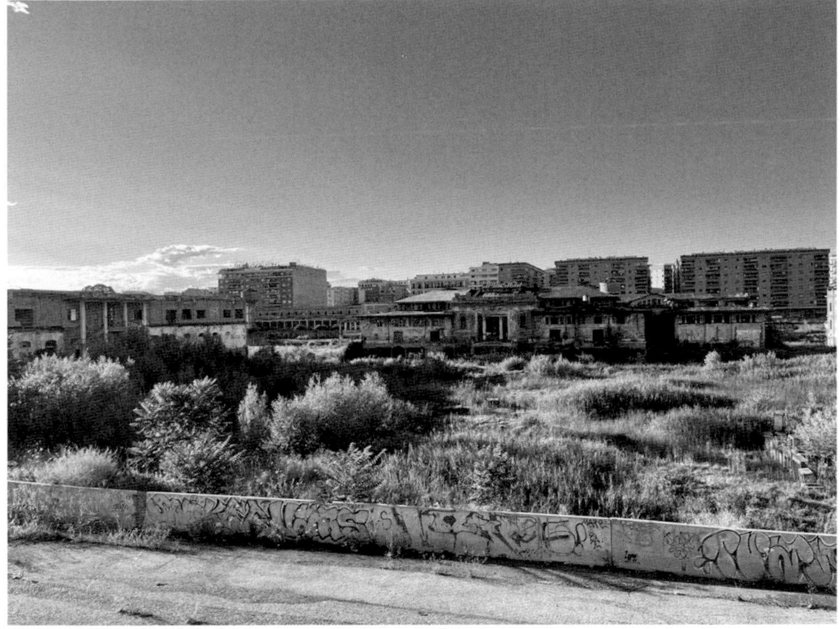

Figure 8.8. The former Wholesale Markets in a state of neglect, Rome. Photograph by author, 2022.

fall of the fascist regime but suffered continuous decline as the facility became increasingly inadequate and outdated for the growing city. Since the decommissioning of the market in 2002, the site has gone through several iterations of planned redevelopment. However, like many former food buildings in Rome, the Wholesale Market exists in a perpetual state of limbo. Over two decades later, it remains an abandoned construction zone, with the former pavilions in varying states of decay (figure 8.8).

When the market activities transferred to a new wholesale facility on the outskirts of Rome, the city soon planned to convert the former Wholesale Market into an area that would be more fitting for the new, ex-industrial Ostiense.[36] Through the engineering and construction company Sviluppo Centro Ostiense, the city held an international competition and selected as the winning entry a proposal by Rem Koolhaas's firm, Office of Metropolitan Architects (OMA). The scheme proposed to transform the Wholesale Market into a commercial and cultural destination by simultaneously restoring original structures and adding new ones. The complex, dubbed by then-mayor Walter Veltroni as "City of Youth," would comprise green streetscape lined with shops and cafes, as well as a cinema, a theater, galleries, and sport and recreational areas.[37] OMA envisioned the project to serve as a vibrant center in a transitioning neighborhood that is also home to Roma Tre, one of Rome's major universities, which has invested heavily into the redevelopment of Ostiense.

However, the different parties involved with the project have not been able to come to an agreement on the program, thus hindering construction progress while squandering funds. Despite OMA's attempts to reach a compromise through revisions to its original competition proposal, including the addition of buildings for student activities, the city and investors continued to squabble, resulting in the architectural firm's eventual departure. Newspaper articles and online blogs ridiculed the city's management of the project and saw it as a consummate example of failed municipal administration.[38] In September 2017, discussion for the conversion project reopened under the new mayoral administration of Virginia Raggi. The proprietor, construction company, and investors reached an agreement with the city to alter the project's programing to include more public spaces, such as moving the complex's thoroughfare from inside the proposed shopping center to an open-air main street that would be accessible at any time. Roman newspapers reported enthusiastically on these developments, noting that the project's name would change from "City of Youth" to the trendy, monosyllabic "Ex," with a planned opening in 2020.[39] Yet the only journalistic accounts on the former Wholesale Market in 2020 were of late-night police raids to remove unhoused people from occupying its ever more derelict structures that were at risk of collapse.[40] Based on the lack of construction progress, it may be another decade before we see the full transformation of Rome's Wholesale Market into a new kind of civic space, one that promotes public health as the city and OMA had originally intended.

Notes

1. On the achievements of Ernesto Nathan as mayor of Rome, see, for example, Romano Ugolini, *Ernesto Nathan: Tra idealità e pragmatismo* (Rome: Edizioni dell'Ateneo, 2003) and Domenico Maria Bruni, *Municipalismo democratico in età giolittiana: L'esperienza della giunta Nathan* (Soveria Mannelli: Rubbettino, 2010). On the municipalization of Rome's public utility system, ACEA, see Stefano Battilossi, *Acea di Roma 1909–2000: Da azienda municipale a Gruppo multiservizi* (Milan: Franco Angeli, 2001).
2. Archivio Storico Capitolino (ASC), Atti, 1907, vol. 3, seduta 13 dicembre 1907, prop. 188, 554–59. The Commission's report, published in 1908, was called the *Relazione Ruini*, named after the author of the report, Bartolomeo Meuccio Ruini (1877–1970).
3. The development of Ostiense was inextricably tied to the relocation of Rome's slaughterhouse from Piazza del Popolo to Testaccio in the 1870s, which was

prompted by considerations of the Tiber's flow and its impact on the city's sanitation. For reference, see Gioacchino Ersoch, *Il Mattatoio e mercato del bestiame costruiti dal Comune negli anni 1888–1891* (Rome: Virano, 1891); Giovanna Franco, *Il mattatoio di Testaccio a Roma: Costruzioni e trasformazioni del complesso dismesso* (Bari: Dedalo, 1998); and Alberto Maria Racheli, "I disegni di architettura dell'archivio di Gioacchino Ersoch: Due progetti inedita, per l'ampiamento del mattatoio di piazza del Popolo," *Bollettino della Biblioteca della Facoltà di Architettura dell'Università di Roma* 19–20 (1978): 11–23. The engineer Paolo Orlando founded the Comitato Nazionale pro Roma Marittima pel Porto di Roma e la Navigazione del Tevere e della Nera in 1904 and had drawn possible schemes that he published in the book, *Roma: Porto di mare* (Rome: Comitato Pro Roma Marittima, 1905). Orlando's proposal for a river port was even incorporated into a study for the development of Ostiense as an industrial zone by the architects Gustavo Giovannoni and Marcello Piacentini in 1916. See Gustavo Giovannoni, "Per lo sviluppo industriale di Roma, dalla Relazione della Commissione comunale," *Annali di Ingegneria e d'Architettura* 32 (1917): 1–8. Orlando's project also led to the building of the Via Ostiense that connected Rome to Ostia Lido (a new town built on reclaimed marshland) and the establishment of Garbatella as a garden-city neighborhood for worker's housing.

4. Essays on the history of these buildings in Ostiense may be found in Enrica Torelli Landini (ed), *Roma, Memorie della città industriale: Storia e riuso di fabbriche e servizi nei primi quartieri produttivi* (Rome: Palombi, 2007).
5. Emilio Saffi, "Il nuovo Mercato generale di Roma," *Annali della Società degli ingegneri e degli architetti italiani* 29, no. 12 (1914).
6. Mario Terlizzi, "I Mercati Generali," *Capitolium* 32, no. 12 (1957): 49.
7. Scholarship on Les Halles is vast. On its architecture, see Christopher Curtis Mead, *Making Modern Paris: Victor Baltard's Central Markets and the Urban Practice of Architecture* (University Park: Pennsylvania State University Press, 2012); and Meredith TenHoor, "Architecture and Biopolitics at Les Halles," *French Politics, Culture and Society* 25, no. 2 (2007): 73–92. On the social history of Les Halles, see, for example, Steven L. Kaplan, *Provisioning Paris: Merchants and Millers in the Grain and Flour Trade* (Ithaca: Cornell University Press, 1984), and Victoria E. Thompson, *The Virtuous Marketplace: Women and Men, Money and Politics in Paris, 1830–1870* (Baltimore: Johns Hopkins University Press, 2000).
8. For a comparison of Italian market halls at the turn of the nineteenth and twentieth centuries, including a section on the structures in Turin and Florence, see Filippo De Pieri, "Mercados cubiertos en la Italia liberal: Una comparación entre cuatro ciudades," *Hacer ciudad a través de los mercados. Europa, siglos XIX y XX*, ed. Manuel Guàrdia and José Luis Oyón (Barcelona: Ajuntament de Barcelona / Institut de Cultura de Barcelona / Museu d'Història de Barcelona, 2010), 197–232. On the architecture of Turin's Porta Palazzo, see Rachel Black,

"The Evolution of a Market," in *Porta Palazzo: The Anthropology of an Italian Market* (Philadelphia: University of Pennsylvania Press, 2012), 25–45.

9. ASC, Contratti, prot. 1912, fasc. 5, tit. 2.
10. E.S., "Il nuovo mercato generale di Roma," *Rivista di ingegneria sanitaria e di edilizia moderna* 11, no. 9 (1915): 101.
11. ASC, Atti, 1919, vol. 3, seduta del 29 novembre 1919, prop. 42, 78–79.
12. The Wholesale Market only permitted licensed and registered vendors, either as producers or brokers, to sell inside. The regulations, approved by the deliberazione governatoriale n. 1176 on March 9, 1934, were outlined in *Testo Unico dei Regolamenti sui mercati* (Rome: Tip. Centenari, 1934). On where the selling occurred for local and extraprovincial produce, see E. S., "Il nuovo mercato generale di Roma," 101.
13. Alberto Manzi-Fè, "I mercati di Roma," *Capitolium* 3, no. 4 (1927): 170.
14. Filippo Cremonesi, "L'Amministrazione straordinaria del Comune di Roma nell'anno 1925," *Relazione del Reale commissario senatore Filippo Cremonesi* (Rome: Tip. Centenari, 1925), 193–95.
15. In papal Rome, the wholesale of chicken primarily took place in the Piazza della Pollarola near Campo de' Fiori. Due to increasingly unhygienic conditions at this location, the market transferred in 1876 to a private property near Porta Angelica. Prior to the market at Via Marconi, lamb arrived in Rome via railway and was sold directly at Termini station. Unlike the many rules governing the processing and vending of beef and pork, few regulations were applied to the slaughtering, sanitation, and commerce of lamb and chicken. The latter types of meat were allowed to travel to the city already slaughtered. *Annuario commerciale, geografico, statistico e amministrativo della città e provinciale di Roma per l'anno 1878* (Rome: Tip. Romana, 1878), 156–57.
16. Prior to the installation of the refrigeration system at the slaughterhouse, butchered meat, like wine, was stored in the caves of Monte Testaccio.
17. Comune di Roma, *Cinque anni di amministrazione popolare*, 1907–1912 (Rome: Tip. Centenari, 1913), 167.
18. The water from the Acqua Paola was for washing of equipment and sewage, and the water from the Acqua Marcia was for drinking and cleaning of foodstuffs. Comitato Pro-Roma marittima, *Roma marittima: Bollettino ufficiale del Comitato* (Rome: Tip. Artero, 1912), 6.
19. "Capitolato generale per l'esecuzione di due serbatoi in cemento armato nei nuovi Mercati Generali a via Ostiense," ASC, Contratti, via Ostiense, Rip. V, Div. III, prot. 1918, fasc. 3–4, 24/4, and "Capitolato speciale per l'esecuzione di un serbatoio in cemento armato nei nuovi Mercati Generali in via Ostiense," ASC, Contratti, Rip. V, Servizio Architettura e Fabbriche, Contratto Bazzani Augusto, prot. 1926, fasc. 2, 21/1.

20. On Rome's gas plant, known as the *fabbrica del gas* or the *gazometro*, see Michele Furnari, *La fabbrica del gas all'Ostiense* (Rome: Gangemi, 2006).
21. Named after the theorist on municipalization Giovanni Montemartini (1867–1913), the thermoelectric power plant was inaugurated in 1912. The building was designed by the engineers M. Carocci and I. degli Abbati under the supervision of Corrado Puccioni.
22. Manzi-Fè, "I mercati di Roma," 170–71.
23. On Italy's food rationing system during World War I, see for example, Matthew Richardson, *The Hunger War: Food, Rations and Rationing, 1914–1918* (South Yorkshire, UK: Pen and Sword Books, 2015), 170–212, and Carol Helstosky, *Garlic and Oil: Politics and Food in Italy* (Oxford: Berg, 2004), 39–62.
24. ASC, Atti, 1913, vol. 2, seduta del 25 giugno 1913, prop. 392, 437–39.
25. ASC, Deliberazioni del Reale Commissario, 1923, vol. 1, 13 marzo 1923, delib. 287, 271–72.
26. Maria I. Macioti, *Ernesto Nathan: Un sindaco che non ha fatto scuola* (Rome: Ianua, 1983), 111.
27. I use the spelling "autarchy" throughout this essay because I believe that it best reflects the fascist Italian concept of *autarchia*, which encompasses both autarky (a national policy of economic self-sufficiency) and autarchy (absolute sovereignty). This is also the spelling that the fascist regime used in its English-language materials.
28. ASC, Deliberazioni del Governatore, 1927, vol. 1, 28 gennaio 1927, delib. 570, 73–74.
29. Istituto Luce, *Roma: Scene dei mercati generali* (1932; Rome, Italy: Istituto Luce, 1932), newsreel.
30. See, for example, Paola Salvatori, *Il governatorato di Roma: L'amministrazione della capitale durante il fascismo* (Milan: Franco Angeli, 2006), 51 and 87–89.
31. ASC, Deliberazioni del Reale Commissario, 1924, vol. 3, 17 novembre 1924, delib. 1602, 466.
32. Lanfranco Maroi, "Prezzi di calmiere nell'Italia centrale," *Capitolium* 3, no. 2 (1927): 102.
33. On fascist Italian price controls, see for example, Henry S. Miller, "Techniques of Price Control in Fascist Italy," *Political Science Quarterly* 53, no. 4 (1938): 584–98; and Roman F. Pitt, "Government Price Fixing in Italy, 1922–1940," *Southern Economic Journal* 8, no. 2 (1941): 218–37.
34. ASC, Consulta di Roma, Verbali, December 5, 1935.
35. Archivio Centrale dello Stato (ACS), Partito Nazionale Fascista (PNF), Segreteria politica, Situazione politica ed economica delle provincie, b. 19, relazione di un informatore, August 25, 1935.
36. On November 23, 2002, Rome moved its food wholesale to the city's outskirts and established the Centro Agroalimentare Roma (CAR) in Guidonia.

37. "Mercati Generali," OMA, accessed December 15, 2020, https://oma.eu/projects/mercati-generali.
38. See for example, Giuliano Longo, "Mercati generali dell'Ostiense, I topi ci ballano e il progetto langue," *Cinque Quotidiano*, May 12, 2017, https://www.cinquequotidiano.it/2017/05/12/mercati-generali-ostiense-topi-ballano-progetto-langue/; and Daniele Autieri, "Grandi incompiute: Così Roma brucia un miliardo di euro," *La Repubblica,* March 12, 2017, https://roma.repubblica.it/cronaca/2017/03/12/news/grandi_incompiute_cosi_roma_brucia_un_miliardo_di_euro-160358721/.
39. See for example, "Roma, riqualificazione ex Mercati Generali: L'inaugurazione nel 2020," *La Repubblica*, September 22, 2017, https://roma.repubblica.it/cronaca/2017/09/22/news/roma_riqualificazione_ex_mercati_generali_campidoglio_inaugurazione_nel_2020_-176203832/.
40. See for example, Giuseppe Pullara, "Roma: Ex Mercati Generali di via Ostiense, la grande beffa," August 20, 2020, https://roma.corriere.it/notizie/cronaca/20_agosto_05/ostiensee-grande-beffa-19947554-d689-11ea-b09b-c444f41468ab.shtml.

Archival Sources

Archivio Centrale dello Stato (ACS), Rome, Italy
  Partito Nazionale Fascista
Archivio Storico Capitolino (ASC), Rome, Italy
  Atti
  Consulta di Roma
  Contratti
  Deliberazioni del Governatore
  Deliberazioni del Reale Commissario

Bibliography

Comitato Pro-Roma marittima. *Roma marittima: Bollettino ufficiale del Comitato*. Rome: Tip. Artero, 1912.

Comune di Roma. *Cinque anni di amministrazione popolare*, 1907–1912. Rome: Tip. Centenari, 1913.

———. *Testo Unico dei Regolamenti sui mercati.* Rome: Tip. Centenari, 1934.

Cremonesi, Filippo. "L'Amministrazione straordinaria del Comune di Roma nell'anno 1925." In *Relazione del Reale commissario senatore Filippo Cremonesi.* Rome: Tip. Centenari, 1925, 193–95.

Istituto Luce. *Roma. Scene dei mercati generali.* 1932; Rome: Istituto Luce, 1932. Newsreel.

Macioti, Maria I. *Ernesto Nathan: Un sindaco che non ha fatto scuola.* Rome: Ianua, 1983.

Manzi-Fè, Alberto. "I mercati di Roma." *Capitolium* 3, no. 4 (1927): 169–79.

Maroi, Lanfranco. "Prezzi di calmiere nell'Italia centrale." *Capitolium* 3, no. 2 (1927): 101–10.

Office for Metropolitan Architecture. "Mercati Generali." Accessed December 15, 2020. https://oma.eu/projects/mercati-generali.

S., E. "Il nuovo mercato generale di Roma." *Rivista di ingegneria sanitaria e di edilizia moderna* 11, no. 9 (1915): 99–101.

Saffi, Emilio. "Il nuovo Mercato generale di Roma." *Annali della Società degli ingegneri e degli architetti italiani* 29, no. 12 (1914).

Terlizzi, Mario. "I Mercati Generali." *Capitolium* 32, no. 12 (1957): 49–50.

Torelli Landini, Enrica (ed). *Roma, Memorie della città industriale: Storia e riuso di fabbriche e servizi nei primi quartieri produttivi.* Rome: Palombi, 2007.

CHAPTER 9

MODERNIZATION AND MOBILIZATION

Parisian Retail Market Halls, 1961–1982

Emeline Houssard

Introduction: Modernization through Reconstruction?

Covered markets appeared in the nineteenth century as one of the paragons of hygienist architecture, lauded for their concern with ventilation and impermeability and their rationalist approach to spaces and flows.[1] Studies published on Parisian ones since then have tended to focus mainly on Baltard's central market halls, known as the Halles de Paris,[2] but fin de siècle Paris was also home to twenty retail covered markets (figure 9.1), several of which were built earlier. Although these two architectural types belong to an overall supply network, their difference in function, based on the distinction between wholesale and retail trade, has led municipal authorities to almost systematically separate the design and management of retail markets from those of central or specialized market halls. In the early twentieth century, such covered markets became commonplace in Europe, often with very similar designs. However, the rise in self-service shopping and other types of commerce led to a gradual decline in footfall, also attributable in part to the poor upkeep of hall structures. Many such markets were demolished or partially converted. Elected officials in Paris often referred to their state of disrepair and numerous architectural projects were launched from the 1930s onward to rid the city of such "hideous buildings" from the previous century and provide more hygienic premises.[3]

Beyond their dilapidated state, the hygienist principles of their nineteenth-century architecture required modernization in light of technological and medical advances. Despite the introduction of penicillin in the 1940s, public health concerns in postwar Parisian public space remained essentially limited to the city's fight against "insalubrity,"[4] as measured by the number of cases of tuberculosis according to the Athens Charter.[5] As a result, public authorities considered that the healthiness of covered markets depended upon their complete reconstruction. This choice became strategic over the years, for

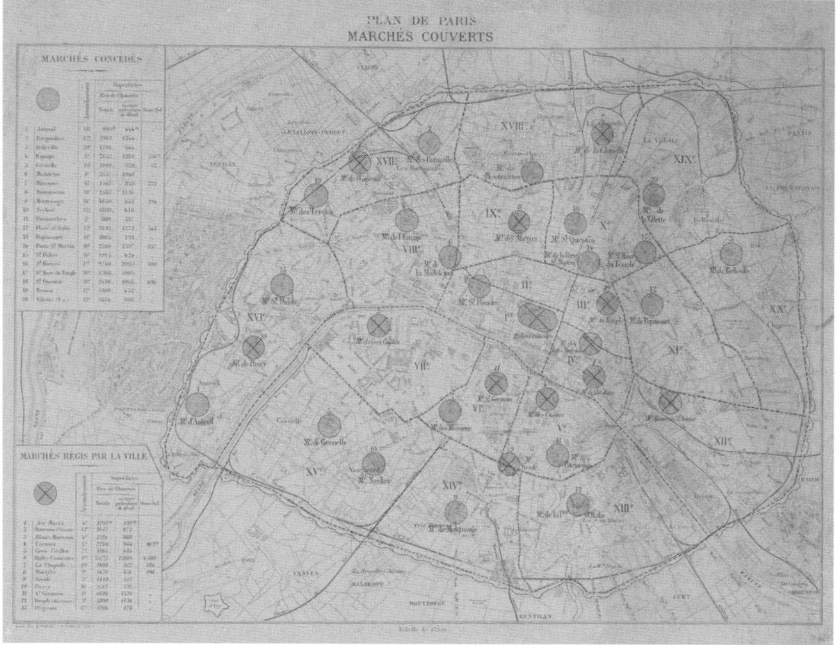

Figure 9.1. *Plan de Paris, marchés couverts*, ca. 1885, 1:25 000, 57,5 × 43 cm. Courtesy of Bibliothèque historique de la Ville de Paris (BHVP), Paris. File G 376.

these new buildings could easily integrate public facilities that were sorely lacking in some districts, such as day-care centers, gymnasiums, and municipal offices. One of the new means favored to ensure the salubrity of such buildings was the generalization of mechanical ventilation, which allowed the restrictions imposed by the natural ventilation of covered markets in the nineteenth century to be overcome.

In postwar Paris, fifteen retail covered markets were still operating, and there were even some signs of a renewed interest in the architectural type, with the reconstruction of the Passy (1st arr.) and Saint-Honoré (16th arr.) ones, located in two of Paris's upscale districts. Both projects had first been mooted long before but then constantly postponed and redesigned, in large part due to World War II. The Saint-Honoré market, designed by Abro Kandjian and Georges Dumont, took up the entire Place Saint-Honoré: it was a superstructure with a reinforced concrete structure and austere elevations as seen on the photograph and cross-section of figure 9.2.[6] Only four of its thirty-two thousand square meters floor area were dedicated to public facilities. The ground-floor market had nearly seventy stands in regularly spaced aisles with an offset central walkway that opened onto the car park access points.[7] Although the

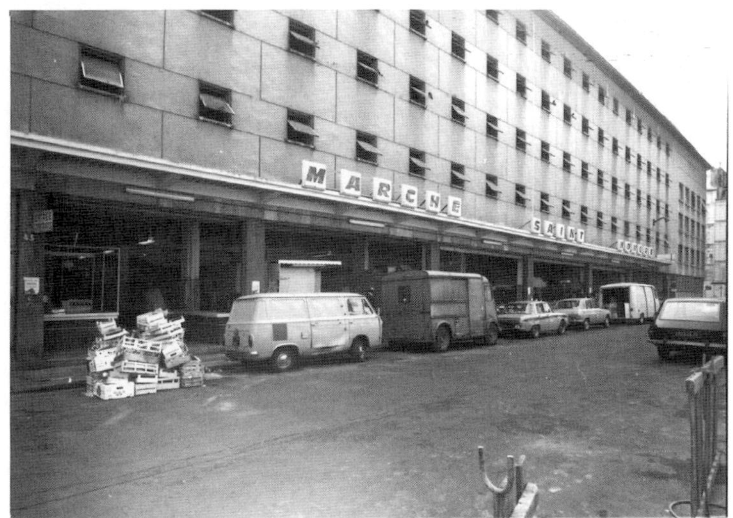

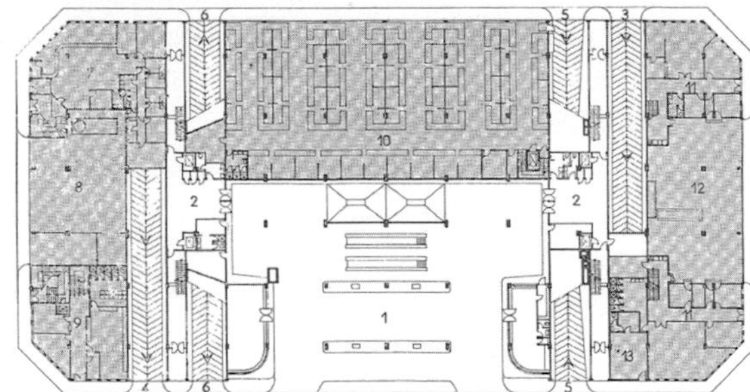

REZ-DE-CHAUSSÉE

En grisé : *Services Publics et divers*

1 - Station-service.
2 - Hall clientèle garage-parking.
3 - Rampe d'entrée du 1er sous-sol.
4 - Rampe de sortie du 1er sous-sol.
5 - Rampes d'entrée garage-parking.
6 - Rampes de sortie garage-parking.
7 - Poste de Police.
8 - Remise du service Nettoiement.
9 - Locaux du service du Nettoiement.
10 - Marché de détail.
11 - Locaux du Poste des Sapeurs-Pompiers.
12 - Remise des Sapeurs-Pompiers.
13 - Magasin.

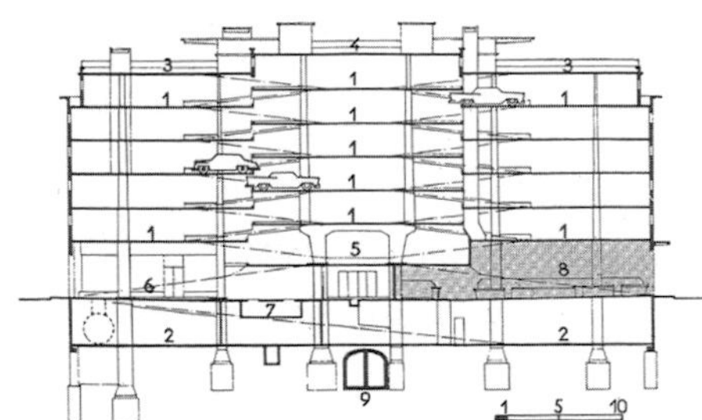

Ci-contre : COUPE TRANSVERSALE (partie centrale).

1 - Garage privé en étages et niveaux.
2 - Parking en 1er sous-sol.
3 - Parking en terrasse.
4 - Plateau d'évolution des Sapeurs-Pompiers.
5 - Premier niveau. Plateau de contrôle entrées et sorties.
6 - Station-Service.
7 - Fosses de graissage.
8 - Marché de détail.
9 - Galerie E.D.F. (existante).

Figure 9.2. Saint-Honoré market, 1955-1959. Above: View from the square, ca. 1975, Photograph, 23,9 × 17,7 cm. Georges Dumont, Abro Kandjian, architects. Courtesy of Direction de l'Urbanisme et du logement/Pavillon de l'Arsenal, Paris. Middle and below: First-floor plan and Section, in *Architecture française*, no. 187–88 (March–April 1958): 35, 38.

building was criticized and modified during the design stage,[8] it came to define the principal aspects of covered market design in the 1960s–1970s: a competition to select the architect, difficult negotiations with private companies to fund new public facilities, and reinforced concrete buildings, often exceeding the heights authorized by the current legislation, with a small ground-floor market. Indeed, during the *Trente Glorieuses* years that preceded the oil crisis in France, retail covered markets became key sites for large real-estate complexes that combined several types of facilities. As this period highlights the different fates of retail markets compared to that of the central Halles,[9] it allows us to redefine the architectural principles underpinning the typology of market design in contrast to supermarkets and shopping centers.

This chapter first demonstrates how French public authorities attempted to rethink the use and appearance of retail covered markets in the 1960s according to the renewed standards of public health. Then, it analyzes the various architectural and technical solutions that were developed in a number of multipurpose projects in the early 1970s in order to respond to these requirements. While this solution allowed for the integration of new social facilities, it also sparked a massive mobilization of protesters led by local heritage associations and a few personalities. Eventually, this chapter echoes the political response given to these protests and their impact on the modernization projects. Following the municipal reform and Jacques Chirac's election as mayor of Paris in 1977, hygiene and modernity tended to be tied to the old market structures, some of which were ultimately listed on the Supplementary inventory of historical monuments (ISMH) in 1982.

1961–1970: Reinventing Covered Markets for the Modern City

Attempts at a City-Wide Planning Vision and the Search for a "Formula for the Future"

The early 1960s were marked by attempts to develop an expansive program of modernization and construction across Paris, similar to what had happened in the nineteenth century. In March 1961, a prefectural decree established a consultative commission on covered markets in Paris.[10] As part of the development of the Plan d'Urbanisme Directeur (PUD) of the city, the Directorate of Economic Affairs planned twenty-two new markets.[11] The lack of specific directives for covered markets in the various documents that made up the PUD of 1959 meant that numerous projects were eventually included in detailed local urban planning programs, called Plans d'urbanisme de détail. Many of them considered the possibility of including covered markets at various stages of their design.[12]

At the same time, there were discussions on the functions and architecture of covered markets: the decade was marked by the search for a new modernity for this architectural type. Covered markets were initially presented as the natural heirs to open-air ones, held to be "outdated" in a city whose streets had been increasingly taken over by cars since the 1950s.[13] Most concerns centered around questions of hygiene. In 1961, the Directorate of Economic Affairs and Auguste Marboeuf, a city councilor for the Paris-Majorité party, presented a report aiming to define a number of basic principles for modern covered markets. Marboeuf argued that market halls were a solution to protect foodstuffs from dust, bad weather, or sunlight, and merchants from the cold or the heat, thanks to the roof and to modern "air conditioning."[14] The new buildings had to include between eighty and one hundred fifty stands depending on the local population density, on a footprint ranging between four and six thousand square meters. The site also had to offer parking for stallholders, telephone access, and even childcare facilities for shoppers. The aim was to rival self-service shopping by installing air conditioning, good lighting, and visible, well-lit, attractive signage while maintaining the advantages of market shopping—human contact and cheap prices.[15]

On the other hand, the councilors went back and forth on the issue of single- vs. multipurpose buildings. The minutes of the City Council debates record their uncertainties: in 1966, the Director of Economic Affairs was still discussing the possibility of "small established markets" and multipurpose buildings.[16] Their locations were not clearly stipulated at this point, even though the tendency was to go for a central position in the heart of block developments or green spaces.[17] Although there were some fears about how consumers would react to these "complex real-estate developments,"[18] this solution was preferred by the authorities due to the pressure from the property market, a lack of public facilities, and lower costs. At this time, the types of facilities gathered within multipurpose buildings still varied considerably. In 1961, some programs preferred the traditional association with housing,[19] while a new program combining a covered market and car park was put forward the following year.[20] The latter became "the preferred model" in the 1970s, despite concerns being voiced as early as 1963 by Bernard Lafay over the sanitary risk posed by the exposure of foodstuffs to car pollution.[21] Although this question gradually came to the fore during the 1960s,[22] it did not influence the development of the covered markets built in Paris during this period.

Moreover, the close relationship of market halls with automobiles was part of a longer tradition. In the nineteenth century, public authorities often created new streets around market halls to facilitate traffic, but this solution did not anticipate the development of cars and soon became inadequate. On the other hand, the economic failure of some markets allowed for their partial or complete conversion into parking lots or garages from the beginning of the twentieth century onward.[23]

The search for a "formula for the future"[24] was built on the Saint-Honoré and Passy markets, which were said to attract more shoppers than older markets,[25] but in reality several approaches were adopted: new markets were created as part of block renovation projects, while old ones on multipurpose sites were modernized. The City of Paris reached individual agreements with social housing landlords as well as private developers. However, only a handful of these numerous projects came to fruition. Indeed, many of them were competing for the same market,[26] which reflects an eagerness to fill large plots spread evenly across the urban fabric. From 1961 to 1970, three projects were completed and became the prototypes for subsequent reconstruction programs in the 1970s.

Detailed Urban Development Plans and a Single Prototype: The Riquet Market (19th arr.)

While most projects for covered markets within blocks were gradually interrupted in favor of other commercial spaces, the Riquet market was in fact built (figure 9.3). It was part of the detailed urban development plan for the Flandre-Riquet-Curial-Mathis block (19th arr.) and was approved by prefectural decree in June 1966.[27] Once completed, the program included not only a covered market, but also 1,816 housing units, a retirement home with eighty housing units, a nursery with occupancy for eighty children, a preschool with eight classes, a youth club with a swimming pool and gym, eleven thousand square meters of offices, five thousand square meters of shops, and eleven thousand square meters of green spaces.[28] An initial agreement was signed as early as 1962 by the City of Paris and the social housing company Foyer du Fonctionnaire et de la Famille (FFF).[29] The market belonged to the second phase of work on the block, following the retirement home. The Council of Paris was asked to collaborate on the program for the market in December 1966 and, budget restrictions notwithstanding, came up with a relatively ambitious plan for the "first truly modern covered market in Paris," choosing "the most attractive" option rather than "the cheapest."[30]

Following the deliberations, a building permit was quickly issued to Maurice-André Favette,[31] a modernist architect who had completed several social housing projects since the late 1950s.[32] The permit came with a brief note on the market, reflecting the ambition and care involved in its design and function. Favette retained the basic principle of a ground-floor market with housing on the upper floors, an association common since the nineteenth century (although Baltard himself had been opposed to it),[33] and widely used in

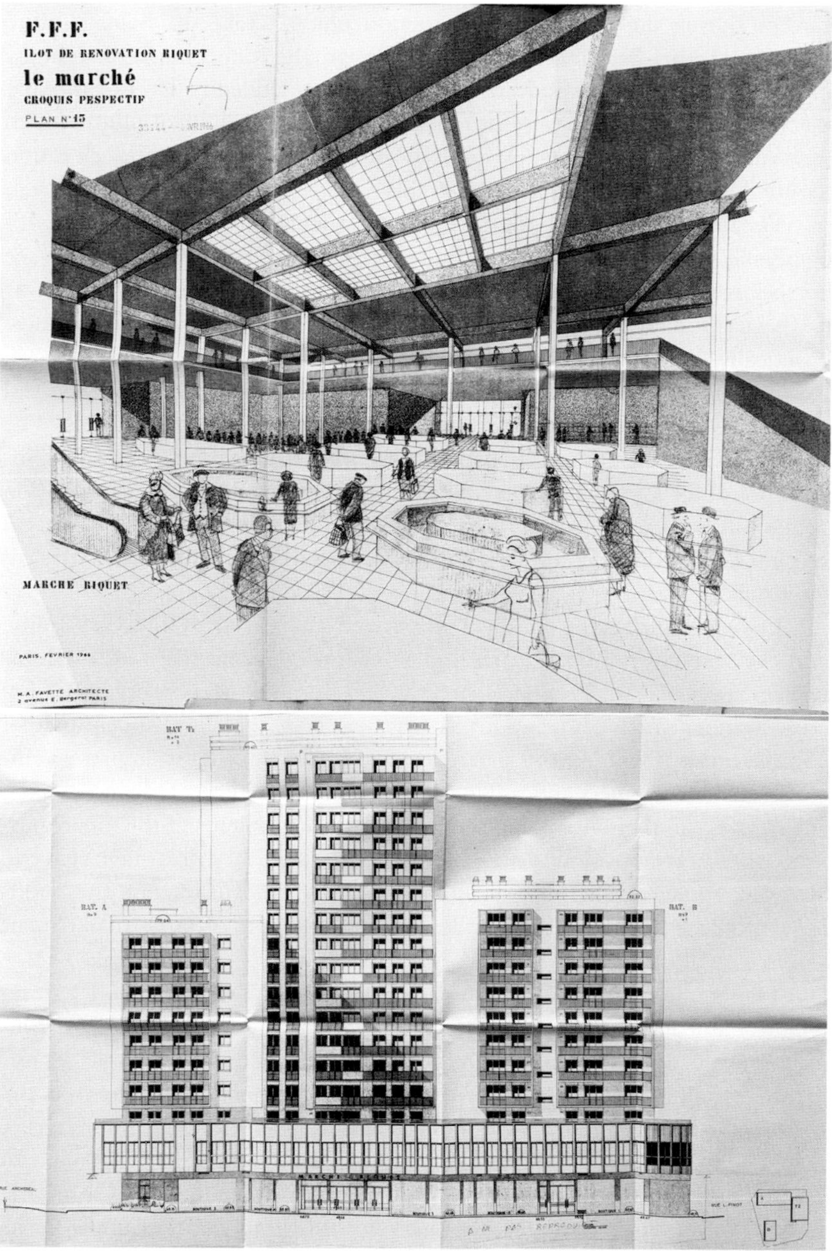

Figure 9.3. Riquet market, 1966-1972. Above: Perspective, 1966. Maurice-André Favette, architect. Courtesy of Archives de Paris, Paris. File 1178W 705. Below: Elevation, 1967. Courtesy of Archives de Paris, Paris. File 1178W 706.

Europe during the postwar reconstruction phase.[34] Like the Saint-Honoré market and other Paris markets of similar design, the Riquet market had housing on the upper floors—indeed, extra floors were added in 1971—but what made it really stand out were its volumes: a sort of individual plinth coifed with three blocks of flats of different heights, as seen in the elevation (figure 9.3).

The market's internal design ensured a hygienic and practical space, with octagonal sets of four stands each that were more accessible to shoppers (see perspective, figure 9.3). These ushered in a new kind of circulation in contrast to the traditional covered market design of rows of quadrangular stands, practically unchanged since the nineteenth century. On the other hand, Favette retained that period's hygienic solution of covering walls, pillars, and stands with washable and impermeable glass blocks and ceramic tiles. The market also included an aerothermal heat pump that ensured a minimal temperature of 14°C and provided the storage facilities with a wall insulation (while non-refrigerated stores were only wire-mesh insulated) and electrical refrigeration, which could regulate temperatures for different types of foodstuffs.[35]

In the meantime, the architect prioritized issues of accessibility, visibility, and the market's power of attraction in the urban fabric. It had three entrances and its façades, set back three meters from the street, were punctuated with independent shops to avoid "the sad, even 'desolate' appearance of covered markets without this particular feature."[36] In order to improve vehicle access for customers and stallholders alike, he also integrated a new street, rue Archereau, thereby solving one of the major problems of the older markets, where car accessibility was often very difficult.[37] At this stage, Favette also gave some consideration to illuminated signs meant to raise the building's profile from the outside, following the example of large department stores.

The Riquet market, as all later ones, was equipped with modern mechanical air conditioning and refrigeration. However, it did not deviate from nineteenth-century principles of hygiene, as it retained impermeable ceramic tiling for all surfaces. Despite the careful attention paid to the design of the market, the building process was nonetheless fraught with internal disagreements that saw Maurice-André Favette replaced by Martin Schulz van Treeck,[38] who reworked the program to incorporate the famous Orgues de Flandre tower blocks. In 1977, the market was held up as an example for its high levels of customer use.[39] However, defects in the flooring, roof lights, and water drainage system required substantial renovations from 1979 to 1981.[40]

The Lure of Private Developers: The Europe and Ternes Markets

The Riquet market was a totally different case from two other markets that were designed in the same period. Indeed, for the Ternes (figure 9.4) and Europe (figure 9.5) markets, the City of Paris worked with private developers and did not follow the traditional tendering process.[41] These companies took advantage of their previous involvement in the two nineteenth-century markets that were located on the same sites and had been partially converted into a garage and a car park in the first half of the twentieth century.[42] In this instance, the modernization lay in the choice of a mixed-use program for a large building, then in vogue in public architecture, rather than in the design of the covered market itself, which took a back seat. The two projects were shaped by major programs combining public and private facilities, principally car parks.[43]

In 1956, the Messine Automobile company, which already operated the parking lot of the former market, proposed a first reconstruction project. Several proposals followed without success until 1968–1973, when the project designed by Olivier Rabaud was finally carried out.[44] In addition to the market, which only occupied 382 square meters of the ground floor and received little attention in the architect's project (as seen in the ground-floor plan of figure 9.5), the program featured a car park, municipal premises, a nursery, a retirement home, and office spaces. Like the Saint-Honoré market, the new building accommodated

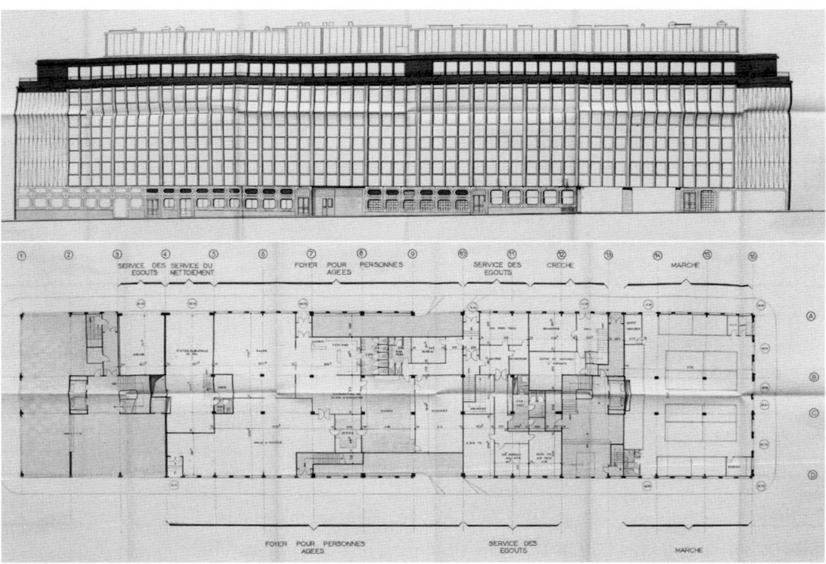

Figure 9.4. Europe/Treilhard market, 1968–1972. Elevation and First-Floor plan, 1970–1971. Olivier Rabaud, architect. Courtesy of Archives de Paris, Paris. File 2407W 7.

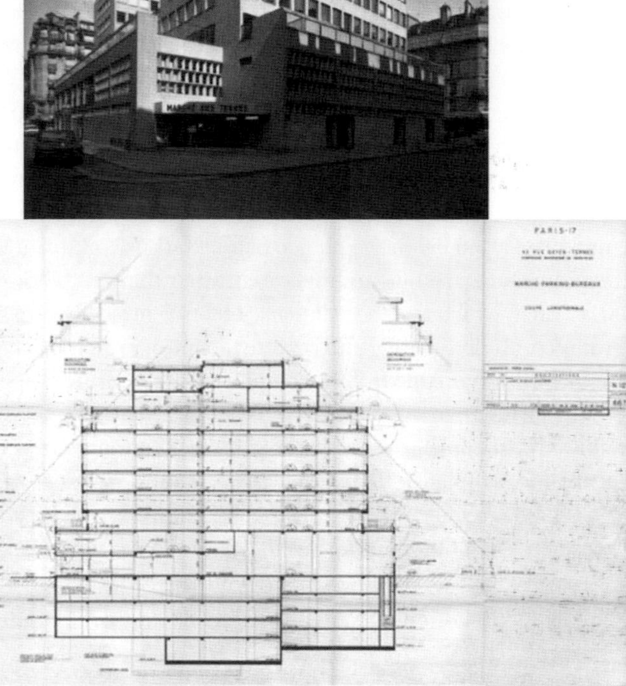

Figure 9.5. Ternes market, 1966–1971. Above: View from the rues Lebon et Torricelli, ca. 1975. Photograph, 23,9 × 17,7 cm. Courtesy of Direction de l'Urbanisme et du logement/Pavillon de l'Arsenal, Paris. Middle and below: Section and First-floor plan, 1968. Pierre Dufau, architect. Courtesy of SIAF/Cité de l'architecture et du patrimoine/Archives d'architecture du XXe siècle, Paris. File 066 Ifa 1149/1.

city departments related to sanitation and sewerage, as if the contracting authorities had seen a correlation between market and salubrity (see figures 9.2 and 9.5). Seen from the outside, the uniform appearance of the curtain walls was nuanced by the alternation of white ceramic cladding and rounded openings on the first level. Contrary to the Riquet market, the Europe market did not open onto the street through large openings and shops but appeared as a small part of a multiuse complex enclosed on its plot. The building, markedly different in design from the rest of the Haussmann-style neighborhood, was given a frosty reception.[45]

Building the Ternes market (17th arr.) took a similar amount of time, but for very different reasons. The Council of Paris profited from both the end of a rental lease in 1961 and the forthcoming end of the market concession to reach an agreement on the rebuilding of the market with a car park.[46] It started working with one company in 1963,[47] before the Compagnie parisienne des parkings (CPP) submitted a study to the city authorities later that same year.[48] On June 29, 1965, the city signed a lease with the CPP for a new building with a ground-floor market with storage space on the ground floor and the mezzanine, eight levels of office space, and four underground parking levels.

The first building permit was signed in 1966 for a design by Pierre Dufau. This was later revoked and a second permit was granted in 1968. As in the case of the new Europe market, the Ternes one played with the legal limits of height and volume, thus requiring several revisions and approval for breaching height restrictions. The agreement with the City of Paris left all the interior features up to the city and the 890.5 square meters of market space were delivered without wall finishes or internal partitions. Given the need to increase the budget to complete the interior, the offer was renegotiated in the spring of 1968 and the architect and his team installed openwork paneling in it.

The three markets built in the late 1960s thus reflect three different approaches employed by the Prefecture and the City of Paris to determine the most appropriate program and financial model to modernize market facilities. In the early 1970s, even before these markets were finished, they were used as examples to argue for or against the modernization program.

1970–1975: Implementing Multi-purpose Complexes and the Rise of Community Activism

Multi-purpose Complexes and Heterogeneity of Form

In the early 1970s, municipal authorities adopted the formula of the multipurpose complex, while at the same time striving to produce buildings of better architectural quality. Once again, they set out to establish broad guidelines for

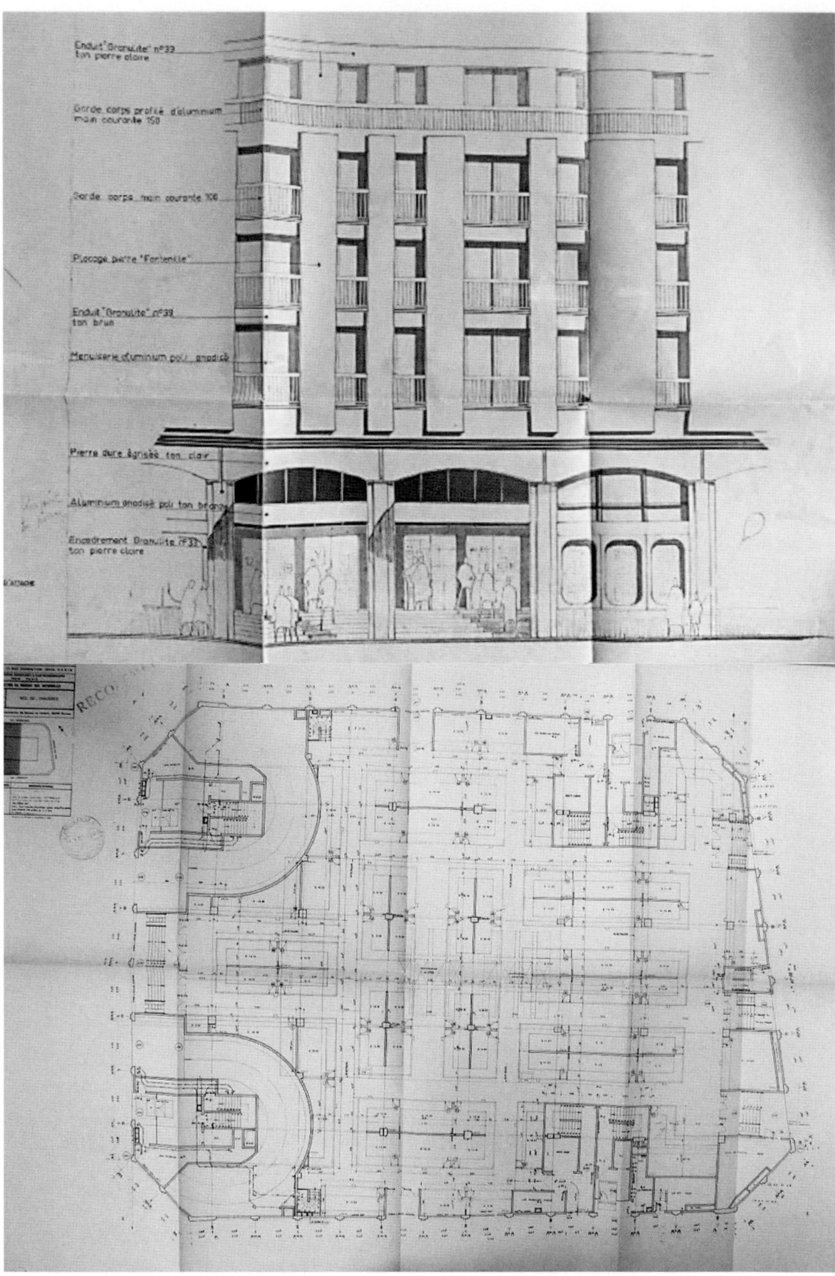

Figure 9.6. Batignolles market, 1975–1979. Elevation and First-Floor plan, 1977. Georges Massé, Fernand Roy, architects. Courtesy of Archives de Paris, Paris. File 1178W 2067.

the modernization of the old markets, thereby speeding up the implementation process. At the end of 1970, funds went into a study for the reconstruction of the Carreau du Temple market,[49] while the City Council discussed developer-led rebuilding projects for the Saint-Germain[50] and Batignolles ones.[51] In this wake, the Council of Paris received a memorandum on the Paris covered markets on November 25, 1971.[52] It summarized the city's recent achievements in building the five new markets of Passy, Saint-Honoré, Ternes, Riquet, and Europe and laid out plans for eleven additional markets at an estimated cost of two hundred and fifty to three hundred million francs. The memorandum only made a few solid recommendations, reflecting the city councilors' considerations on covered markets since the start of the 1960s. It referenced both the need to keep them open for locals and traders and doubts over their economic viability. While the memorandum welcomed the possibility of adding more facilities to the market plots, it did not come down firmly on either side of the issue of public financing or private developers.[53] As a result, the economic solutions chosen for later projects differed. Public funds fully financed market projects built in the city center, where the arrondissements were under the control of the council majority, such as Saint-Germain (6th arr.) and Carreau du Temple (3rd arr.). On the contrary, private developers funded such projects in less central areas, controlled by the council opposition, like Saint-Quentin (10th arr.) and Batignolles (17th arr.).

The Batignolles project (figure 9.6), designed by Georges Massé and Fernand Roy for the Moines-Batignolles property management company and Lemercier-Brochant LLC, proved to be a turning point: it was the last market rebuilt during this period. Modest in size, it combined a ground-floor market with housing, a senior citizen's club, and parking facilities.[54] Massé, who like Van Treeck and Favette had worked with Ginsberg on some ten projects,[55] offered a modernist reinterpretation of the arcaded building by playing on the polychromy of the wall-paneling.[56] The quadrangular block had four stories over the ground floor and four underground levels, with the sixty-stall market taking up most of the ground floor. The design featured four entry points, one on each façade, echoing the geometrical layout of the stands and perpendicular aisles. The levels were arranged around a central void so that the market benefited from zenithal lighting. There were also roof terraces as in the Riquet market. Massé provided a space for unloading merchandise in the basement, in order to avoid congestion on adjacent streets. He also included mechanical ventilation in masonry ducts and electrical access to each market stall and storeroom. Finally, Massé introduced floor coverings made of epoxy, an impervious component whose use began to spread in the 1960s.[57]

A similar approach was planned to light the market and reuse the roof at the Saint-Quentin market (10th arr., figure 9.7), designed by André Korniloff.

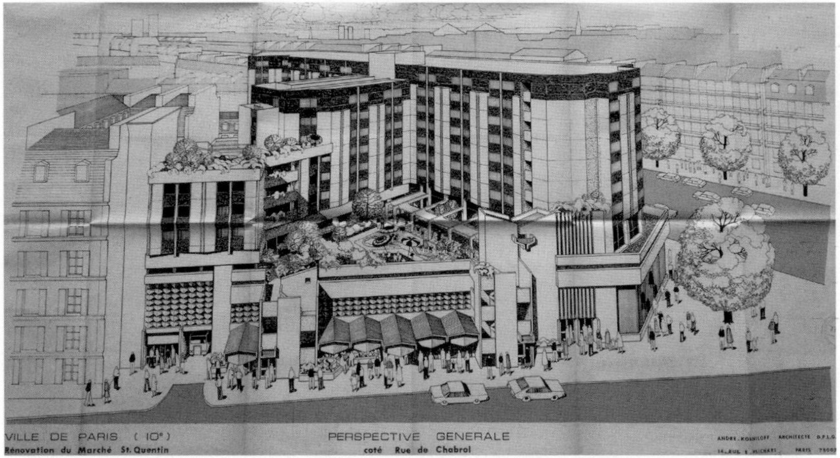

Figure 9.7. Project for the Saint-Quentin market (unrealized), 1974. Perspective. André Korniloff, architect. Courtesy of Archives de Paris, Paris. File 1178W 4217.

The project, which in the end was never built, was for a complex with a three-star hotel with three hundred and fifty bedrooms, a garden terrace, a restaurant, meeting rooms, a nursery, a sports hall, and parking for fifty-three vehicles.[58] Like the Ternes and Europe markets, this massive project also benefited from special waivers regarding its height and land use. It also proposed an involuntary synthesis of these earlier designs: the ground floor served as a base for the elevations, as in the Riquet market (figure 9.3), and the openwork partitions were similar to those chosen by Pierre Dufau to decorate the ground floor (figure 9.4). The latter contrasted with the vertical treatment of the elevations, according to the rhythms already seen in the Soissons hospital completed by Korniloff around the same time.[59] Indeed, Korniloff was mainly known for designing hospitals,[60] which made him the ideal candidate to ensure the hygiene of this building.

Almost at the same time, the Prefecture had applied for building permits for two covered markets that reflect the great gap between two generations of architects after May '68. On the one hand, the Carreau du Temple project (3rd arr.) is a monumental complex in a modernist and almost sculptural style commissioned from Louis Arretche (figure 9.8), who had attracted the attention of the jury during the Halles design competition.[61] In addition to the market, the project incorporated a nursery, a preschool, a gymnasium, a library, and a retirement home. The building, which had been refurbished several times, offered about sixty honeycomb-shaped stands in a very elaborate modernist style.[62] On the other hand, the Saint-Germain market (6th arr., figure 9.9) is the work of the young architects Pierre Colboc (a student of

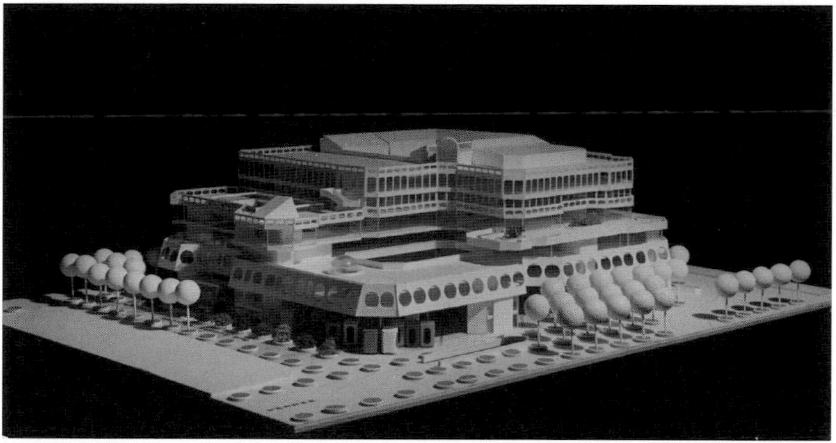

Figure 9.8. Project for the Carreau du Temple market (unrealized), 1973–1977. Model. Louis Arretche, architect. Photograph by Haphong. Courtesy of Académie d'architecture/Cité de l'architecture et du patrimoine/Archives d'architecture du XXᵉ siècle, Paris. File 258 AA 238/2.

Arretche),[63] Renaud Bardon, and Jean-Paul Philippon,[64] as well as Philippe-Georges Lamy.[65] Its hybrid design associating a new iron and glass structure to the old market façade, came rather opportunely at the point where one architectural trend was giving way to another. Indeed, this project stands between a radically new modernist approach and a return to heritage design.

The highly ambitious reconstruction project of the Saint-Germain market intended to emphasize its ancient structure, built in 1811 by the architect Jean-Baptiste Blondel, the last one from the period of the French Empire still in operation.[66] The project took an extremely long time to come to fruition, eventually being inaugurated in the mid-1990s.[67] Work began on pre-projects and studies in 1963 and the decision to rebuild was agreed upon in principle in 1970, combining the market with a swimming pool, a gymnasium, a service for children with special needs, a mental health center, a nursery with room for sixty children, and a senior citizen's club.[68] An anonymous competition open to architects across the Paris region was held, attracting forty-four submissions. Five winners were selected in January 1973, including very young architects who had not yet made a name for themselves, while leading architects like Guillaume Gillet were not chosen.[69] Once the results had been announced, an exhibition opened in the Saint-Jean Room at Paris City Hall, where another on Les Halles had taken place six years earlier.[70] Of the five winning designs, three kept parts of Blondel's arcades, while the others were deliberately at odds with the architecture of the market and the surrounding

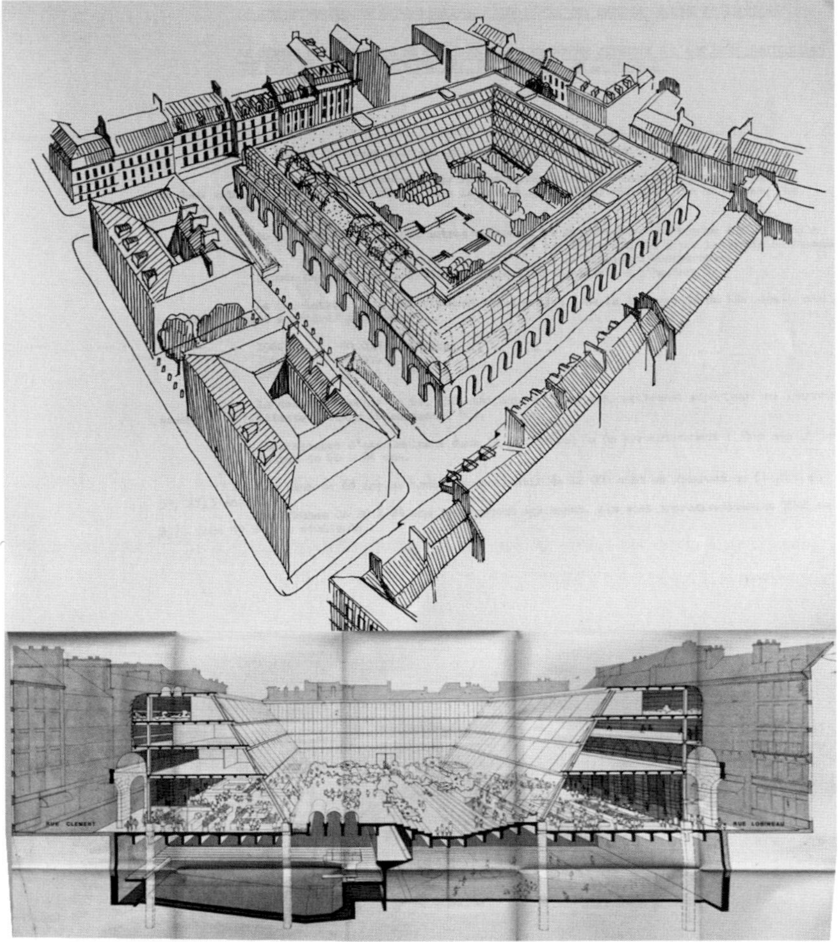

Figure 9.9. Project for the Saint-Germain market (modified and partly realized), 1972–1981. Perspective and Section, 1976. Pierre Colboc, Renaud Bardon, Jean-Paul Philippon, Philippe-Georges Lamy, architects. Courtesy of Archives de Paris, Paris. File 1178W 4273.

buildings. These differences reflect the jury's indecision after the Ministry was called upon to decide the market's fate in 1970 and put forward two completely different options—classifying the market as a historical monument or agreeing to demolish it "on serious grounds."[71] The terms of the competition only vaguely referred to "a design appropriate for a neighborhood protected by a number of measures under historical monuments and sites legislation."[72]

The winning project broke with the approach of earlier Paris market buildings by keeping all the external arcades: the metal and glass elevations formed a striking contrast with the original stonework while echoing the shape of the round arches below (as seen in the perspective of figure 9.9).

The market itself seemed to nod to self-service shopping by creating islands with a central void for the traders at their various stands. To ensure the preservation and cleanliness of the foodstuffs, each stand was provided with access to both water and electricity. According to Jean-Paul Philippon, the architects took only a passing interest in typologies of market design.[73] The explanatory note accompanying the building permit even stated that the specialist market furniture would be "low" to "preserve the transparency between the arcades and the inner courtyard."[74] Public health concerns remained essentially limited to the search for better thermal control of the building. The architects were praised for a less-polluting heating system, choosing tinted glass and steam-based district heating for the storage areas. However, the temperature of the market itself was to be regulated with highly consuming infrared heat lamps installed on each stand.[75]

Pierre Colboc had discovered advocacy planning in the United States and the importance of involving local communities in project development.[76] He and his team set out to develop the market's public face by bringing the inner courtyard of the Blondel market, which had been covered over in the early twentieth century, back into use and pedestrianizing some of the abutting streets. The idea of a "forum" was then fashionable in Berlin shopping centers.[77] The perspective generated new connections with Claude Vasconi and Georges Pencreac'h's Forum des Halles, whose façade borrowed the final 1976 version of the Saint-Germain market's round metal arch elevations. The various project managers also listened to traders to some extent.[78] At their request, they added a mezzanine for a new kind of self-service shopping that heralded today's cooperatives and direct sales.

The Rise of Community Activism

Faced with these new projects and the need to prevent their implementation, local communities, supported by public figures, formed protest groups. The argument went back and forth for many years, until eventually the Batignolles market was rebuilt, while the Saint-Germain and Saint-Quentin market proposals were thoroughly reworked, and the latter underwent several modifications from both users and commissioners.

In the 1960s, anxiety over the projects became palpable among locals. In 1962, a written question was asked to the city council about the alleged loss

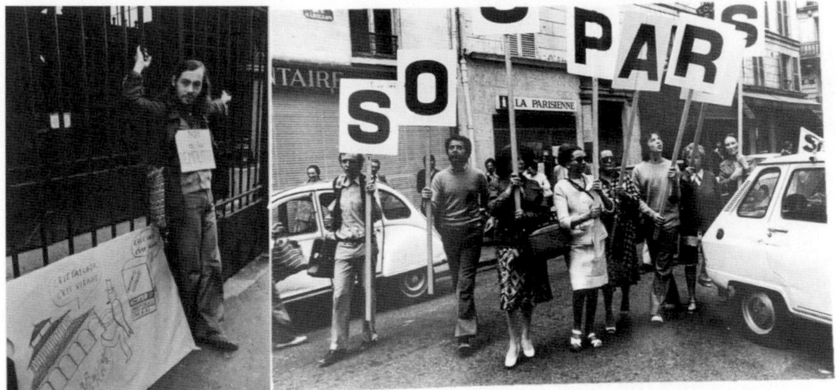

Figure 9.10. Left: Batignolles market. Demonstration by PSU activists in defence of the market, 1975. Léon-Claude Vénézia. Photograph, 18 x 24 cm. Courtesy of Bibliothèque historique de la Ville de Paris (BHVP)/Roger Viollet, Paris. File 80890-1. Right: *Marché Saint-Germain*, Demonstration, 1975. Photograph. Courtesy of Private Archives of Michèle Prouté, Paris.

of the Ternes market, to be replaced by a "supermarket." The rumor was denied by the Prefect for the Seine department,[79] but it nonetheless indicates that locals were taking an interest in the question and were keen to protect their traditional markets from the increasingly dominant self-service model. The first true signs of community activism began with a new reconstruction project for the Europe market. Although the mobilization went relatively unnoticed outside the local district, it was already soliciting a variety of appeals and arguments that were to be used ten years later against other market projects. The locals presented a petition to the local council on March 14, 1964. At the same time, the 7th arrondissement branch of the Union féminine civique et sociale and the nonprofit organization Vivre à Paris, founded just a few months earlier, sought to cancel the project on the grounds that it would threaten the neighborhood's appearance and architectural coherence.[80] Likewise, The Syndicat de Défense des riverains du marché de l'Europe was founded in 1964.[81] These different bodies distributed handouts, contacted the Ministry for Construction, and made use of the various urban planning and historical monument protection regulations to support their statements and invalidate the building permit, which had already benefited from a number of exemptions. Initially, they succeeded in cancelling the reconstruction, but in December 1968, the project managers and contracting authorities brought out a similar project which was quickly approved and completed in 1971.

However, this episode did not attract significant attention and it was not until the Halles de Paris scandal in the early 1970s that the issue led to major protests.[82] The same names spearheaded the movements against Les Halles and the covered markets—Michel Guy for the political authorities and André Fermigier for the intellectual and public spheres[83]—when some architects put forward projects for both Les Halles and retail markets, such as Louis Arretche and Pierre Colboc. Retail covered markets became a topic for debate in their own right,[84] regularly covered in the national and even international press.[85]

In the meantime, the main protests were driven by nonprofit organizations, many set up specifically to address the issue.[86] They proved highly effective, organizing demonstrations (figure 9.10), petitions,[87] studies by various experts,[88] press conferences and publications,[89] and even putting forward alternative architectural projects.[90] They were also supported by other nonprofit organizations such as the local-interest groups Comité des habitants du 3e arrondissement and SOS Paris and the heritage body of the Société pour la Protection des Paysages et de l'Esthétique de la France (SPPEF). With the help of lawyers,[91] they managed to suspend or even overturn several building permits for the Batignolles,[92] Saint-Germain,[93] and Carreau du Temple markets.[94] The protests often took a similar course but with differing motivations and results. Initially, activists protested against the terms and conditions of these projects—on the grounds of their privatization, their height, their density of use, and even their appearance—rather than against the demolition of old buildings per se. For instance, the Plateforme des associations de participation à l'urbanisme announced in 1972 that it planned to set up "information and activity centers for the local community" on the sites of covered markets scheduled for demolition and only criticized the participation of private developers in the case of the completed Europe and Ternes markets.[95] Later, the Association des habitants et des commerçants du 3e pour la défense du projet d'équipement socio-culturel et commercial sur l'emplacement du Carreau du Temple[96] argued against the proposals put forward to save the market by the Association Sauvons le Carreau du Temple, founded one year earlier.[97] Broadly speaking, these nonprofit organizations, working with local councilors favorable to their cause, rejected the Modernist architectural vocabulary that was fashionable in early 1960s supermarket design, including elements such as escalators, roundly criticized in the projects for Batignolles[98] and Saint-Germain markets.[99] Specialists lent their support to the criticism, such as André Fermigier's 1975 virulent article in *Le Monde* on the new covered markets in Paris.[100] Gradually, as the Halles were demolished, the movement to save original markets grew. Further, legal opportunities to revoke planning permission could also be seen as a factor.

In this context, the Association de défense du marché Saint-Germain-des-Prés is emblematic in a number of ways.[101] It was the first nonprofit organization specifically founded to save the market in February 1971, one month after the publication of Pierre Branche's article announcing the project.[102] The association organized an exhibition on the market, presenting the project designed by the firm Dynamique urbaine and its École Spéciale d'Architecture (ESA) graduate architects Alain Oudin and Lionel de Segonzac, in March 1972, even before the design competition was officially launched in October that same year.[103] In an article published in *Le Monde,* Pierre Branche had even suggested to the city that the exhibition should be held at the 6th arrondissement town hall rather than at Paul Prouté's art gallery.[104] Once the competition results were announced in October 1973, Michèle Prouté began to contact the historical monuments department to request heritage protection for the building. Her determination and extensive network put her in touch with the highest authorities, including the Senate[105] and even the president himself.[106] From 1971 to 1977, many requests were submitted to revoke building permits for the Saint-Germain, Batignolles, and Carreau du Temple markets, generating numerous changes of direction and stoking tensions between councilors, architects, and local inhabitants. Faced with the resonance of this conflict and in the electoral context of the mid-1970s, the debate on the future of covered markets became highly politicized.

1977–1982: Seeking Compromise and Supporting Preservation of Original Structures

Retail Covered Markets and Electoral Issues

The 1975 law on the reform of the administrative structures of the Paris region and the status of the city of Paris, followed by the 1977 election of Jacques Chirac as the new mayor, profoundly changed the debate around Parisian retail covered markets. From the mid-1970s onward, political parties, especially left-wing ones such as the Parti socialiste unifié (PSU), the Parti communiste (PC), and the Parti socialiste (PS) (figure 9.10), began to join nonprofit organizations and produce posters and handouts making the case for the preservation of the markets.[107] The focus of political debate on this question was evident at the time of the 1977 municipal elections. Several articles in *Le Monde* discussed the issue,[108] and Françoise Giroud, a candidate for the Giscard d'Estaing list defeated in the 15th arrondissement, attempted to destabilize Chirac by bringing up the Saint-Germain market.[109] The front-runners Michel d'Ornano[110] and Chirac[111] eventually included covered markets in their manifestos. A similar trend was apparent within specific arrondissements: when the 3rd arrondissement town hall changed hands, Georges Dayan, a Parti socialiste councilor, explicitly linked the result to the Carreau du Temple market.[112]

Jacques Chirac and the Art of Compromise

One of Jacques Chirac's first actions as mayor was to organize a "tour of the markets" to soothe tensions between councilors, architects, stallholders, and users.[113] He met traders from the Secrétan,[114] Carreau du Temple,[115] and Saint-Quentin[116] markets, as well as the architects of the project for the Saint-Germain market.[117] Facing criticism from his opponents, who held some forty seats on the City Council,[118] Chirac pushed the administration[119] and partners outside city hall,[120] seeking quick and efficient compromises. He often brought in local councilors, though some felt as if he was acting outside his remit.[121] The impact of the market defense associations led to a change of direction, with councilors now almost systematically referring to the opinions of market users and the organizations representing them,[122] demanding that users should be kept abreast of project developments to avoid challenges to the completed design.[123] Chirac initially lent his support to Paul Bas and the architects who came up with the winning design to rebuild the Saint-Germain market, while at the same time trying to persuade them to alter it and come closer to the defense organizations' requirements.[124] Compromise proved impossible and the project was reduced to the completion of underground levels with parking facilities and a swimming pool.[125]

With regard to the Carreau du Temple market project in the 3rd arrondissement, back in Parti socialiste hands, the decision to interrupt the work and cancel the entire project was taken in May 1977, despite the outlay for a temporary market structure that had only just been completed when the decision was taken.[126] Again, Chirac and the City Council as a whole tried to follow the needs of market users, who presented a white paper in 1976 arguing that Jules de Molinos's structure was "one of the market's major assets."[127]

The policy led to uncertainty for the Saint-Quentin market.[128] Following the setbacks of the Saint-Germain market, a less expensive design competition was organized to rebuild the Saint-Quentin market in 1978, taking the wishes of the traders into account.[129] The new rebuilding program had been launched prior to Chirac's election in June 1976. Six finalists were selected from one hundred and twenty-six entrants,[130] including Michel Duplay, François-Noël Deffontaines, and Ramzi Mahallawi, young architects who had taken part in the international competition to design the Centre Pompidou seven years earlier.[131] The finalists handed in their detailed pre-projects a few months later. Of the six projects, only two retained the original façades, including the winning

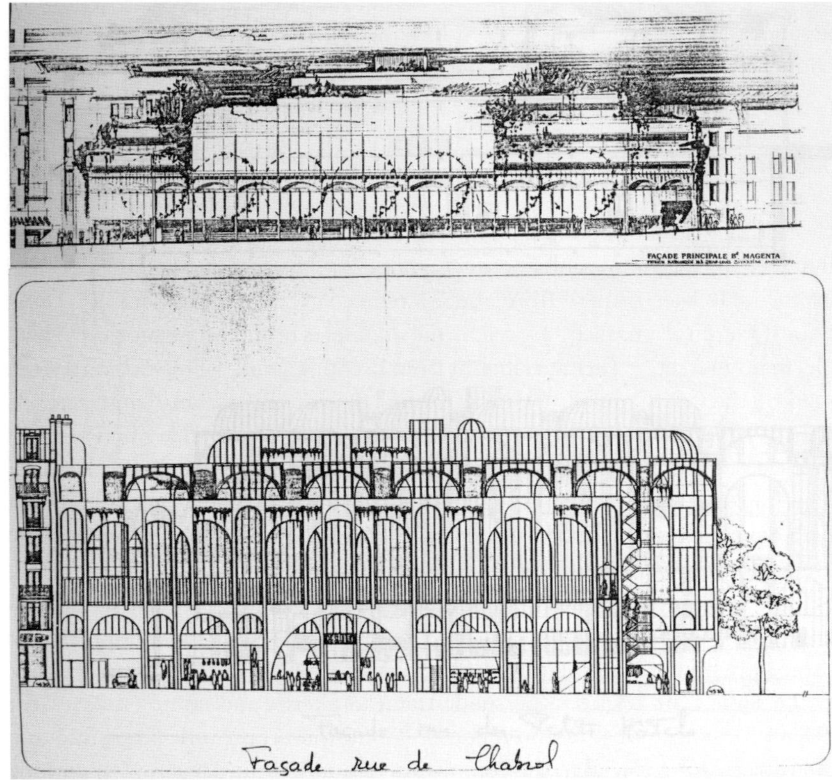

Figure 9.11. Competition for the Saint-Quentin market, 1977–1979. Above: Elevation from the Boulevard Magenta (10th arr.). Patrick Rabourdin, Jean-Louis Sivadjian (Winning Project), architects. Below: Elevation from the rue Chabrol, 1977. Michel Duplay, François-Noël Deffontaines (Third-Prize Winner), architects. Courtesy of Archives de Paris, Paris. File 1436W 85-1.

design by Patrick Rabourdin and Jean-Louis Sivadjian, which punctuated the curtain wall elevations with rounded arches and other sets of curves in dialogue with those of the nineteenth-century building (figure 9.11). In the end, however, the challenging economic climate meant that the project was canceled by the authorities, who took quite some time to communicate the decision.[132] A meeting with the fifty or so stallholders made it possible to accept the principle of a straightforward renovation of the façade. Given the lack of response from the authorities, the stallholders directly contacted the winning architect, Patrick Rabourdin, to establish a rehabilitation project. A few months later, and with a somewhat forced hand, the Paris city hall officially tasked Patrick Rabourdin with renovating the market, to avoid any further conflict with both users and architects.[133] At a cost roughly in line with earlier market rebuilds, the metal structures were renovated, the floor was lowered to street level to improve access, and goods lifts were added to bring stock up from the basement storage area. Electricity, water supply, and drainage were also completely overhauled and under-floor water pipes were installed for heating and to prevent freezing.[134] The architect, working closely with the local community, broke with the legibility of a regular, straight visitor flow typical of nineteenth-century covered markets and sought instead to create a more leisurely impression, giving shoppers the feeling of strolling around the stands. Indeed, from the 1980s onward, markets had come to be seen not only as places to shop for essentials but as leisure and even tourist destinations in their own right.

Market Rehabilitation and Heritage Enhancement

Following the major protests of 1975, the debate and decisions of the City Council tended to take the view that existing buildings should be maintained—though the planning process still proved convoluted. From December 1976, an initial study conducted by the Atelier parisien d'urbanisme (APUR) with a view to restoring the Secrétan market (19th arr.) was discussed by the councilors. Once elected, Jacques Chirac asserted a "comprehensive policy" for the restoration of the Parisian markets.[135] In 1977, work began on renovating the Carreau du Temple and Secrétan ones.

At the same time, the possibility of listing the various Paris markets as heritage buildings was studied from 1975 onward. On November 14, 1977,[136] the Délégation permanente et commission supérieure des monuments historiques approved listed status for the oldest and best-preserved markets with the aim of protecting a range of their styles. The Saint-Germain market, which had been partly dismantled, was listed by the Commission des sites in 1981. The Carreau du Temple one was listed on the Supplementary inventory of historical monuments (ISMH) by a decree dated January 14, 1982, followed on March 8 by the Enfants-Rouges, Beauvau, La Chapelle, and Secrétan markets. This even predated the listing of the Pavillon Baltard, which was moved to Nogent-sur-Marne, just east of Paris, on October 20, 1982.[137]

In 1982, Chirac commissioned his friend Clément-Olivier Cacoub to design a new project for the Saint-Germain market, which was supposed to respect the surviving original structure. The latter produced multiple designs leading up to the one realized in the 1990s. They were criticized by the market protection organizations and the Commission des sites, as a result of which Cacoub increasingly tried to hide the new additions beneath reconstituted brick roofs or in the old market courtyard. For unprotected markets such as Saint-Didier[138] and

Saint-Quentin,[139] the question of reconstruction arose in these years but was finally ruled out in both cases between 1979 and 1980 in favor of rehabilitation, as was also the case for the La Chapelle one.[140] Thus the late 1970s and early 1980s heralded a new chapter in the history of Parisian retail covered markets. Since then, the public authorities have been trying to preserve the nineteenth-century buildings,[141] which have undergone the necessary modernization.[142]

Conclusion

From the late 1960s to the early 1980s, Paris repeatedly tried and failed to develop a clear plan for its covered markets. During this period, one new market was created, five were rebuilt after their demolition, and another five were rehabilitated. These projects demonstrate the interest of public authorities for this type of facility: in Paris, like elsewhere, hygiene was strongly associated with the renewal of old buildings rather than the modernization of their structure. Following a broader trend in public architecture, these reconstructions gradually shifted from large, tall multipurpose buildings to lower-rise buildings, or even simple renovations of the original structure. Simultaneously, community involvement, media, and public interest reflected how fond Parisians were of their markets and their architecture, extending far beyond Baltard's Halles. Despite the setbacks faced by councilors involved in attempts to rebuild the markets, and though some of them were eventually listed on the Supplementary inventory of historical monuments, the 1990s saw what might be described as a resurgence of the past with the completion of the Saint-Germain and Saint-Martin markets, both modern pastiches that preserved elements of the original building. The most telling example, however, remains the Enfant-Rouges market (3rd arr.). A project to rebuild it was eventually canceled due to increasing public protests and the 1995 municipal elections that saw Jacques Dominati lose his position as mayor of the 3rd arrondissement. Today, the increasing number of *Inventer* competitions has brought retail covered markets back into multipurpose buildings, as evidenced by David Chipperfield's design for the former Préfecture Morland building, which includes a ground-floor covered market alongside nine other functions.[143]

Acknowledgements

I am grateful to the Centre André Chastel (UMR 8150) for the financial support provided for the translation of this chapter and the copyrights.

Notes

1. See the numerous monographs on covered markets, as for instance Préfecture du Département de la Seine, *Rapport sur les marchés publics en Angleterre, en Belgique, en Hollande et en Allemagne* (Paris: Vinchon 1846); Georg Osthoff, *Die Markthallen für Lebensmittel* (Leipzig: Karl Schotze, 1894); Marc'Aurelio Boldi, *Per i mercati coperti* (Turin: Bertolero, 1899).
2. With the exception of a few brief articles in specialist European journals related to the building in the nineteenth and twentieth century. See also Jean-Michel Roy, "Les marchés alimentaires parisiens et l'espace urbain du XVIIe au XIXe siècle" (PhD diss., Université Panthéon-Sorbonne, 1998). On the topic of hygiene, see Meredith TenHoor, "Architecture and Biopolitics at Les Halles," *French Politics, Culture & Society* 25, no. 2 (Summer 2007): 73–92.
3. "hideuses bâtisses," Conseil de Paris, Session of April 13, 1967, *Bulletin municipal officiel de la Ville de Paris* (henceforth *BMOVP)*, 86, no. 74 (April 13, 1967): 706.
4. Bruno Vayssière, *Reconstruction-déconstruction, le hard French ou l'architecture française des Trentes Glorieuses* (Paris: Picard, 1988), 56, 67.
5. Albert Levy, "L'impératif sanitaire dans la Charte d'Athènes (1933)," in *Ville, urbanisme et santé, les trois révolutions*, ed. Albert Levy (Paris: Pascal, 2012), 160.
6. A similar design had previously been used for the municipal market in Hussein-Dey, Algeria, by the architect Dupin: see "Marché couvert à Hussein-Dey (Algérie)," *Architecture d'aujourd'hui* 11, no. 3–4 (1940): 56.
7. "Garage-parking du marché Saint-Honoré. G. Dumont et A. Kandjan, architectes," *Architecture française,* no. 187–188 (March–April 1958): 32–39.
8. Conseil de Paris, Session of July 5–6, 1956, *Bulletin municipal officiel de la Ville de Paris, Débats* (henceforth *BMOVP Débats)* 76, no. 13 (July 18, 1956): 663.
9. On this subject, see for instance Meredith Tenhoor, "Markets and the Food Landscape in France, 1940–72," in *Food and the City: Histories of Culture and Cultivation,* ed. Dorothée Imbert (Cambridge, MA: Harvard University Press, 2015).
10. Conseil de Paris, First extraordinary session of 1965, April 8–9, 1965, *BMOVP Débats* 85, no. 4 (April 21, 1965): 35.
11. They are located across Paris in the 5th, 9th, 11th, 13th, 14th, 15th, 16th, 17th, 18th, and 20th arrondissement. See Conseil de Paris, Session of March 9, 1961, *BMOVP Débats* 81, no. 2 (March 18, 1961): 36–37.
12. These include the block developments, called *ilôts*, at Saint-Eloi (12th arr.), no. 13 (17th arr.), Plaisance (14th arr.), Gros-Boulainvilliers (16th arr.), passage Thiéré (11th arr.), later, Lahire (13th arr.), and Saint-Blaise (20th arr.). See, respectively, Conseil de Paris, Session of July 8, 1960, *BMOVP Débats* 80, no. 12ter (July 25, 1960): 552–57; Conseil de Paris, Session of July 6–7, 1961, *BMOVP Débats* 81, no. 13bis (July 25, 1961): 544; Conseil de Paris, Session of

December 14, 1961, *BMOVP Débats* 81, no. 25 (December 29, 1961): 1044; Conseil de Paris, Session of April 4–5, 1963, *BMOVP Débats* 83, no. 16 (April 19, 1963): 548–52; Conseil de Paris, Session of December 8, 1966, *BMOVP Débats* 86, no. 24 (December 24, 1966): 944; Conseil de Paris, Session of July 6, 1967, *BMOVP Débats* 87, no. 10bis (July 26, 1967): 417–20. It was eventually replaced by a street market, *BMOVP Débats* 90, no. 37 (January 28, 1971): 1517; Conseil de Paris, Session of July 6, 1967, BMOVP Débats 87, no. 10bis (July 26, 1967): 421–26.

13. Mathieu Flonneau, "Rouler dans la ville. Automobilisme et démocratisation de la cité: Surprenants équilibres parisiens pendant les 'Trente Glorieuses'," *Articulo, Journal of Urban Research*, special issue no. 1 (2009).
14. Conseil de Paris, Session of March 9, 1961, *BMOVP Débats* 81, no. 2 (March 18, 1961): 36–37.
15. In France, self-service chains such as Leclerc began to replace local stores at the end of the 1940s. In Paris, the first supermarket opened in 1957. See Alain Chatriot, Marie-Emmanuelle Chessel, "L'histoire de la distribution: Un chantier inachevé," *Histoire, économie et société* 25, no. 1 (2006): 75.
16. "hallettes fixes," Conseil de Paris, Session of December 8, 1966, *BMOVP Débats* 86, no. 24 (December 24, 1966): 943.
17. Conseil de Paris, Session of December 8, 1966, *BMOVP Débats* 86, no. 24 (December 24, 1966): 941.
18. "ensembles immobiliers complexes," Conseil de Paris, Session of April 13, 1967, *BMOVP* 86, no. 74 (April 13, 1967): 706–07.
19. Conseil de Paris, Session of March 9, 1961, *BMOVP Débats* 81, no. 2 (March 18, 1961): 36.
20. Conseil de Paris, Session of April 11, 1962, *BMOVP* 81, no. 83 (April 11, 1962): 946.
21. Conseil de Paris, Session of July 11–12, 1963, *BMOVP Débats* 83, no. 23bis (July 26, 1963): 919.
22. See Stéphane Frioux, "La pollution de l'air, un mal nécessaire? La gestion du problème durant les 'Trentes polluеuses,'" in *Une autre histoire des "Trentes Glorieuses." Modernisation, contestations et pollutions dans la France d'après-guerre*, 2nd ed, ed. Céline Pessis, Sezin Topçu, and Christophe Bonneuil (Paris: La Découverte, 2015), 99–115.
23. Subsequently, in 1917, a report considered turning all Parisian covered markets into car parks and garages in response to the rapid increase in car use in the city. The proposal was rejected, since the author considered the nineteenth-century buildings to be too cramped. See Conseil de Paris, *Rapport au nom de la 2e Commission, relatif à l'exploitation en régie des camions automobiles achetés par la Ville de Paris présenté par M. Fiancette, conseiller municipal,* annexe 2, no. 69 (July 11, 1917): 21, 26. Similarly, in 1961, a city counselor suggested raising each market to house

additional car parks. Conseil de Paris, Session of November 23, 1961, *BMOVP Débats* 81, no. 83 (April 11, 1962): 946.

24. "*formule d'avenir*," Conseil de Paris, Session of April 13, 1967, *BMOVP* 86, no. 74 (April 13, 1967): 706–7.
25. Ibid.
26. Multiple projects for various facilities were put forward for the same sites, for instance the Gros-Caillou market in 1964 and 1965, *BMOVP Débats* 84, no. 28 (January 23, 1965): 21 (minutes for 1964); *BMOVP Débats* 84, no. 13 (November 29, 1965): 422. In the 1960s, other reconstruction projects were considered for the markets Wagram, Batignolles, Carreau du Temple, Saint-Martin, Saint-Quentin, Secrétan, Saint-Germain, Aligre, La Chapelle, and Nicot.
27. Conseil de Paris, Session of December 22, 1966, *BMOVP Débats* 86, no. 28 (January 14, 1967): 1124.
28. Mairie de Paris, Direction de l'aménagement urbain, bureau des opérations d'aménagement, *Zones de Rénovation Urbaine, Programmation, État d'avancement des travaux* (Paris: n.p., 1988), 35–36.
29. FFF, now the Groupe Immobilier 3F. Conseil de Paris, Session of December 19–20, 1966, *BMOVP Débats* 83, no. 35 (January 9, 1964): 1430–31.
30. "premier marché couvert parisien vraiment moderne," "la plus attrayante," "la plus économique," although it did not choose to include a shopping arcade, Conseil de Paris, Session of December 22, 1966, *BMOVP Débats* 86, no. 28 (January 14, 1967): 1124.
31. Explanatory note, 1967, Building permit for the Riquet market, 1966-1981, File 1178W 706, "Dossiers d'autorisation d'urbanisme: permis de construire," 1963-1980 ("Permis de construire," 1963-1980), Archives de Paris, Paris.
32. Most notably for the FFF in Versailles and in Étampes, where he worked with Jean Ginsberg and Martin Schulz van Treeck. See *Chacun cherche son toit: Le logement social à Versailles du début du XXe siècle à la fin des Trente glorieuses*, ed. Corinne Hubert (Versailles: Archives communales de Versailles, 2011), Exhibition catalogue; and "Ensemble de logements 'La Croix de Vernailles', Étampes (Essonne)," 1965, File GINJE-B-65-01, vox 100 Ifa, Fonds Ginsberg, Jean (1905–1983), Centre d'archives d'architecture du XXe siècle, Paris.
33. Victor Baltard, *Complément à la monographie des Halles de Paris* (Paris: Ducher, 1873; repr. Paris: L'Observatoire, 1994), 138. Citations refer to the L'Observatoire edition.
34. A letter dated January 20, 1953, from the director of the Vienna Market Office to the Augsburg Market Office, Germany, demonstrates the interest in this postwar system, described on a study visit by elected municipal officials. "Markthalle VII, 7, Burggasse 78-80/Neustiftgasse," 1952-1974, File 1.3.2.641.106.A12, "Magistratabteilungen," Wiener Stadt- und Landesarchiv,

Vienna. Likewise, the Conseil de Paris was interested in a similar solution for the Pré-Saint-Gervais market, *BMOVP* 81, no. 2 (March 18, 1961): 36.

35. Building permit for the Riquet market, 1966–1981, File 1178W 705, "Permis de construire," 1963–1980, Archives de Paris, Paris.
36. "l'aspect triste et même 'désolé' des marchés couverts n'offrant pas cette particularité," Building permit for the Riquet market, 1966–1981, File 1178W 706, "Permis de construire," 1963–1980, Archives de Paris, Paris.
37. The plans included parking for five large delivery lorries, and the two first basement floors had loading bays for up to ten lorries at once and parking for thirty lorries. These features, which were not included in subsequent projects for the Ternes and Batignolles markets, proved to be crucial for good market performance. *BMOVP Débats* 98, no. 12 (November 10, 1978): 640.
38. The name Martin Schultz van Treeck appears on a description of the market project dating from 1969. See also Estelle Thilbaut, "Martin Schulz van Treeck: Les Orgues de Flandre 1967–1976, Paris 19e," *Le Moniteur architecture*, no. 116 (May 2001): 82–89.
39. According to Jean Diard, a Communist councilor for the 19th arrondissement, Conseil de Paris, Session of December 10, 1976, *BMOVP Débats* 96, no. 30 (January 17, 1977): 1461–63.
40. "Marché Riquet. Construction, ouverture, attribution des places, fonctionnement, problèmes divers," 1969–1982, File 85-7, Box 2, Dossiers d'affaires, 1436W, Archives de Paris, Paris.
41. Conseil de Paris, Session of July 6–7, 1964, *BMOVP* 84, no. 14 (July 21, 1964): 599.
42. Emeline Houssard, "Le destin des marchés couverts parisiens, entre obsolescence et renaissance, de 1883 à nos jours" (Master's thesis, Université Paris-Sorbonne, 2015), 28.
43. This was the sole angle taken by an article on the project published in 1963: Guy Muller, "Le Conseil municipal se prononce sur le tracé de l'axe nord-sud," *Le Monde*, June 25, 1963, https://www.lemonde.fr/archives/article/1963/06/25/le-conseil-municipal-se-prononce-sur-le-trace-de-l-axe-nord-sud_2231730_1819218.html.
44. Building permit for the Europe market, 1969–1973, File 1178W 1815-1816, "Permis de construire," 1963–1980, Archives de Paris, Paris. This little-known architect lived very close to the market
45. André Fermigier, "Les Batignolles avec le cœur en écharpe," *Le Monde*, June 14, 1975, https://www.lemonde.fr/archives/article/1975/06/14/les-batignolles-avec-le-c-ur-en-echarpe_2578027_1819218.html.
46. Conseil de Paris, Session of March 23--24, 1961, *BMOVP Débats* 81, no. 6 (April 10, 1961): 188–89.

47. Conseil de Paris, Session of July 11--12, 1963, *BMOVP Débats* 83, no. 23 (July 25, 1963): 901–02.
48. Hugo Massire, "Pierre Dufau architecte (1908–1985): Un libéral discipliné. Parcours, postures, produits" (PhD diss., Université de Tours, 2017), 3:338. I am thankful to the author for sharing his unpublished dissertation with me.
49. Conseil de Paris, Session of December 22, 1970, *BMOVP Débats* 90, no. 37 (January 28, 1971): 1497–98.
50. *BMOVP Débats* 90, no. 37 (January 28, 1971): 1494.
51. Conseil de Paris, Session of December 22, 1970, *BMOVP Débats* 90, no. 37 (January 28, 1971): 1497–98; Conseil de Paris, Session of November 20, 1970, *BMOVP Débats* 90, no. 24 (December 9, 1970): 1002–03.
52. Memorandum from the Préfecture de Paris to the Conseil de Paris and the Direction des Finances et des Affaires économiques, signed Virenque, November 25, 1971, "Dossier concernant les marchés couverts de Paris," 1964–1979, File 19860612/34, "Direction de l'aménagement foncier et de l'urbanisme," 1967–1980, Archives nationales de France, Pierrefitte-sur-Seine.
53. Ibid.
54. Building permit for the Batignolles market, 1976–1981, File 1178W 2067, "Permis de construire," 1963–1980, Archives de Paris, Paris.
55. Philippe Dehan, *Jean Ginsberg: la naissance du logement moderne* (Paris: Éditions du Patrimoine, 2019), 33.
56. He and Jean Ginsberg had already revisited an eighteenth-century private mansion at 19 rue du Docteur Blanche (16e arr.). Dehan, *Jean Ginsberg*, 68.
57. Building permit and certificate of conformity, 1976–1977, File 1178W 4417, "Permis de construire," 1963–1980, Archives de Paris, Paris.
58. Building permit for the Saint-Quentin market, 1974, File 1178W 4217, "Permis de construire," 1963–1980, Archives de Paris, Paris.
59. "Hôpital, Soissons (Aisne)," 1965–1975, File FORPI-G-65-2, Box 063 Ifa, "Fonds Forestier, Pierre (1902–1989)," Centre d'archives d'architecture du XXe siècle, Paris. Pierre Forestier, chief architect, André Korniloff, André Szivessy (Sive), Gérald Allée, Jean Péry, Paul Phelouzat, and Robert Lebret, architects.
60. Jean Lefèbvre, "André Korniloff, architecte hospitalier, 1934–1988," *Techniques hospitalières*, no. 512 (May 1988): 5.
61. Arretche was involved in the different stages of the project in 1967 and 1974 and designed the public garden in the late 1970s. See Dominique Amouroux, *Louis Arretche* (Paris: Éditions du Patrimoine, 2010): 178.
62. Building permit for the Carreau du Temple market, 1976–1977, File 1178W 4458, "Permis de construire," 1963–1980, Archives de Paris, Paris. It seems that this project has never been the subject of any real study, not even in the monograph by Renée Davray-Piekolek [et al.], *Le Carreau du Temple* (Paris: N. Chaudun, 2014).

63. Moreover, the Arretche and Colboc families were very close, according to Thierry Roze in "Louis Arretche architecte (1905–1991)" (Master Diss., Université Paris I – Panthéon Sorbonne, 1997: 5).
64. These are the future founders of ACT architecture.
65. Building permit for the Saint-Germain market, 1976–1982, File 1178W 4273, "Permis de construire," 1963–1980, Archives de Paris, Paris.
66. Of the original four, only the Blancs-Manteaux market, converted in the early twentieth century, remains today. Curiously, it was never mentioned by those in favor of rebuilding the Saint-Germain market or by advocates of the old market.
67. This can be explained in part by the changes in architectural approach brought about by the impact of May '68, the succession of three distinct presidents of the French Republic, the structural reform of municipal organization, and the evolution of urban planning rules with the new POS, voted in 1977 but applied in advance since 1974.
68. "service pour l'enfance inadapté," "centre d'hygiène mentale." The authorities also wanted to add a parking, a sports hall, and a meeting room and to improve road access. Pavillon de l'Arsenal, Photothèque de la Direction de l'urbanisme, numbers on the back of photographs 108649 to 108660, Competition program, on-site reconstruction of the Saint-Germain market and development of various public facilities, 1973.
69. "Planche de présentation du projet: coupes," "Marché Saint-Germain, Paris 6e," reconstruction," 1972–1973, File GILGU-F-72-04, Box 152 Ifa 163, "Fonds Gillet, Guillaume (1912–1987)," Centre d'archives d'architecture du XXe siècle, Paris.
70. The display then moved to the 6th arrondissement town hall for just under a month.
71. "pour des raisons sérieuses," Letter from Michel Denieul, Delegate Director of Architecture to the Prime Minister, to the Paris Prefect, 27 November 1970, "Projet de rénovation du marché, menaces de démolition," 1970–1973, File 1991/025/0002, Box 159, "Avis de Jean Trouvelot (1897–1985), Inspecteur général des monuments historiques sur des travaux Paris, Région Paisienne, Indre-et-Loire," Médiathèque de l'architecture et du patrimoine, Charenton-le-Pont.
72. "recherche appropriée à un quartier qui fait l'objet de diverses mesures de protection au titre de la législation des monuments historiques et des Sites," Competition programme, on-site reconstruction of the Saint-Germain market, and development of various public facilities, 1973, Photographs 108649-108660, Photothèque de la Direction de l'urbanisme, Pavillon de l'Arsenal, Paris.
73. Jean-Paul Philippon, interview with the author, Paris, March 4, 2020.
74. "afin de réserver la transparence entre les arcades et la cour intérieure," Building permit for the Saint-Germain market, 1976–1982, File 1178W 4273, "Permis de construire," 1963–1980, Archives de Paris, Paris.

75. The Compagnie parisienne du chauffage urbain (CPCU), active since the late 1920s, ensured the system.
76. Jean-Paul Philippon considers this theoretical reference to be essential for understanding both their project and their incredulity in the face of the virulent criticisms voiced by some inhabitants of the neighborhood. See also Pierre Colboc, "Advocacy planning: Échec ou réalité de la démocratie directe," *L'Architecture d'aujourd'hui*, no. 153 (December–January 1970): 34–37.
77. Especially the Steglitz Forum, which received widespread coverage in European architectural journals in the early 1970s.
78. Conseil de Paris, Session of March 21, 1975, *BMOVP Débats* 95, no. 9 (May 6, 1975): 429–33.
79. Conseil de Paris, Session of April 21, 1962, *Réponse à une question écrite, BMOVP* 81, no. 92 (April 21, 1962): 1035.
80. Conseil de Paris, Session of July 6–7, 1964, *BMOVP Débats* 84, no. 14 (July 21, 1964): 598–605.
81. An independent association under the law of 1901; *JO*, October 9, 1964, 9320.
82. This was to prove a reference point for both market advocates and opponents. Other examples fed into their respective arguments, such as Covent Garden Market in London and the Halles de l'île in Geneva.
83. Other public figures actively defended the Saint-Germain market in a letter to Michel Guy, May 20, 1975, signed by Ionesco, Leiris, Chastel, Levis-Strauss, and many others. Later, on April 27, 1985, the Association Suisse d'Historiens d'Art also wrote to the mayor of Paris and to the French president. Files about the Saint-Germain market, 1970–1986, Michèle Prouté Private Archives, Paris. Michel Guy and André Fermigier were both close to the Prouté family, which was very active in the Association de défense du marché Saint-Germain-des-Prés.
84. Some architectural journals published articles on this subject: Odile Fillon, "Bataille rangée pour les marchés couverts," *Créé*, no. 41 (May-June 1975): 64–69; "Reconstruction du marché Saint-Germain dans le 6e," *Techniques et architecture*, no. 317 (December 1977): 98–99.
85. For instance, almost one hundred articles were printed on this issue in *Le Monde* between the years 1971 and 1998. Thomas W. Gaehtgens, "Zerstörung des Marché Saint-Germain in Paris?," *Neue Zürcher Zeitung*, April 19–20, 1975, 61; "City and Citizens Battle over Fate of Historic Market," *Passion*, no. 45 (February–March 1986): 6.
86. A nonexhaustive list includes the Association de défense du marché Saint-Germain-des-Prés, founded in 1971, the Association de défense du marché des Batignolles, founded in 1975, and the Association Sauvons le Carreau du Temple, founded in 1976.
87. The first, organized by the Association de défense du marché Saint-Germain-des-Prés, received forty-five hundred signatures in 1972. It continued throughout

the 1970s and 1980s: each petition was authenticated by a bailiff. Files about the Saint-Germain market, 1970–1986, Michèle Prouté Private Archives, Paris.

88. For instance, the Compagnons du Devoir were called on to examine the wooden frame of the Saint-Germain market.

89. Comité des habitants du 3e arrondissement, *Livre blanc du Carreau du Temple* (Paris, 1976); Michèle Prouté (ed), *Le marché Saint-Germain* (Paris: Association pour la sauvegarde et l'embellissement des sites du marché Saint-Germain-des-Près et de Saint-Sulpice, 1980).

90. Projects by Oudin and de Segonzac for the Saint-Germain market, 1972–1976.

91. The first president of the Association de défense du marché Saint-Germain-Des-Prés, Gérard Lolivier, was a lawyer. Thereafter, Michèle Prouté and her entourage had their own lawyer to conduct legal proceedings.

92. Decree on the implementation of the building permit issued on 3 July 1975 for the Batignolles market, Conseil d'État, 2/6 SSR, March 17, 1976, No. 00756, unpublished in *Recueil Lebon*, https://www.legifrance.gouv.fr.

93. Implementation decree in July 1975, then cancellation for formal defects in January 1976 by the Tribunal Administratif de Paris, in Prouté, *Le marché Saint-Germain*, 21–22.

94. Jean Perrin, "La rénovation du Carreau du Temple, le permis de construire est annulé," *Le Monde,* February 12, 1977, https://www.lemonde.fr/archives/article/1977/02/12/la-renovation-du-carreau-du-temple-le-permis-de-construire-est-annule_3084663_1819218.html.

95. "des centres d'information et d'animation au service de la population", "Les associations d'habitants veulent 'reconquérir' les marchés couverts," *Le Monde*, March 10, 1972, https://www.lemonde.fr/archives/article/1972/03/10/les-associations-d-habitants-veulent-reconquerir-les-marches-couverts_2379893_1819218.html.

96. Declared on June 19, 1977, it represented locals and traders who sought to replace the Carreau du Temple market with a social and cultural center.

97. *JO*, July 29, 1976: 4640. Created in 1973, it supported the proposals and actions of the Comité des Habitants du 3e arrondissement: *JO*, December 9, 1973: 13091.

98. Conseil de Paris, Session of March 18, 1976, *BMOVP Débats* 96, no. 5 (April 29, 1976): 257–60.

99. Conseil de Paris, Session of December 20, 1973, *BMOVP Débats* 93, no. 31bis (January 31, 1974): 1469–70.

100. Fermigier, "Batignolles."

101. *JO*, February 27, 1971, 1997.

102. Pierre Branche, "Le marché Saint-Germain pourrait être remplacé par un ensemble immobilier moderne," *Le Monde*, January 13, 1971, https://www.

lemonde.fr/archives/article/1971/01/13/le-marche-saint-germain-pourrait-etre-remplace-par-un-ensemble-immobilier-moderne_2456865_1819218.html.

103. Both had devoted their graduation project at the ESA to the market; their new project was presented at the Paul Prouté Gallery after solicitations from the two architects. Alain Oudin, email correspondence with the author, April 28, 2020.
104. Pierre Branche, "Quand les riverains prennent en main la restauration du marché Saint-Germain," *Le Monde*, September 30, 1971, https://www.lemonde.fr/archives/article/1971/09/30/quand-les-riverains-prennent-en-main-la-restauration-du-marche-saint-germain_2447771_1819218.html.
105. According to Michèle Prouté, it was partly through her actions that Christian Langlois, architect attached to the Senate, proposed an alternative project around 1976. Files about the Saint-Germain market, 1970–1986, Michèle Prouté Private Archives, Paris.
106. Letter-petitions were sent to Valéry Giscard d'Estaing in 1975, Prouté, *Le marché Saint-Germain*, 21.
107. Michèle Prouté's private archives contain numerous PC, PSU, Union de Gauche, and PS handouts.
108. "Le marché Saint-Germain dans la bataille électorale," *Le Monde*, February 7, 1977, https://www.lemonde.fr/archives/article/1977/02/07/le-marche-saint-germain-dans-la-bataille-electorale_2876350_1819218.html.
109. "Le maintien de la candidature de M. Jacques Chirac à la Mairie de Paris. Mme Giroud, M. Chirac et le marché Saint-Germain", *Le Monde*, January 29, 1977, https://www.lemonde.fr/archives/article/1977/01/29/le-maintien-de-la-candidature-de-m-jacques-chirac-a-la-mairie-de-paris-mme-giroud-m-chirac-et-le-marche-saint-germain_3081390_1819218.html.
110. Michel d'Ornano wished to "systematically protect the covered markets," in "'La Bataille de Paris.' M. d'Ornano veut protéger les artisans et les petits commerçants victimes des opérations de rénovation," *Le Monde*, February 23, 1977, https://www.lemonde.fr/archives/article/1977/02/23/la-bataille-de-paris-m-d-ornano-veut-proteger-les-artisans-et-les-petits-commercants-victimes-des-operations-de-renovation_3084620_1819218.html.
111. Chirac wished to maintain the support of Pierre Bas and therefore took a more nuanced stance.
112. Conseil de Paris, Session of May 2, 1977, *BMOVP Débats* 97, no. 4 (May 23, 1977): 65–69.
113. "*tour des marchés*," ironic statement by Pierre Guidoni, a Parti socialiste councilor in the 19th arr.: *BMOVP* 98, no. 7 (July 18, 1977): 253.
114. Conseil de Paris, Session of May 2, 1977, *BMOVP Débats* 97, no. 4 (May 23, 1977): 65–69.
115. Ibid.

116. Conseil de Paris, Session of June 23, 1977, *BMOVP Débats* 98, no. 7 (July 18, 1977): 253.
117. Conseil de Paris, Session of November 7, 1977, *BMOVP Débats* 97, no. 13 (December 3, 1977): 574–75. Substantiated by Jean-Paul Philippon, interview with the author, Paris, March 4, 2020.
118. Marc Ambroise-Rendu, *Paris-Chirac, Prestige d'une ville, ambition d'un homme* (Paris: Plon, 1987): 11.
119. Bernard Billaud, one of Chirac's closest collaborators wrote a note to the Director of Finance and Economic Affairs dated July 20, 1979, testifying to the direct reports of the mayor and stallholders, at the Riquet market in this case, which lead to a decision by the mayor. Archives de Paris, 1436W carton 2, 85.7, marché Riquet 1969–82.
120. Chirac's surprise visit to the Secrétan market stallholders was heavily criticized by Henri Fiszbin, a left-wing politician and former candidate for the municipal elections. *BMOVP Débats* 97, no. 4 (May 23, 1977): 65–69. Similarly, Jean-Paul Philippon, a young architect at the time, admitted that he was taken aback by the request to modify the project for the Saint-Germain market and the addition of "stone." Jean-Paul Philippon, interview with the author, Paris, March 4, 2020.
121. *BMOVP Débats* 97, no. 4 (May 23, 1977): 65–69.
122. For example, Pierre Guidoni boasted that he was "in permanent contact with the Saint-Quentin market traders' association," adding that his colleague "Mr. Marcu, deputy of the 10th arrondissement, is in permanent contact with the association that was created between users and traders for the reconstruction of the market." *BMOVP Débats* 98, no. 7 (July 18, 1977): 253.
123. Conseil de Paris, Session of November 7, 1977, *BMOVP Débats* 98, no. 13 (December 3, 1977): 574–78.
124. Ibid.
125. "At that time, we did some hybrid projects that I'm not at all proud of, to try to meet this demand. Our project was coherent and it was quite difficult to falsify it in this way—even though we kept the principles, it was quite watered down. … This attitude was criticized, including by the Director of the APUR, Ligen, who criticized us for getting into this game." Jean-Paul Philippon, interview with the author, Paris, March 4, 2020.
126. Conseil de Paris, Session of May 2, 1977, *BMOVP Débats* 97, no. 4 (May 23, 1977): 65–69.
127. "un des atouts majeurs de ce marché," Comité des habitants du 3e arrondissement, *Livre Blanc*, 15.
128. After the building permit for Korniloff's project was revoked and while a reconstruction project was being drawn up, councilors were forced to approve urgent renovation work to keep the market open: Conseil de Paris, Session of June 25, 1975, *BMOVP Débats* 96, no. 14 (July 31, 1976): 761–63.

129. The competition did not require a highly detailed study at the first stage, since unsuccessful entrants were not paid. The prize panel only selected six competitors who had to draft a proposal. *BMOVP Débats* 98, no. 13 (December 3, 1977): 574–78; "Reconstruction du marché Saint-Quentin," 1977–1983, File 85-1, Box 1, "Dossiers d'affaires," 1436W, Archives de Paris, Paris.
130. Ibid.
131. *Projet soumis au jury du concours international pour la réalisation du Centre Beaubourg* (Paris: n.p., 1970), 136, 143.
132. The project was canceled in June 1979 and the decision was published in the 10th arrondissement journal before the architects were officially notified. The file also contains letters from several candidates urging the city to seek compensation. "Reconstruction du marché Saint-Quentin," 1977–1983, File 85-1, Box 1, "Dossiers d'affaires," 1436W, Archives de Paris, Paris.
133. The 1979 memorandum on the various rehabilitation options still considered the nineteenth-century structure unsuitable for a modern market: Ibid.
134. Conseil de Paris, Session of March 24, 1980, *BMOVP Débats* 100, no. 3 (April 17, 1980): 215.
135. "politique d'ensemble," Conseil de Paris, Session of May 2, 1977, *BMOVP Débats* 97, no. 4 (May 23, 1977): 65–69.
136. The Saint-Martin, Saint-Didier and Gros-Caillou markets were turned down from being listed. "Extrait du procès verbal de la Délégation Supérieure des Monuments, séance du 14 novembre 1977," "Paris 10 (Paris). Marché de la Porte Saint-Martin," 1975–1977, File E/81/7510/8-32, "Restauration des édifices de Paris (10e arrondissement)," Médiathèque de l'architecture et du patrimoine, Charenton-le-Pont.
137. In France, only a few market halls from the second half of the nineteenth century were listed before this date. These include markets in Sens, Nevers, and Dijon that were listed in 1975.
138. Improvement of the Saint-Didier market, 1979–1981, File 85-4, Box 2, "Dossiers d'affaires," 1436W, Archives de Paris, Paris.
139. Reconstruction of the Saint-Quentin market, 1977–1983, File 85-1, Box 1, "Dossiers d'affaires," 1436W, Archives de Paris, Paris.
140. Refurbishment of the La Chapelle market, 1983, File 85-6, Box 2, "Dossiers d'affaires," 1436W, Archives de Paris, Paris.
141. With the exception of the Saint-Martin market, rebuilt at the end of the 1980s.
142. As early as 1980, the Communist councilors were preoccupied with the project of rebuilding the Enfants-Rouges market and were already vehemently opposed to the idea: "Aussi veillerons-nous à ce qu'elle soit abandonnée," Conseil de Paris, Session of December 15–16, 1980, *BMOVP Débats* 100, no.12 (February 16, 1981): 931.

143. Pavillon de l'Arsenal, *Réinventer Paris: Appel à projets urbains innovants* (Paris: Pavillon de l'Arsenal, 2016), Exhibition catalogue, 400.

Archival Sources

"Avis de Jean Trouvelot (1897–1985), Inspecteur général des monuments historiques sur des travaux Paris, Région Paisienne, Indre-et-Loire." Médiathèque de l'architecture et du patrimoine, Charenton-le-Pont.

"Direction de l'aménagement foncier et de l'urbanisme," 1967–1980. Archives nationales de France, Paris.

"Dossiers d'affaires." Archives de Paris, Paris.

"Dossiers d'autorisation d'urbanisme: Permis de construire," 1963–1980. Archives de Paris, Paris.

Files about the Saint-Germain market, 1970–1986. Michèle Prouté Private Archives. Paris.

"Fonds Forestier, Pierre (1902–1989)." Centre d'archives d'architecture du XXe siècle, Paris.

"Fonds Gillet, Guillaume (1912–1987)." Centre d'archives d'architecture du XXe siècle, Paris.

"Fonds Ginsberg, Jean (1905–1983)." Centre d'archives d'architecture du XXe siècle, Paris.

"Magistratsabteilungen." Wiener Stadt- und Landesarchiv, Vienna.

"Photothèque de la Direction de l'Urbanisme." Pavillon de l'Arsenal, Paris.

"Restauration des édifices de Paris (10e arrondissement)." Médiathèque de l'architecture et du patrimoine, Charenton-le-Pont.

Bibliography

Ambroise-Rendu, Marc. *Paris-Chirac, Prestige d'une ville, ambition d'un homme.* Paris: Plon, 1987.

Amouroux, Dominique. *Louis Arretche.* Paris: Éditions du Patrimoine, 2010.

"Les associations d'habitants veulent 'reconquérir' les marchés couverts." *Le Monde,* March 10, 1972. https://www.lemonde.fr/archives/article/1972/03/10/les-associations-d-habitants-veulent-reconquerir-les-marches-couverts_2379893_1819218.html.

Baltard, Victor. *Complément à la monographie des Halles de Paris.* Paris: Ducher, 1873. Reprinted with preface by Patrice de Moncan, *Baltard, les Halles de Paris.* Paris: L'Observatoire, 1994. Citations refer to the L'Observatoire edition.

Boldi, Marc'Aurelio. *Per i mercati coperti.* Turin: Bertolero, 1899.

"'La bataille de Paris'. M. d'Ornano veut protéger les artisans et les petits commerçants victimes des opérations de rénovation." *Le Monde*, February 23, 1977. https://www.lemonde.fr/archives/article/1977/02/23/la-bataille-de-paris-m-d-ornano-veut-proteger-les-artisans-et-les-petits-commercants-victimes-des-operations-de-renovation_3084620_1819218.html.

Branche, Pierre. "Le marché Saint-Germain pourrait être remplacé par un ensemble immobilier moderne." *Le Monde*, January 13, 1971. https://www.lemonde.fr/archives/article/1971/01/13/le-marche-saint-germain-pourrait-etre-remplace-par-un-ensemble-immobilier-moderne_2456865_1819218.h%E2%80%A6.

———. "Quand les riverains prennent en main la restauration du marché Saint-Germain." *Le Monde*, September 30, 1971. https://www.lemonde.fr/archives/article/1971/09/30/quand-les-riverains-prennent-en-main-la-restauration-du-marche-saint-germain_2447771_1819218.html.

Chacun cherche son toit: Le logement social à Versailles du début du XXe siècle à la fin des Trente glorieuses. Edited by Corinne Hubert. Versailles: Archives communales de Versailles, 2011. Exhibition catalogue.

Chatriot, Alain, Chessel, Marie-Emmanuelle. "L'histoire de la distribution: Un chantier inachevé." *Histoire, économie et société*, 25, no. 1 (2006): 67–82.

"City and Citizens Battle over Fate of Historic Market." *Passion*, no. 45 (February–March 1986): 6.

Colboc, Pierre. "Advocacy planning: Échec ou réalité de la démocratie directe." *L'Architecture d'aujourd'hui*, no. 153 (December–January 1970): 34–37.

Comité des habitants du 3e arrondissement. *Livre blanc du Carreau du Temple*. Paris: Association pour la sauvegarde et l'embellissement des sites du marché Saint-Germain-des-Près et de Saint-Sulpice, 1976.

Conseil de Paris, *Bulletin municipal officiel de la Ville de Paris* (BMOVP). 81, no. 83 (April 11, 1962).

Conseil de Paris, *BMOVP* 81, no. 92 (April 21, 1962).

Conseil de Paris, *BMOVP* 84, no. 14 (July 21, 1964).

Conseil de Paris, *BMOVP* 86, no. 74 (April 13, 1967).

Conseil de Paris, *BMOVP* 98, no. 7 (July 18, 1977).

Conseil de Paris, *Bulletin municipal officiel de la Ville de Paris. Débats* (*BMOVP Débats*) 76, no. 13 (July 18, 1956).

Conseil de Paris, *BMOVP Débats* 80, no. 12ter (July 25, 1960).

Conseil de Paris, *BMOVP Débats* 81, no. 2 (March 18, 1961).

Conseil de Paris, *BMOVP Débats* 81, no. 6 (April 10, 1961).

Conseil de Paris, *BMOVP Débats* 81, no. 13bis (July 25, 1961).

Conseil de Paris, *BMOVP Débats* 81, no. 25 (December 29, 1961).

Conseil de Paris, *BMOVP Débats* 81, no. 83 (April 11, 1962).

Conseil de Paris, *BMOVP Débats* 83, no. 16 (April 19, 1963).

Conseil de Paris, *BMOVP Débats* 83, no. 23 (July 25, 1963).

Conseil de Paris, *BMOVP Débats* 83, no. 23bis (July 26, 1963).
Conseil de Paris, *BMOVP Débats* 83, no. 35 (January 9, 1964).
Conseil de Paris, *BMOVP Débats* 84, no. 14 (July 21, 1964).
Conseil de Paris, *BMOVP Débats* 84, no. 28 (January 23, 1965).
Conseil de Paris, *BMOVP Débats* 85, no. 4 (April 21, 1965).
Conseil de Paris, *BMOVP Débats* 84, no. 13 (November 29, 1965).
Conseil de Paris, *BMOVP Débats* 86, no. 24 (December 24, 1966).
Conseil de Paris, *BMOVP Débats* 86, no. 28 (January 14, 1967).
Conseil de Paris, *BMOVP Débats* 87, no. 10bis (July 26, 1967).
Conseil de Paris, *BMOVP Débats* 90, no. 24 (December 9, 1970).
Conseil de Paris, *BMOVP Débats* 90, no. 37 (January 28, 1971).
Conseil de Paris, *BMOVP Débats* 93, no. 31bis (January 31, 1974).
Conseil de Paris, *BMOVP Débats* 95, no. 9 (May 6, 1975).
Conseil de Paris, *BMOVP Débats* 96, no. 5 (April 29, 1976).
Conseil de Paris, *BMOVP Débats* 96, no. 14 (July 31, 1976).
Conseil de Paris, *BMOVP Débats* 96, no. 30 (January 17, 1977).
Conseil de Paris, *BMOVP Débats* 97, no. 4, (May 23, 1977).
Conseil de Paris, *BMOVP Débats* 98, no. 7 (July 18, 1977).
Conseil de Paris, *BMOVP Débats* 97, no. 13 (December 3, 1977).
Conseil de Paris, *BMOVP Débats* 98, no. 12 (November 10, 1978).
Conseil de Paris, *BMOVP Débats* 100, no. 3 (April 17, 1980).
Conseil de Paris, *BMOVP Débats* 100, no.12 (February 16, 1981).

Davray-Piekolek, Renée, Meunier, Florian, Charpy, Manuel and Simon, Philippe. *Le Carreau du Temple*. Paris: N. Chaudun, 2014.

Dehan, Philippe. *Jean Ginsberg: La naissance du logement moderne*. Paris: Éditions du Patrimoine, 2019.

Fermigier, André. "Les Batignolles avec le cœur en écharpe." *Le Monde*, June 14, 1975. https://www.lemonde.fr/archives/article/1975/06/14/les-batignolles-avec-le-c-ur-en-echarpe_2578027_1819218.html.

Fillon, Odile. "Bataille rangée pour les marchés couverts." *Créé*, no. 41 (May–June 1975): 64–69.

lonneau, Mathieu. "Rouler dans la ville. Automobilisme et démocratisation de la cité: Surprenants équilibres parisiens pendant les 'Trente Glorieuses'." *Articulo, Journal of Urban Research*, special issue no. 1 (2009).

Frioux, Stéphane. "La pollution de l'air, un mal nécessaire? La gestion du problème durant les 'Trentes polluеuses.'" In *Une autre histoire des "Trentes Glorieuses." Modernisation, contestations et pollutions dans la France d'après-guerre*, edited by Céline Pessis, Sezin Topçu, and Christophe Bonneuil, 99–115. 2nd ed. Paris: La Découverte, 2015.

Gaehtgens, Thomas W. "Zerstörung des Marché Saint-Germain in Paris?" *Neue Zürcher Zeitung*, April 19–20, 1975.

"Garage-parking du marché Saint-Honoré. G. Dumont et A. Kandjan, architectes." *Architecture française*, no. 187–188 (March–April 1958): 32–39.
Houssard, Emeline. "Le destin des marchés couverts parisiens, entre obsolescence et renaissance, de 1883 à nos jours." Master's thesis, Université Paris-Sorbonne, 2015.
Lefèbvre, Jean. "André Korniloff, architecte hospitalier, 1934–1988." *Techniques hospitalières*, no. 512 (May 1988): 5.
"Le maintien de la candidature de M. Jacques Chirac à la Mairie de Paris. Mme Giroud, M. Chirac et le marché Saint-Germain." *Le Monde*, January 29, 1977. https://www.lemonde.fr/archives/article/1977/01/29/le-maintien-de-la-candidature-de-m-jacques-chirac-a-la-mairie-de-paris-mme-giroud-m-chirac-et-le-marche-saint-germain_3081390_1819218.html.
Levy, Albert. "L'impératif sanitaire dans la Charte d'Athènes (1933)." In *Ville, urbanisme et santé, les trois révolutions*, edited by Albert Levy, 157–72. Paris: Pascal, 2012.
Mairie de Paris, Direction de l'aménagement urbain, bureau des opérations d'aménagement. *Zones de Rénovation Urbaine, Programmation, État d'avancement des travaux*. Paris: n.p., 1988.
"Marché couvert à Hussein-Dey (Algérie)." *Architecture d'aujourd'hui* 11, no. 3-4 (1940): 56.
"Le marché Saint-Germain dans la bataille électorale." *Le Monde*, February 7, 1977. https://www.lemonde.fr/archives/article/1977/02/07/le-marche-saint-germain-dans-la-bataille-electorale_2876350_1819218.html.
Massire, Hugo. "Pierre Dufau architecte (1908–1985): Un libéral discipliné. Parcours, postures, produits." PhD diss., Université de Tours, 2017.
Moncan, Patrice de, ed. *Baltard, les Halles de Paris*. Paris: L'Observatoire, 1994.
Muller, Guy. "Le Conseil municipal se prononce sur le tracé de l'axe nord-sud." *Le Monde*, June 25, 1963. https://www.lemonde.fr/archives/article/1963/06/25/le-conseil-municipal-se-prononce-sur-le-trace-de-l-axe-nord-sud_2231730_1819218.html.
Osthoff, Georg. *Die Markthallen für Lebensmittel*. Leipzig: Karl Schotze, 1894.
Pavillon de l'Arsenal. *Réinventer Paris: Appel à projets urbains innovants*. Paris: Pavillon de l'Arsenal, 2016. Exhibition catalogue.
Perrin, Jean. "La rénovation du Carreau du Temple, le permis de construire est annulé." *Le Monde*, February 12, 1977. https://www.lemonde.fr/archives/article/1977/02/12/la-renovation-du-carreau-du-temple-le-permis-de-construire-est-annule_3084663_1819218.html.
Préfecture du Département de la Seine. *Rapport sur les marchés publics en Angleterre, en Belgique, en Hollande et en Allemagne*. Paris: Vinchon, 1846.
Projet soumis au jury du concours international pour la réalisation du Centre Beaubourg. Paris: n.p., 1970.

Prouté, Michèle, ed. *Le marché Saint-Germain.* Paris: Association pour la sauvegarde et l'embellissement des sites du marché Saint-Germain-des-Près et de Saint-Sulpice, 1980.

"Reconstruction du marché Saint-Germain dans le 6e." *Techniques et architecture,* no. 317 (December 1977): 98–99.

Roy, Jean-Michel. "Les marchés alimentaires parisiens et l'espace urbain du XVIIe au XIXe siècle." PhD diss., Université Panthéon-Sorbonne, 1998.

Roze Thierry. "Louis Arretche architecte (1905–1991)." Master's thesis, Université Paris I – Panthéon Sorbonne, 1997.

TenHoor, Meredith. "Architecture and Biopolitics at Les Halles." *French Politics, Culture & Society,* 25, no. 2 (Summer 2007): 73–92.

———. "Markets and the Food Landscape in France, 1940–72." In *Food and the City. Histories of Culture and Cultivation,* edited by Dorothée Imbert, 333–58. Cambridge, MA: Harvard University Press, 2015.

Thilbaut, Estelle. "Martin Schulz van Treeck: Les orgues de Flandre 1967–1976, Paris 19e." *Le Moniteur architecture,* no. 116 (May 2001): 82–89.

Vayssière, Bruno. *Reconstruction-déconstruction, le hard French ou l'architecture française des Trentes Glorieuses.* Paris: Picard, 1988.

CHAPTER 10

FINDING FOOD AT TORVEHALLERNE

Market Halls in Copenhagen between Gastrosexual Consumerism and the Coronavirus Pandemic

Henriette Steiner

Torvehallerne, built in 2011 in the center of Copenhagen, comprise two large glass-covered food market halls. Boasting high-end produce, takeaway food, and cafés, the site has become a main hub for the city's booming foodie scene, catering to the "gastrosexual" consumer, a figure that has been on the rise in Denmark in recent years. In Copenhagen, the gastrosexual emerged alongside a booming restaurant scene—spearheaded by people such as Claus Meyer, whose restaurant Noma opened in 2003—in parallel with the city's economic upswing and its consumer- and livability-oriented urban restructuring since the early 2000s. According to the Danish Language Council, the term gastrosexual, *gastroseksuel* in Danish, first emerged in 2013 in Denmark to describe a person excessively obsessed with good food. The term also involves a play on the word "metrosexual," which during the early years of the millennium referred to heterosexual men who were obsessed with good looks and fashion—British soccer player David Beckham being a famous example.[1]

Until recently, Copenhagen might have been characterized as a gastronomic desert, where high-end produce and gourmet experiences were largely unavailable. But this has changed with the economic upswing beginning in the late 1990s, the emergence of the New Nordic food scene, and places such as Torvehallerne. A unique type on the Danish food consumption scene, food market halls have found a foothold, and other Danish cities now also wish to build covered market halls, or sometimes more specifically "food halls." Indeed, this trend has become so pronounced that we can speak of a "market hall effect" in Denmark: market halls have been built not only in cities such as Odense but also in less dense urban settings such as Bornholm, a tourist island that actively uses high-end food to attract visitors.[2]

These market halls have become the symbol of a new consumerist urban culture in Copenhagen oriented around the purchase of high-end food and produce. They provide a dense, lively environment wherein people flow in and

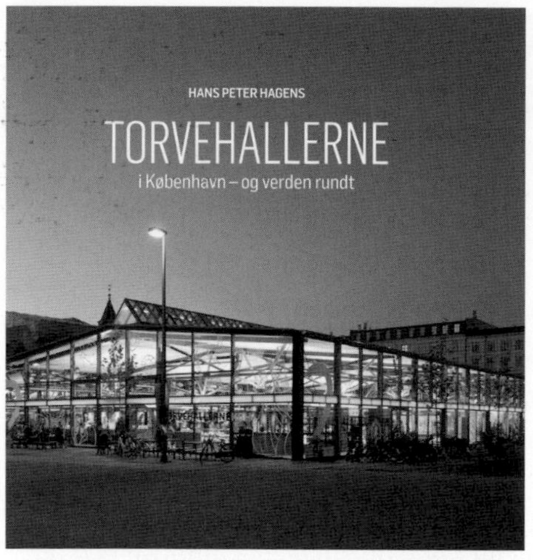

Figure 10.1. Torvehallerne pictured on the front page of a book by the architect. Courtesy of Strandberg Publishing.

out, flocking around the small restaurants and stalls. Even during the COVID-19 pandemic, when the government forced restaurants and some shops to suspend business in mid-March 2020, Torvehallerne remained partially open, as food shopping was considered essential. While the life of Copenhagen's city center temporarily slowed down and thinned out, the public space next to Torvehallerne was never quite deserted; nor was the market hall culture suspended. Denmark's lockdown measures (to date, in July 2020) never restricted people's movement outdoors, and it seemed to be business as usual around Torvehallerne, even if the flow of people was reduced and the dense gathering of large groups was prohibited. Speaking about the first year of the pandemic, its comparatively gentle impact on Denmark's culture and economy did not seem to diminish either Torvehallerne's gastrosexual consumerist culture or the urban livability paradigm.

This chapter investigates the recent architectural history of Denmark's covered market halls and their intimate links with a specific experience-oriented urban food culture and economic urban planning logic that belong to Copenhagen's most recent urban past. As an urban regeneration measure, Torvehallerne have arguably become successful at the cost of the more heterogeneous urban culture they displaced. Nevertheless, the chapter will consider what possibilities exist for civic life in the segmented twenty-first-century Western city, and the role of food—and indeed of the covered market hall as a type—in this process. It will also consider Torvehallerne's position in light of the recent restructurings of urban space due to the COVID-19 pandemic. At the time of writing it is not possible to draw any firm conclusions about whether Copenhagen's affluent new urban consumer culture will survive the economic and societal effects of the pandemic. But for the time being, Danish culture, and this site in particular, seems relatively unaffected. If the pandemic has been a time for cultural reflection, this new type of urban culture seems to have been deemed "essential."

History of the Site

Torvehallerne were built on a section of the former rampart area, a military zone outside the historical perimeter of Copenhagen that was largely undeveloped until the city's fortifications were decommissioned in the 1860s. In 1889, a large vegetable market opened on this site, and it remained an important commercial location until a larger market was constructed in the suburb of Valby in the late 1950s. Originally called Linnés Torv (Linnaeus's Square, after the Swedish botanist), in 1968 the site was renamed Israels Plads (Israel's Place) to mark the twenty-fifth anniversary of the events of October 1943, when the majority of Denmark's Jews fled the German occupation and escaped to Sweden. Nevertheless, for decades the site continued to exist only rather vaguely in the minds of the population, tucked away as it is behind Nørreport, one of the city center's busiest railway stations, which funnels people primarily into the large pedestrian shopping streets of Copenhagen's medieval core, rather than in the direction of Israels Plads. Subsequently, Torvehallerne opened in 2011, and in 2015 the rest of the square was renovated into a combined playground, ballpark, skater zone, and recreation area. Since then, the vagueness and obscurity of the area has been replaced by a strong paradigm of quality food consumption and urban life in general.

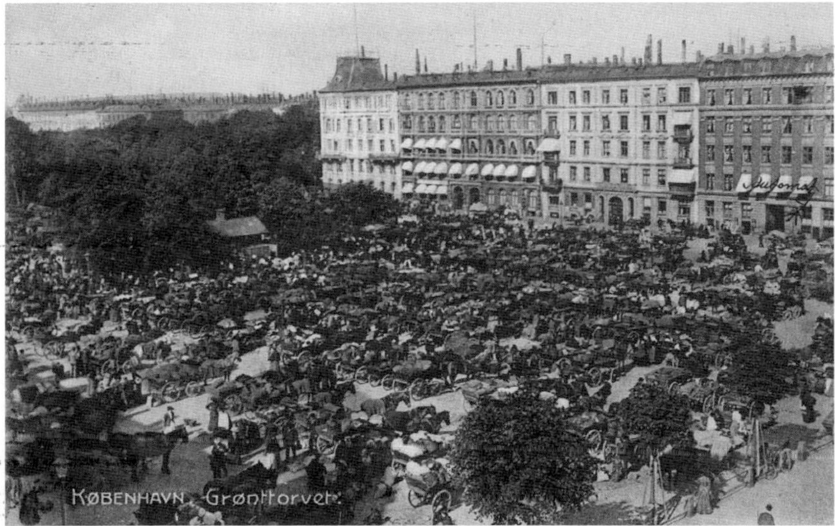

Figure 10.2. The vegetable market on Grønttorvet, Copenhagen, 5 October 1963. Photographer unknown. Courtesy of Mogens Falk-Sørensen, Stadsarkivets fotografiske Atelier, Copenhagen City Archives, 6854.

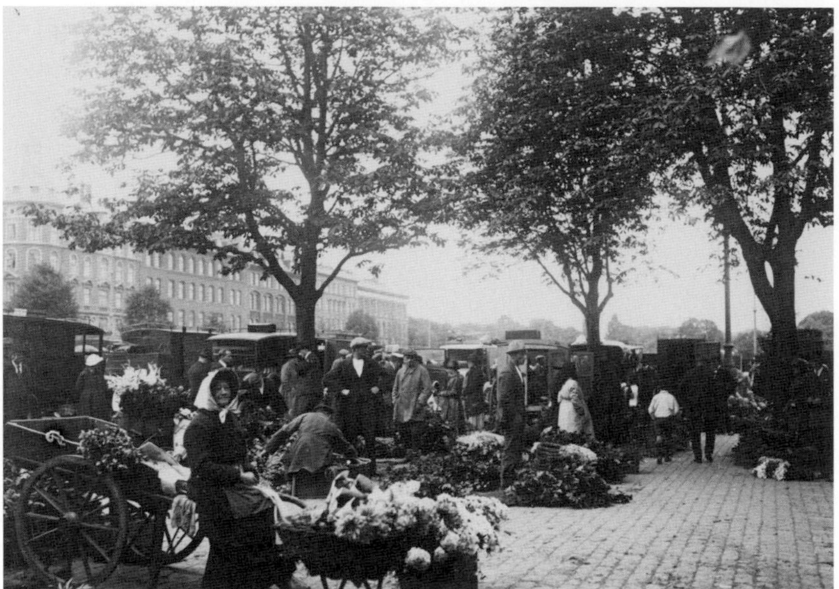

Figure 10.3. The vegetable market on Grønttorvet on the site where Torvehallerne stands today, 1890–1930. Photographer unknown. Courtesy of Copenhagen City Archives (public domain).

Architecturally speaking, Israels Plads and the area around it belong to Copenhagen's expansive late nineteenth-century development. This is visible in the way the large square is lined with five-story nineteenth-century urban blocks, with stuccoed façades fretted with historical motifs, as well as in the way the site edges one of the city's green spaces, Ørstedsparken—perhaps the finest example of a park from the early phase of Copenhagen's expansion beyond the ramparts during the 1870s.[3] With its hilly terrain and deep lakes, Ørstedsparken is a direct reminder of the defensive ramparts that surrounded the city during the seventeenth century. When it was laid out, the park (named after Danish physicist H.C. Ørsted) allowed bourgeois salon culture to spill over into the open space: couples from the burgeoning economic elite were meant to stroll along the winding paths and bump into each other in social encounters staged by the park's topography.[4] The still, reflective surface of the lake around which these paths swirl animates a strong "swan lake" motif.[5] A fetishized relationship to the swan was a powerful current in nineteenth-century Danish culture, represented in Hans Christian Andersen's 1843 tale "The Ugly Duckling." The story is an allegory of Andersen's own life, from his arrival in the city as a poor and awkward child from the countryside to his social and cultural rise to become a famous writer. A tale of sublime genius set against

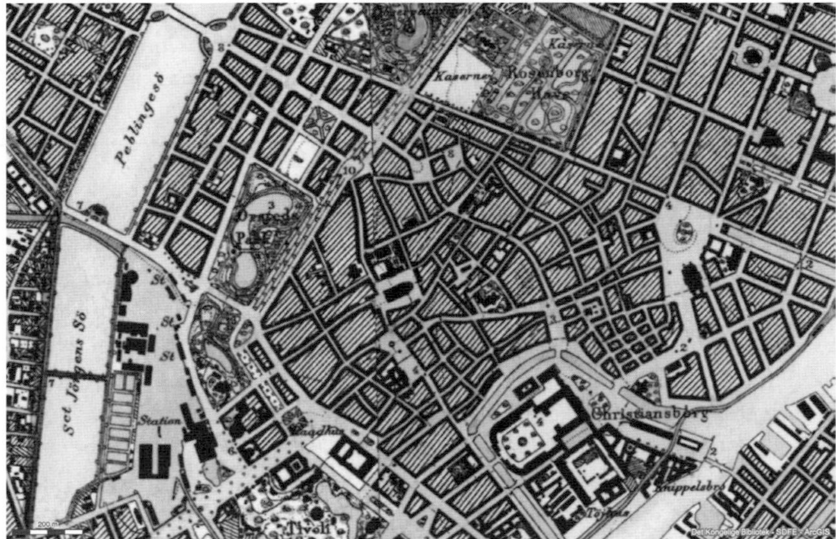

Figure 10.4. Map of Copenhagen as the city began expanding around 1880. The swirling lakes and paths in the park marked number 3 is H.C. Ørstedsparken and the site next to it—the white square and the square with the paths marking a cross is the site of Israels Plads, the latter marking the current site of Torvehallerne. Map dated 1885.Courtesy of the Danish Royal Library.

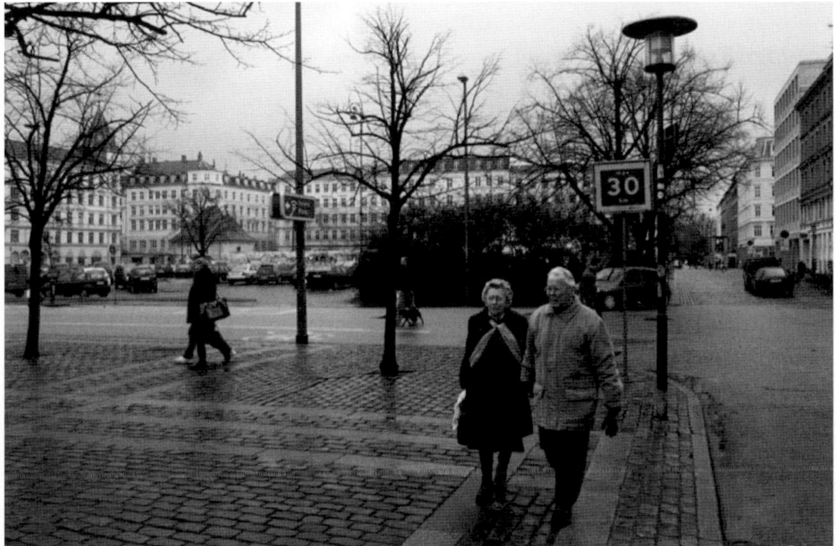

Figure 10.5. The windswept atmosphere of Israels Plads before the advent of Torvehallerne. Matthias Arni Ingimarssn, Israels Plads, 2008. Courtesy of Matthias Arni Ingimarssn (Wikimedia Commons).

the backdrop of an introverted, provincial city, "The Ugly Duckling" is not altogether complimentary to Copenhagen. Nevertheless, this chapter will return to the figure of the ugly duckling in relation to the more recent story of the Torvehallerne project, which in some ways offers an analogous narrative for the Danish architectural scene at the turn of the millennium.

After the large vegetable market on Israels Plads closed in the 1950s, the site remained a heterogeneous one. A visitor to Israels Plads in the 1990s would have found it laid out in a functional way, with a gas station, ball game areas, and relatively sparse planting. During this period Israels Plads was little more than a passageway to the swan lake in Ørstedsparken, or a place where children from the nearby schools, kindergartens, and residential blocks could play ball games. Moreover, the area had enough shrubs and bushes to be regarded as fairly rough at night, as a place known to attract homeless people and adjacent to Ørstedsparken's queer cruising grounds. In one corner of Israels Plads, a small outdoor vegetable and flower market nevertheless continued its unobtrusive existence. Improvised stalls typically sold cheap produce, punctuated by the atmospheric cries of the vendors, who toward the end of a cold, windy day would announce special offers to passers-by—a reminder of the city's bygone traditional open-air food markets. It was around this time that the site, with its almost-forgotten market culture, caught the imagination of the visionary architect Hans Peter Hagens.

Toward Torvehallerne

In the 1990s Copenhagen was nearly bankrupt, and the inner city was rundown, poor, and dirty. While Europe prospered south of the border, Denmark was still in political and economic recovery following the 1980s, a period of austerity named the "potato diet" by the Conservative prime minister Poul Schlüter. Copenhagen seemed to be the vacuous center of the crisis, and the exodus of people from the inner city throughout the 1980s had left it on the brink of economic breakdown; eventually it had to be economically administered by the Ministry of Internal Affairs during 1993–94.[6] By the end of the decade, Copenhagen was considered an inappropriate living environment for middle-class families, a fact that contributed in turn to soaring unemployment in the city. Poor-quality housing, a lack of jobs, and bad infrastructure were compounded by an inadequate relationship with the rest of Europe and the world, as the relatively low-capacity airport was separated off from the city center, with no proper public transportation or expressway.

Schlüter believed that the capital city could not continue in this condition if Denmark wanted to experience an economic upturn in the near future. In

1989 he therefore set up a commission, which published a report titled *Hovedstaden, hvad vil vi med den?* (The Capital City: What Do We Want from It?).[7] Visitors to Copenhagen in recent years will have seen some of the fruits of the report's infrastructural suggestions: the airport is now the largest in Scandinavia; it is connected to the city by railroad, metro, and an expressway that culminates in a bridge to neighboring Sweden; and the entire area between the city and the airport, known as Ørestaden—the development of which was intended to co-finance some of these infrastructures—is a new urban area with funky architecture in the twelve-story range, including landmarks such as the 8 House by Bjarke Ingels and his company BIG.[8]

But in 1991, before all this construction took place, Schlüter was forced to resign as prime minister due to a political scandal. He was replaced by the Social Democrat Poul Nyrup Rasmussen. The Social Democrats' "third way" continued the neoliberal economic focus, but it also had a more explicit urban-cultural agenda, epitomized in the huge effort behind Copenhagen's bid to become the 1996 European Capital of Culture. A spirit of progressiveness and a metropolitan urban lifestyle began to take form in the city, setting the stage for Hagens's vision of covered market halls on Israels Plads: the idea of Torvehallerne was born. At the time, Copenhagen had no such halls, and food shopping was then (and indeed remains) primarily restricted to discount supermarket chains. Hagens challenged the Copenhageners and municipal politicians who believed that covered food markets belonged only in southern European cities. Why not in Copenhagen, he asked, when such markets were already thriving in other northern cities such as Helsinki, Stockholm, and Gothenburg?[9] While Copenhagen had historically had outdoor food markets, the city's cool and windy climate seemed to cry out for the construction of covered market halls.

Given this context of optimism, the slow but steady economic upturn, and the rebranding of Copenhagen as a northern European economic and cultural center, Copenhageners might have been expected to greet Hagens's vision with cheers. But in fact this did not happen, and it took Hagens fourteen years of hard work in the context of controversy and resistance before the Torvehallerne covered food market opened in September 2011. Since then, however, the project has been an overwhelming success, with more than five million annual visitors, aided by the extended renovation of Israels Plads as a huge skater-park-style public space that opened in 2015. The success of the Torvehallerne project situates it as more than just a food market: it is a multisensuous experience-oriented place, not only for the consumption of food but also for a particular urban lifestyle, establishing an eclectic consumerist universe where global delicatessen meets "New Nordic" authenticity.[10] Indeed, Torvehallerne have it all—including what are allegedly Europe's best tacos,

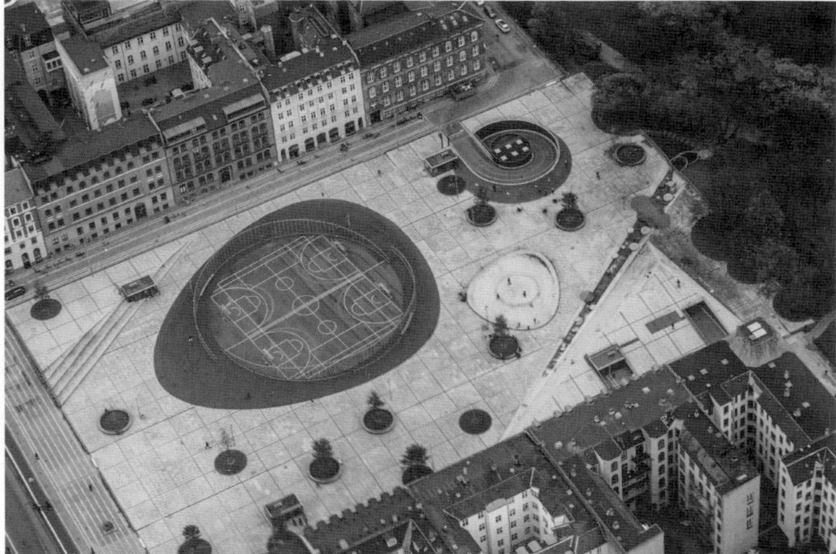

Figure 10.6. Aerial image of Torvehallerne with the new play areas and open space in the center, and Ørstedsparken at the bottom of the picture. Photograph by Rasmus Hjortshøj. Image courtesy of Rasmus Hjortshøj – COAST.

served by Noma's former dessert chef Rosio Sanchez—and the place has even caught the attention of the *New York Times*.[11]

This progressive, upbeat, and explicitly marketed picture of Copenhagen as a rising global tourist and food destination has almost obliterated the city's previous image as poor, dirty, peripheral, and even backward. At the time when Hagens was making his pitch for Torvehallerne, Copenhagen was so "unmetropolitan" that it was hard to go out to eat after 9 p.m., and the city's prime culinary destinations were the overpriced beer bodegas along the canal in Nyhavn. Hagens's vision and persistence were as spectacular as those of Andersen, the "ugly duckling" who wanted to bring a spark of genius to the Danish literary scene. Torvehallerne's transparent glass and steel architecture now stands like a swan on the white stone surface that replaced the dark asphalt of Israels Plads. Nowadays this place is an emblem of Copenhagen as attractive and "livable," a picture-perfect city where smartly dressed millennials lead the way with their bicycles, baby strollers, smartphones, paper coffee cups, and sourdough loaves, the price of which would have bought a full hot lunch in one of the area's dimly lit cafés at the time when Hagens was setting out his vision.

Clearly, none of this is any less relevant, accommodating, or indeed urban than what was there before. However, when market halls offer a particular range of high-end and heavily branded products,[12] and when only certain

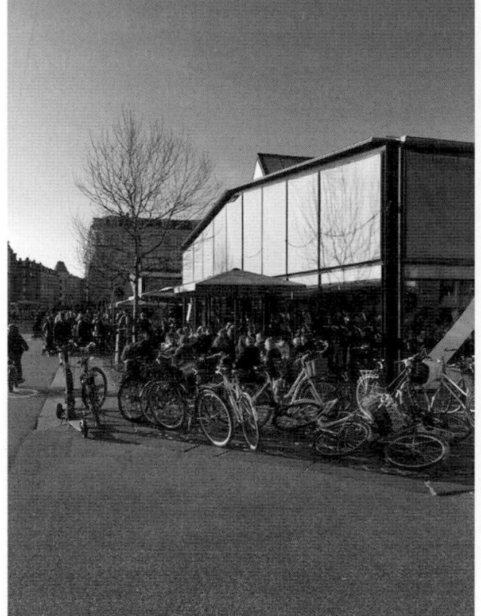

Figure 10.7. Torvehallerne, Copenhagen. Photograph by author, March 29, 2019.

Figure 10.8. Israel's Place, Copenhagen. Photograph by author, March 29, 2019.

segments of the population have the personal finances to pay for those products, then something crucial has gone missing. Moreover, Hagens never intended to attune Torvehallerne to Copenhagen's neoliberal branding. It is therefore necessary to reconsider the market halls' success against the backdrop of their "unintended" aspects. Doing so yields an important insight: a successful urban project can simultaneously be a failed project when it is seen in relation to the vision that originally brought it into being. In the case of Torvehallerne, this becomes evident in relation to the changing urban ethos and politics, and people's changing financial abilities and consumerist desires, over the last twenty years. Today, Torvehallerne do not cater to those who longed for a more multicultural and vivid urban scene in Copenhagen in the 1990s. Instead, they serve a gastrosexually oriented segment of the population. This does not chime well with the vision according to which the project was conceived.

Foodies, Tourists, and Body Politics in the Livable City

This argument becomes more nuanced if one considers practices of bodily experience in interactions with food in and around Torvehallerne. The market is packaged as luxurious in a way that speaks to all the senses—through the smells, the colors, and the noise of the people, as well as the food production and preparation that takes place in front of the visitors on-site. But this packaging brackets an everyday practice. The consumption of food, and the interaction between cities and their hinterlands through the retail of produce, has of course always been part of that everyday urban practice. However, Torvehallerne's new sensuous "packaging" speaks to a touristification of everyday life, to borrow a phrase from sociologist John Urry.[13] At Torvehallerne, this touristification of everyday life—given in the experience of the city through the lens of "livability"[14]—is elevated into a seamless notion whereby the experience of the covered market rises above the city's actual everyday food culture. This is the case even though the kind of food on offer at Torvehallerne is bracketed as the form of the everyday for which Copenhagen would like to be known as part of its livability paradigm.

The concept of livability is often associated with the Danish architect and urban planner Jan Gehl. It entails an argument against the separation of functions in the modernist urban planning paradigm, to which livability offers an alternative. From the 1960s onward, Gehl proposed that architects should turn their attention to people's behavior in the open spaces of the city—to life between buildings, as suggested by the title of one of his famous books. Architects, he argued, ought to consider how buildings and urban structures influence people's lives, and the aim of the architect and urban planner should be to create cities not for infrastructural visions but for people. According to Gehl, the aim was therefore to create urban spaces whose use would make people happier, taking account of safety and weather conditions no less than urban design measures.[15]

What could be more appealing than the humanist aim of creating cities where people like to spend time in open spaces and participate in urban culture? Yet the concept of livability also has a starkly anthropocentric, consumerist, and experience-oriented strain. If the architect focuses on making cities for "people," where does that leave all the other actors, agents, and systems in the city—plants, animals, or the material world, our relationships with which we must take into account in light of the current ecological crisis? Gehl's approach does not accord with more complex understandings of sustainability. Even though it is situated within a framework of antagonism toward modernist architects' infrastructural and top-down planning, it essentially shares their anthropocentric approach, narrowly focused on the needs of humans.

In recent years, Copenhagen's planning department has leaned toward this concept of urban livability. However, it is notable that the experience-oriented and gastrosexual consumerist culture that results from that concept is not entirely dominant around Torvehallerne. Denmark's less gourmet, more everyday food culture is still strongly present in the area's small, unobtrusive discount supermarket chains, which point to the broader context of Danes' relationship with food. After all, Denmark is also known in the food world for its highly

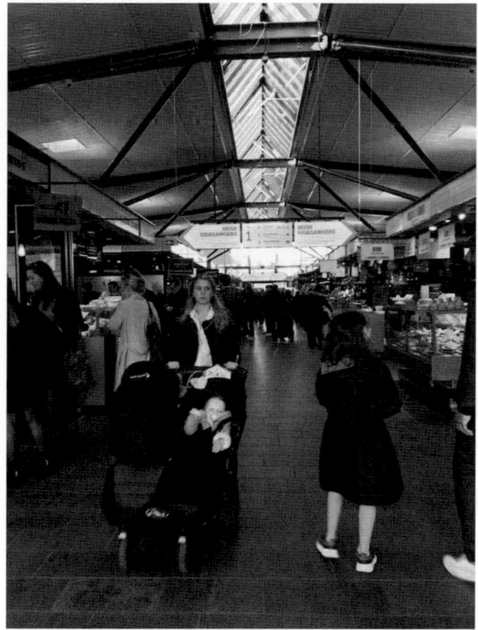

Figure 10.9. Interior view of Torvehallerne, Copenhagen. Photograph by author, March 29, 2019.

industrialized pork production, which sometimes comes at great cost in terms of meat quality and the use of antibiotics. One might be forgiven for thinking that the good pork is all sold abroad, while the Danes themselves are left with endless shelves of cheap supermarket pâté. If this is everyday life in the livable city of Copenhagen, it also indicates the "limits of the livable city," in the words of architectural theorists Maros Krivy and Leonard Ma.[16] These limits reflect not just the way we *look* at the city, through the aestheticized gaze explored by Urry;[17] they are limits we physically consume through our interactions with food.

This is what makes Torvehallerne such a strong symbol of Copenhagen's most recent urban and architectural history. If Torvehallerne were intended to be the center of a food culture where small businesses would sell their produce according to a paradigm of "authenticity"—a paradigm that harks back to the late nineteenth-century marketplace culture, where farmers' wives would carry their produce into the city on foot—then Torvehallerne have failed. What has emerged instead—and become incredibly successful—is a branded and experience-oriented version that caters to a "New Nordic" cuisine and style, using local and national narratives to elevate particular forms of produce, taste, and packaging. There exists a cultural paradigm that associates good food with cosmopolitanism or multiculturalism, where different countries' food cultures can be acknowledged and appropriated in sites such as Torvehallerne. The global attention the "New Nordic" brand has garnered emphasizes that the arrow also goes "the other way," pointing outward from Denmark rather than in.

As described at the start of this chapter, high-end food markets and covered market halls have become popular and widespread in Denmark, to such an extent that one can speak of a "market hall effect" analogous to the Bilbao effect or the High Line effect.[18] Torvehallerne have arguably become so successful as an urban regeneration measure that they are accepted as an absolute good, in a way that brackets more complex understandings of how they might influence urban culture or produce wider, potentially more problematic effects. Like the High Line park in New York City, for example, they come at the cost of the more heterogeneous urban culture they displaced, foregrounding an idea of urban-cultural authenticity that is a rather recent addition to Copenhagen.[19] The market halls themselves, and the part they have played in recent neoliberal urban development, are not an isolated phenomenon in Copenhagen, or even Denmark. Indeed, they can be tied to the "new metropolitan mainstream" proposed by Swiss sociologist Christian Schmid as a way to explain the (in many ways successful) postindustrial developments in cities around the globe, mainly in Western contexts.[20]

As Schmid argues, following the widespread dismantling of industrial production in the Western world from the 1970s onward, many cities experienced economic downturns and saw massive population declines.[21] Once this process had taken hold, he argues, the underlying planning aspirations associated with the new metropolitan mainstream responded by attempting to stimulate growth through the creation of urban environments that were attractive to the wealthier segments of the population, even in former industrial areas. Such aspirations concerned the desire to revitalize cities in light of the dwindling industrial heritage that had conditioned metropolitan culture. But they relied on urban forms of industrial production, in part through the repurposing of old factory buildings as offices or dwellings, albeit without the pollution, noise, and working-class culture that had accompanied them. Torvehallerne are an example of such a project, falling between the remains of the industrially driven expansion of the city as a European metropolis and the heavily branded new mainstream of the livable Danish city. Aesthetically, as a stylistic paradigm, the glass and steel structure also closely resembles the new metropolitan mainstream. The market halls employ an architecture that is modernist and functional in the way it makes visible the buildings' joints and structural properties; there is almost something historicist in the structure, so that one might be led to think that this is an old, modern construction that has been repurposed, whereas in fact the buildings were constructed from scratch.

This chapter's critique of the Torvehallerne project thus springs from its status as a product of Copenhagen's most recent urban history. This issue is not that Torvehallerne are added to the city's food culture, or that they are insufficiently urban. The issue is that they rely on a branding that makes them urban in a sense that speaks only to particular wealthy segments of society. The project does indeed emerge like a white swan against a provincial backdrop. But at the same time, it evokes ambiguous feelings, because of its one-sided focus on one kind of urban livability: the kind that lies behind the urban planning goal to "copenhagenize"[22] (i.e., to export Copenhagen's well-known cycling culture); the kind that can be branded as part of a tourist regime (whether by locals or by actual visitors from abroad). Despite the project's refreshing focus on sensory experience and the consumption of high-quality food, it welcomes only a certain kind of controlled body, one that dares to be on display and can match the crafted and high-end produce on offer. It resists the parts of urban culture that do not fit its over-aestheticized vision and what the livability paradigm might regard as an eyesore.

This discussion thus taps into questions about what possibilities exist for civic life in wealthy twenty-first century Western cities, and about the role of food—and indeed the covered market hall as a type—in that process. As Krivy and Ma conclude, the livable city is not without its appeal to civic culture, as it "goes along" with conversations and with being social; but as the "urbanity of the livable city [is] produced, consumed, and produced again," it requires active participants as "a distinct type of unwaged surplus labor."[23] While the transformation of Copenhagen took off from welfare state politics, which in Denmark have traditionally been tied to *qualitative* concerns (with well-being), it also indicates a movement that is increasingly preoccupied with *quantitative* concerns (with wealth),[24] and it therefore implies a certain ontological leveling between the human and fiscal cultures of the city. This is perhaps nowhere more deeply intertwined than in the food culture at Torvehallerne, which is therefore particularly good at silencing its own underlying economic and biopolitical effects. The implicit and inevitable co-generation of value involved in this urban culture—a culture marked by decades of neoliberal urban politics—is transforming not only the city's architecture but also its people. It can therefore be said that these politics, and this paradigm of urban life, are transforming civic life itself into a reservoir and generator of economic value and value accumulation.

This argument may perhaps seem to be marked by nostalgia for the vague, windswept, asphalted, and partially scruffy cruising areas around Israels Plads. If so, it is nostalgia not in a reparatory sense, but as a longing for a form of meaning making in civic culture where the involvement is vaguer and more open, rather than fused with the body-political agendas of neoliberal urban governmental forms.

Coda: Torvehallerne in the Time of Coronavirus

Spring 2020 saw the nationwide lockdown of Danish institutions and businesses in light of the rapid spread of the new coronavirus, COVID-19. What happened to Torvehallerne? From March 11 onward, people in Denmark were asked to stay at home, public institutions and workplaces made most employees work from home, children were kept out of schools, and nurseries and public gatherings of more than ten people were prohibited. With the rapid economic downturn that followed, did people's priorities shift from high-end coffee and bakery goods to more stringent financial concerns? Were Torvehallerne deserted?

During most of the pandemic in 2020, Torvehallerne seemed as vibrant as ever. After the hard lockdown in March, the area around Israels Plads quickly regained its sense of public life. During the early phase of lockdown there was some media speculation that "the time of the city" was coming to an end, because people would no longer be willing to pay soaring rents and house prices in order to be crammed together in a dense environment; the opportunities for experience and consumption that that city had to offer were about to pass away. For a moment, there was a feeling that people would use the experience of the pandemic to reconsider their priorities and move to the countryside.[25] But that quickly faded with the arrival of summer, as Denmark's coronavirus crisis declined into latency and the number of infections remained low. Indeed, good coffee, bread, specialty teas, and the opportunity to hang out amid the bright surfaces of Israels Plads remained attractive. Children continued to

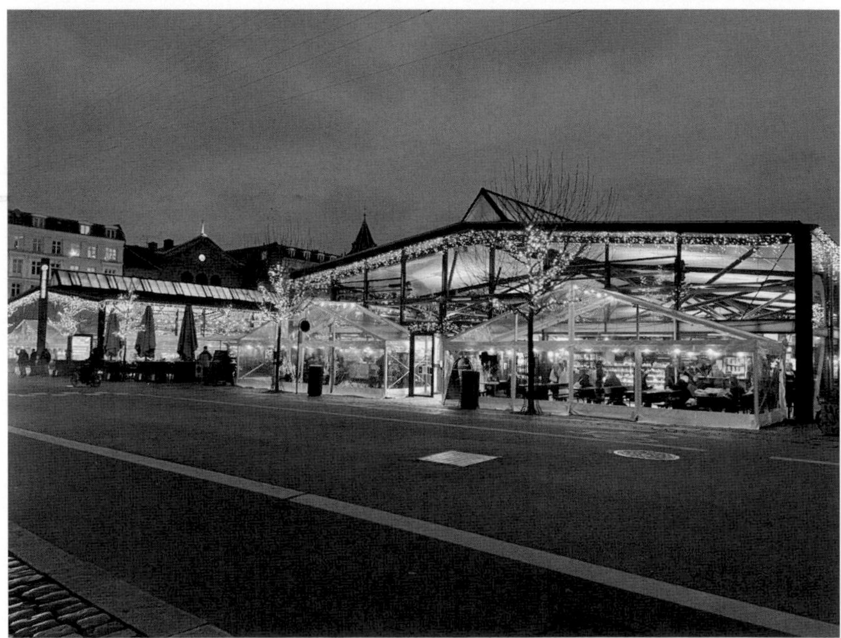

Figure 10.10. Torvehallerne, Copenhagen, pictured open during the COVID-19 pandemic as well as on the day Copenhagen was preparing for the second lockdown. Photograph by author, December 7, 2020.

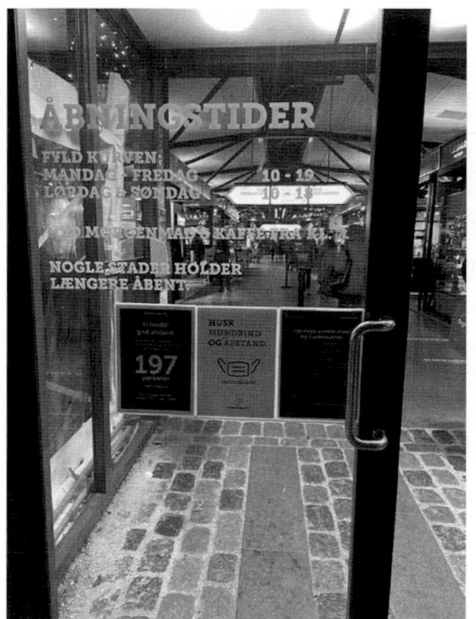

Figure 10.11. Entrance of Torvehallerne. From the early autumn of 2020, visitors were required to wear masks inside Torvehallerne. Photograph by author, December 7, 2020.

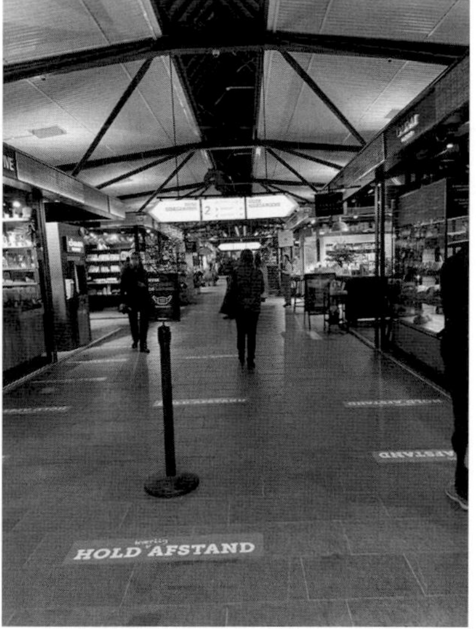

Figure 10.12. As Denmark was on the brink of the second COVID-19 lockdown, people still came to do their shopping and hang out inside Torvehallerne, enjoying the last days when cafes were open prior to a month-long lockdown. Photograph by author, December 7, 2020.

play, and people enjoyed the sunshine and the view of Torvehallerne's shiny glass boxes, where the sparkling clean design seemed to conform to the new focus on hygiene. During the later summer and autumn of 2020, as infection numbers rose in Denmark, however, Torvehallerne remained open for business but people were asked to wear face masks inside the buildings. From December 9, 2020, the restaurants and cafes at Torvehallerne but not the shops were closed in a second lockdown. However, on the eve of Monday, December 7, as the second lockdown had just been announced with effect from the upcoming Wednesday, the atmosphere was pleasant and people were enjoying food and drinks as well as shopping. What would happen during the rest of the winter, time would tell, but certainly, with the pretty Christmas decorations, Torvehallerne did their best to light up the spirit of Copenhageners in the dark pandemic winter.

Notes

1. See Dansk Sprognævn, "Nye ord i 2013," *Dansk Sprognævn*, January 10, 2014, https://dsn.dk/nyt/nyheder/2013/nye-ord-i-2013-1.
2. The architect and originator of Torvehallerne, Hans Peter Hagens, notes in an interview that there is potential for building forty or fifty similar market halls in other Danish cities. Thomas Møller Larsen, "Arkitekt: Der er potentiale for torvehaller i 40–50 danske byer," Foodculture.dk, May 31, 2016, https://foodculture.dk/tema/marked/2016/torvehaller-spreder-sig/arkitekt-der-er-potentiale-for-torvehaller-i-40-50-danske-byer. Although it is unclear whether this number is realistic, cities elsewhere in the country already have planned developments. Christian Nobel, "Nu vil Frederiksberg også have torvehaller," *Politiken*, October 26, 2017, https://politiken.dk/ibyen/byliv/art6176424/Nu-vil-Frederiksberg-også-have-torvehaller; Alfred Rosenfeldt, "Odense får torvehaller," *TV2/Fyn*, July 1, 2016, https://www.tv2fyn.dk/artikel/odense-faar-torvehaller. See also "Torvehal Bornholm," accessed August 26, 2020, http://www.torvehalbornholm.dk/.
3. Birgitte Kortegaard, "Københavns Parkhistorie," *Landskab* 7–8 (1997): 150.
4. Sven-Ingvar Andersson, "Havekunsten i Danmark," *Arkitektur DK* 4 (1990): 161.
5. Andersson, "Havekunsten i Danmark," 161–63.
6. The journalist Gudrun Marie Schmidt has written an amusing account in the newspaper *Politiken* of this bad image of Copenhagen—and of how hard it is to imagine now, only two decades later. Gudrun Marie Schmidt, "Da København var Udskudsdanmark," *Politiken*, July 1, 2015, https://politiken.dk/magasinet/feature/art5581467/Da-København-var-Udskudsdanmark.
7. Kirsten Stallknecht and Initiativgruppen om Hovedstadsregionen, *Hovedstaden, hvad vil vi med den?* (Copenhagen: Statsministeriet, 1989).
8. By and Havn, *Godt begyndt: Et tilbageblik over Ørestads udvikling* (Copenhagen: KLS Grafisk Hus A/S, 2010).
9. See e.g. Søren Saften Overgaard, "Torvekultur skal genskabes," *Information*, March 30, 2001, https://www.information.dk/2001/03/torvekultur-genskabes.
10. See my discussions of related themes in Henriette Steiner, "Café Chairs, Bar Stools and Other Chairs We Sit on When We Eat: Food Consumption and Everyday Urban Life," in *Food and Architecture at the Table*, ed. Samantha Martin-McAuliffe (London: Bloomsbury Academic, 2016); Henriette Steiner, "H.C. ANDERSEN WAS (not) HERE," *Scandinavica* 55, no. 1 (2016); Henriette Steiner, "Welche Sorte Tourist bist Du?" *Baumeister: Das Architektur Magazin*, December 2017.
11. Seth Sherwood, "An Open Invitation to Eat in Copenhagen," *The New York Times*, September 30, 2011, https://www.nytimes.com/2011/10/02/travel/torvehallerne-is-culinary-hot-spot-in-copenhagen.html.

12. Sometimes these are called "food halls" rather than "market halls" and are oriented more toward takeaway food. An example is the upmarket Tivoli Food Halls, which recently opened on the corner of Tivoli Gardens.
13. John Urry, *The Tourist Gaze* (London: Sage, 1990); Steiner, "Welche Sorte Tourist."
14. See, e.g., the work and writing of the Danish urban planner Jan Gehl. Jan Gehl, *Life between Buildings: Using Public Space* (Copenhagen: Danish Architectural Press, 2010).
15. Gehl, *Life between Buildings*. See also Jan Gehl, "Cities for People in the 21st Century," lecture, Aalto University, February 21, 2017, https://www.youtube.com/watch?v=882rELJMHt8.
16. Maros Krivy and Leonard Ma, "The Limits of the Livable City: From Homo Sapiens to Homo Cappuccino," *Avery Review* 30 (2018).
17. Urry, *Tourist Gaze*.
18. See, e.g., the exhibition *Architecture Effects*, Guggenheim Bilbao Museum, December 5, 2018–April 28, 2019, https://architectureeffects.guggenheim-bilbao.eus.
19. Natalie Gulsrud and Henriette Steiner, "When Urban Greening Becomes an Accumulation Strategy: Exploring the Ecological, Social and Economic Calculus of the High Line," *JoLA: Journal of Landscape Architecture* 19, no. 3 (2019).
20. Christian Schmid, "Henri Lefebvre, the Right to the City and the New Metropolitan Mainstream," in *Cities for People, Not for Profit: Critical Urban Theory and the Right to the City*, ed. Neil Brenner, Peter Marcuse, and Margit Mayer (London: Routledge, 2012). See also Henriette Steiner and Kristin Veel, *Tower to Tower: Gigantism in Architecture and Digital Culture* (Cambridge, MA: MIT Press, 2020), chapter 3.
21. Schmid, "Henri Lefebvre."
22. "Copenhagenize," accessed August 26, 2020, https://copenhagenize.eu.
23. Krivy and Ma, "Livable City," online publication, no pagination.
24. Lasse Horne Kjældgaard, *Meningen med velfærdsstaten: Da litteraturen tog ordet—og politikerne lyttede* (Copenhagen: Gyldendal, 2018).
25. "Corona kan få os til at flytte på landet," *Home*, April 18 2020, https://home.dk/bolignyt/flere-artikler/april-2020/corona-kan-faa-os-til-at-flytte-paa-landet/.

Bibliography

Andersson, Sven-Ingvar. "Havekunsten i Danmark." *Arkitektur DK* 4 (1990): 133–170.

By and Havn. *Godt begyndt: Et tilbageblik over Ørestads udvikling*. Copenhagen: KLS Grafisk Hus A/S, 2010.

Dansk Sprognævn. "Nye ord i 2013." *Dansk Sprognævn*, January 10, 2014. https://dsn.dk/nyt/nyheder/2013/nye-ord-i-2013-1.

Gehl, Jan. "Cities for People in the 21st Century." Lecture, Aalto University, February 21, 2017. https://www.youtube.com/watch?v=882rELJMHt8.

———. *Life between Buildings: Using Public Space*. Copenhagen: Danish Architectural Press, 2010.

Gulsrud, Natalie, and Henriette Steiner. "When Urban Greening Becomes an Accumulation Strategy: Exploring the Ecological, Social and Economic Calculus of the High Line." *JoLA: Journal of Landscape Architecture* 19, no. 3 (2019): 38–43.

Hagens, Hans Peter. *Torvehallerne og Verden Rundt*. Copenhagen: Strandberg Publishing, 2015.

Home. "Corona kan få os til at flytte på landet." *Home*, April 18, 2020. https://home.dk/bolignyt/flere-artikler/april-2020/corona-kan-faa-os-til-at-flytte-paa-landet/.

Kjældgaard, Lasse Horne. *Meningen med velfærdsstaten: Da litteraturen tog ordet–og politikerne lyttede*. Copenhagen: Gyldendal, 2018.

Kortegaard, Birgitte. "Københavns Parkhistorie." *Landskab* 7–8 (1997): 149–56.

Krivy, Maros, and Leonard Ma. "The Limits of the Livable City: From Homo Sapiens to Homo Cappuccino." *Avery Review* 30 (2018): online publication, no pagination.

Møller Larsen, Thomas. "Arkitekt: Der er potentiale for torvehaller i 40–50 danske byer." *Foodculture.dk*, May 31, 2016. https://foodculture.dk/tema/marked/2016/torvehaller-spreder-sig/arkitekt-der-er-potentiale-for-torvehaller-i-40-50-danske-byer.

Nobel, Christian. "Nu vil Frederiksberg også have torvehaller." *Politiken*, October 26, 2017. https://politiken.dk/ibyen/byliv/art6176424/Nu-vil-Frederiksberg-også-have-torvehaller.

Overgaard, Søren Saften. "Torvekultur skal genskabes." *Information*, March 30, 2001. https://www.information.dk/2001/03/torvekultur-genskabes.

Rosenfeldt, Alfred. "Odense får torvehaller." *TV2/Fyn*, July 1, 2016. https://www.tv2fyn.dk/artikel/odense-faar-torvehaller.

Schmid, Christian. "Henri Lefebvre, the Right to the City and the New Metropolitan Mainstream." In *Cities for People, Not for Profit: Critical Urban Theory and the Right to the City*, edited by Neil Brenner, Peter Marcuse, and Margit Mayer, 42–62. London: Routledge, 2012.

Schmidt, Gudrun Marie. "Da København var Udskudsdanmark." *Politiken*, July 1, 2015. https://politiken.dk/magasinet/feature/art5581467/Da-København-var-Udskudsdanmark.

Sherwood, Seth. "An Open Invitation to Eat in Copenhagen." *The New York Times*, September 30, 2011. https://www.nytimes.com/2011/10/02/travel/torvehallerne-is-culinary-hot-spot-in-copenhagen.html.

Stallknecht, Kirsten, and Initiativgruppen om Hovedstadsregionen. *Hovedstaden, hvad vil vi med den?* Copenhagen: Statsministeriet, 1989.

Steiner, Henriette. "Café Chairs, Bar Stools and Other Chairs We Sit on When We Eat: Food Consumption and Everyday Urban Life." In *Food and Architecture at the Table*, edited by Samantha Martin-McAuliffe, 223–38. London: Bloomsbury Academic, 2016.

———. "H.C. ANDERSEN WAS (not) HERE." *Scandinavica* 55, no. 1 (2016): 106–17.

———. "Welche Sorte Tourist bist Du?" *Baumeister: Das Architektur Magazin*, December 2017, 82–87.

Steiner, Henriette, and Kristin Veel. *Tower to Tower: Gigantism in Architecture and Digital Culture*. Cambridge, MA: MIT Press, 2020.

Urry, John. *The Tourist Gaze*. London: Sage, 1990.

CHAPTER 11

PANDEMICS AND MARKETPLACES

A Coda from Viareggio, Italy

Andrea Borghini & Min Kyung Lee

Starting in January 2020, journalists sensationally reported that the Huanan wet market of Wuhan was the origin of COVID-19. Images of a crowded, dark, and loud market intended to illicit shock were broadcast around the world. Subsequent reports and scientific studies have suggested a far more complex story to the transmission of the virus to humans. However, its initial connection to a food marketplace poses consequential questions about public spaces, cultural practices, and food systems in a future that will contend with new global contagions. As the virus spread beyond China to Korea, and other parts of Asia, to Europe, Australia, and eventually to the rest of the world, strict quarantines were mandated. Here in our small Tuscan coastal city of Viareggio, residents remained confined to their homes from March through May 2020, only to be subjected to another quarantine with the virus's second wave in November 2020. These spatial restrictions have stressed the cultural and political values of one of the most essential elements of social and personal life: food provisioning.

One of the few permitted outings during the months of the quarantine was to the grocery store. Before COVID-19, there were several options to source food, including large supermarkets, weekly farmers markets, bakeries, specialty shops, the pier, and the central marketplace. However, under lockdown, only one person per household was allowed to provision food; one had to remain within the limits of the town. Furthermore, only grocery stores were allowed to remain open. All other sources were closed. This was a dramatic disruption in the sociability of Italian life, which consists of fresh bread bought daily from a bakery, perishables and produce bought directly from farmers, butchers, cheese and fishmongers multiple times of the week, and where people regularly travel to neighboring towns and areas, especially in the countryside, to provision olive oil, wine, and other essentials. With these patterns come the familiar sounds of people greeting and chatting as they wait in line, butchers calling out orders, the clink of espressos being drunk at the bar while people shop, fishermen announcing their catch of the day, and vendors stuffing paper bags of tomatoes and seasonal vegetables. All of these public spaces went silent.

The central market of Viareggio, Il Piazzone, is one of the city's major public monuments, dating from 1924 and designed in the Liberty style by architect Alfredo Belluomini. It is located at the center of town at Piazza Cavour, along the main axis from the train station to the sea. It occupies two square city blocks, but peripheral vendors extend the lived space of the market into the neighboring streets. Its Mediterranean climate-adapted design includes four built structures, with ample covered outdoor space and open areas between, the largest including two towers. The buildings allow for each vendor to occupy an interior store space that faces outward to the open areas. These generous spaces permit circulation both of customers and deliveries, and in recent years have seen many new independent kiosks managed by immigrants selling inexpensive goods such as plastic beach toys, clothing, and mobile phone covers.

What is the civic role of a marketplace during this era of pandemics? We offer here a few brief comments on how a marketplace and the different actors who inhabit its spaces have been and will be affected in this era of COVID-19. Our thoughts emerge from direct observations and conversations we had during the lockdown, which linked our experience to other marketplaces we have routinely used. Because the quarantine measures restricted food shopping to grocery stores, important characteristics specific to the value of our particular marketplace became evident. We outline these values under four themes: autonomy, provisioning, knowledge exchange, and borders.

Autonomy

Markets and supermarkets afford radically different dwelling experiences, which can be cast in terms of the autonomy and subjectivities of both vendors and customers.

The repetitive spaces of chain supermarkets limits subjectivity to a logic of standardization. The building and its interior spaces represent a uniform and systematized design. Cartons of milk, boxes of pasta, and bottles of oil are all readily available in abundance and appear stocked on identical shelves. Specific questions about the food's geographic origins and the people and the methods of their production are subordinated (sometimes eclipsed) by their location on a shelf and their posted price. The movement of shoppers is linear, proceeding down parallel and unvarying aisles. This organization discourages the shopper from taking breaks, interacting with others, or taking time to be curious. The reigning values in a supermarket are the performed assurance of modernity, hygiene, and safety, signaled by a legible environment surveilled under bright white lights.

The typology of a marketplace, with many independent and heterogeneous vendors, leaves more room for consumers to design their own visit. In the spaces between two shops, or even within a shop, visitors can take the time to smoke a cigarette, get a coffee, sit down, or have a conversation. Dwelling is encouraged and tends to be less centralized. Moreover, many central marketspaces were designed before germ theory but addressed a concern regarding air circulation and access to natural light, basic hygienic principles that are essential even now in our contemporary COVID-19 world.

Marketplaces afford also more autonomy for vendors, in terms of differentiation and curation. Depending on the season, personal connections, or the taste of customers, the order and display of goods can change, and the goods themselves can change in value. Each vendor can decide not only what to sell and how to provision it but also how to organize their spaces. The lack of standardization across the different vendors also requires an engagement with each vending space and demands accountability on the part of the vendor and the customer to adjust to changing spatial expectations.

Supermarkets, owned and managed by a spectrum from large companies to families, are private spaces; marketplaces owned by a government entity and even if managed by a private company, are public places. Accordingly, the people and the ways in which they serve others have important civic consequences. Corporations treat provisioning as a consumer good, in which economic measures drive all corporate decisions, from agricultural production to the arrangement of goods in a store. Most importantly, corporations are concerned with the identity of the company as a brand, which is abstract from the place where the stores are located. In contrast, independent family-owned grocery stores operate based on a different logic of consumerism that draws on site-specific meanings and social norms. Thus, they contribute to the specific identity and culture of a neighborhood, town, and city where they mediate the relationship between customers and producers. A market typically occupies a central square or a major street and arranges patterns of circulation of people and vehicles around it. A marketplace is, in other words, directly connected to the civic life of a community, and its concentration of independent stores in a framework supported and maintained by a town plays a part in defining the community's public life. Procedures for allocating slots to vendors tend not solely to promote capitalistic consumerism but must also confront questions of fairness, equality, cultural values, and public goods, as conceived in the public sphere.

The autonomy of markets also means the autonomy from the space of others. In Viareggio, during the pandemic, it allowed people to control their distance from each other. Natural air ventilation, direct sunlight, open spaces—all elements of modernist architecture—found their design justification again. When the social distancing regulations were outlined by the government, they did not prescribe all details for each site. The laws had to be interpreted for each specific situation, and because of the spatial flexibility that the market spaces offered, the vendors and customers could adapt. People controlled the space and their responses. Thus, the autonomy that the market affords also provides the possibility for a controlled response during contagions.

Provisioning

For a shopper at a supermarket or grocery store, trust is located in external factors, such as government regulations, labeling and food packaging, and the reputation of the corporation. The abundance and variety that is offered in this space is possible because the elements of trust extends beyond a relationship with the producer. The supermarket serves as a proxy.

In a market, the supply chain is much shorter. Vendors of vegetables, meat, and fish, are often also the producers and can speak directly to the methods of food production. In a country where geography and identity are still tightly bound, knowing whether the produce is from the next town or from another country is a significant distinction. Trust is located in a place and a human relationship.

Trust became a major issue during the COVID-19 quarantine. With the closing of many central markets, Italians were forced to shop at grocery stores. In large cities, where a plethora of small ethnic grocery stores surfaced in a recent past, this became a social opportunity of encounter among different ethnic communities sharing the same neighborhood. Shoppers could examine the food choices of their "local" stores and the enterprises of immigrant vendors took on a new civic meaning and social role.

Yet for the many small towns that dot the country, the only available option was a large chain supermarket. Not accustomed to sourcing produce from these companies, many organized individual deliveries directly from farmers, who were given permits to continue to work during the lockdown. This value of trust, in all stages of food production, distribution, and consumption, based on particular relationships to specific people and terrains, was reduced in policy decisions to a mere quantitative matter of food sourcing.

Knowledge Exchange

Vendors in a marketplace are key agents of culinary cultures and of public health issues related to dieting. For instance, a vegetable stand may function as the collective authority over the execution of certain recipes (e.g., a pasta with pesto), or may insist on maintaining seasonality for safeguarding the quality of products, or may suggest dietary habits (e.g., by indicating quantities as well as pairings). A butcher will not only offer appropriate portions and cuts depending on the recipe but may also offer knowledge about methods of meal preparation and suggestions about accompanying foods.

Marketplaces also tend to have specific times and days of operation. They normalize the rhythms and (more or less implicitly) the means for storing, preparing, and consuming foods. The knowledge cultivated through markets, then, also promotes specific long-term dietary patterns. By contrast, supermarkets rely on the idea of food freedom: one may shop, prepare, and consume whenever and as much as one wants. At the same time, it is left up to the shopper to secure adequate knowledge not to waste resources and time and to promote culinary values and pleasures.

By enforcing norms for provisioning, preparation, and consumption, vendors orient the complex mechanisms that give shape to a community. During the lockdown, when we struggled to find new and meaningful forms to organize our daily lives, the marketplace in Viareggio offered a social anchor. At the same time, the difficulty for many small vendors in provisioning the usual supplies of food and in sufficient amounts heightened the sense of disorientation and the erosion of those same social structures.

What does it mean for the supermarket to become that social anchor for a community? On the one hand, for an ethnically and culturally diversifying community, the supermarket offers an alternative to the often-excluding social interactions of a central market. Yet what might be lost when relying solely on a supermarket are the ways in which a shared and public space, such as a marketplace, can offer another kind of freedom not dictated by a private corporation. If the freedom of a supermarket lies in the convenience of being able to shop when you want and buy what you want, the freedom offered in a public marketspace is the right to exist in a shared space alongside others. It is a space defined by the social plurality and relationality among people, rather than relations with consumer products. In this sense, knowledge exchange about pesto is not merely about sharing recipes. It could also stand for a tolerance for differences, alternatives, and the tug and pull of cultural adaption over time.

Borders

While a marketplace is built on a relationship between the countryside, where food is produced, and a central civic space, where it is sold, supermarkets reframe such distinction (when they do not suppress it) in terms of point of production and point of purchase. Supermarkets are set up to offer homogeneous shopping experiences regardless of their location in a city, region, or country. They abstract from the specificities of their surroundings, whether a city center, a suburban landscape, or the open countryside. The supply chains sustaining their economies eclipse distances and site-specific properties.

Supermarkets and marketplaces rely on different distribution systems and establish different geographies of food. They also cut through social spaces in radically different ways in terms of how they represent and sustain a community's collective identity. The places they occupy have opposite civic meanings figuratively and sometimes physically: central (marketplace) or peripheral (supermarkets). Their social contributions go in opposite directions: supermarkets disaggregate community norms, while marketplaces sustain them. The former promotes homogeneity in a segregated social space, the other encourages individual entrepreneurship within a community space. There are many variations between these two poles, and in those cases, it begs the question of what kinds of civic and cultural activities is a municipality ceding to a private company in framing the social practice of food provisioning.

During the lockdown, the human face of each individual employee of the supermarket emerged more vividly, as their role as custodians of civic cultures was heightened and they were recognized as essential workers. In this respect, the social relationship between the workers in the supermarket and in the fields became apparent, as they shared health risks to provide public necessities during the quarantine. Social awareness was also informed by the obligation to cook food that was normally bought, such as bread. The labor of baking at home became part of a shared consciousness of not only the essential place of bakeries in the civic life of a town but also the shared practice of making a basic Italian staple. In those months, social media outlets became inundated with images of homemade baking results and the sharing of recipes. The pandemic offered clarity as to how geographic distances often obscure social connections among different people and tied them together through the food network.

During the COVID-19 pandemic, we missed the opportunity of dwelling in a marketplace, and not only for the missed opportunity of shopping for certain goods. We longed for the sociality, the rhythms, the sociopolitical agency that a marketplace conveys by virtue of its very structure, at least in Viareggio. In the end, we are left with a fundamental question regarding the cultural and political legacy of marketplaces. Assuming that supermarkets (and even online ones) can offer a safer model for shopping during pandemics, how can we recuperate some of the values offered by marketplaces, which are otherwise lost? More generally, which politics and policies can foster the civic values of marketplaces?

Acknowledgments

This research was funded by the Department of Philosophy 'PieroMartinetti' of the University of Milan under the Project 'Department of Excellence 2018–2022' awarded by the Ministry of Education, University and Research (MIUR).

Bibliography

Black, Rachel. *Porta Palazzo: The Anthropology of an Italian Market*. Philadelphia: University of Pennsylvania Press, 2014.

Borghini, Andrea, and Min Kyung Lee. "Dwelling in Times of Quarantine." *Platform*, April 6, 2020. http://https://www.platformspace.net/home/tag/quarantine.

Cabannes, Yves and Cecilia Marocchino (ed). *Integrating Food into Urban Planning*. London: UCL Press, 2018.

Imbert, Dorothée (ed). *Food and the City: Histories of Culture and Cultivation*. Cambridge, MA: Harvard University Press, 2015.

Oldenburg, Ray. *The Great Good Place*. Cambridge, MA: Da Capo Press, 1989.

Seale, Kirsten. *Markets, Places, Cities*. New York: Routledge, 2016.

ABOUT THE AUTHORS

Dr. Samantha L. Martin is an Associate Professor in the School of Architecture, Planning and Environmental Policy at University College Dublin. Her principal research and teaching interests lie in the reciprocity between ethics and urban order, as well as the intersections of food and architecture. She is the editor of *Food and Architecture: At the Table* (New York: Bloomsbury Academic, 2016), and co-editor of *New Research Directions in the Study of Ancient Urban Planning in the Mediterranean* (London: Routledge, 2017). She was a Mellon Fellow at Dumbarton Oaks in 2021. She received her PhD in Architecture from Cambridge University and is a graduate of Smith College.

Ashley Rose Young is the Historian of the American Food History Project at the Smithsonian's National Museum of American History. She earned her PhD and MA in History from Duke University and her BA in History from Yale University. As a cultural and social historian of the United States, Dr. Young's research explores the intersection of race, ethnicity, and gender in American food culture and economy. Her first book, *Nourishing Networks: The Public Culture of Food in New Orleans, 1800–1950* (in progress), examines how diverse communities of New Orleanians exercised agency and built community through the daily work of provisioning a city, work which was always about more than just sustenance.

Daniel Williamson is Professor of Architectural History at the Atlanta campus of the Savannah College of Art and Design. He holds a Master's in Architectural History from the University of Virginia and a PhD in the History of Art and Archaeology from the Institute of Fine Arts, New York University. His research is focused on Colonial and Postcolonial architecture in India, with particular interest in the cities of Mumbai and Ahmedabad. He is the author of *Modern Architecture in Ahmedabad: Global Networks and Local Contexts* (forthcoming).

Zhengfeng Wang is currently a Postdoctoral Research Fellow at University College Dublin, where she obtained her PhD in Art History. Her chapter in this volume is adapted from her dissertation "Institutionalizing Modern Consumption: Market Buildings and Department Stores in Chinese Cities, 1930s–1950s."

Dr. Nkatha Gichuyia is currently a Lecturer at the Architecture and Building Science department of the University of Nairobi, where she teaches Building Physics masters courses as well as design and research undergraduate courses in Architecture. She is deeply involved as well in drawing both the Kenya national government and international policy frameworks and strategies, in her other various capacities as a knowledge broker, Gates Cambridge Scholar, practicing architect, researcher and urban development consultant. Dr. Gichuyia holds an MPhil in Environmental Design and a PhD in Architecture, both from the University of Cambridge in England. Before commencing her PhD, she worked in multiple architectural firms in Nairobi and as a Tutorial fellow at the University of Nairobi.

Leila Marie Farah is an Associate Professor at Toronto Metropolitan University's Department of Architectural Science. Her research focuses on ecology, design, and the supply of cities. In 2019, she was named Chevalier dans l'Ordre des Palmes académiques de la République française. Other recent recognitions include: a Dean's Scholarly Research and Creative Activities Award 2021 from her Faculty; a Merit award for excellence by the International Making Cities Livable (co-recipient); an Outstanding Paper/Design Award from the 26th International Union of Architects World Congress; a National Urban Design Award (member of lead team) by the Royal Architectural Institute of Canada / Canadian Institute of Planners / Canadian Society of Landscape Architects. She holds a professional degree in Architecture from l'Ecole Nationale Supérieure d'Architecture Paris-Malaquais, and a M.Arch and PhD from McGill University, where she was awarded a Jonathan King Medal for Excellence in Architectural and Environmental Research and a Canadian Centre for Architecture Collection Research Grant.

Xusheng Huang is an Associate Professor at the Department of Architecture, Southeast University. He received his doctoral degree from ETH Zurich and worked as a postdoctoral researcher at the Singapore-ETH Center. His writings have been published in *Architectural Theory Review*, *Urban History*, *Architectural Journal*, etc. His current research examines urban modernization and the history of urban space in the first half of the twentieth century.

Ruth Lo is Assistant Professor of Architectural History in the Art History department at Hamilton College. She received her PhD in the History of Art and Architecture from Brown University, and she was a fellow at the American Academy in Rome and the Italian Academy at Columbia University. Her research connects food in fascist Italy to discourses of social and racial hygiene, and she explores the reciprocal relationship between agricultural breeding and medical genetics to analyze the architecture and landscape of Italy and Italian East Africa.

Emeline Houssard is a PhD student in Art History at Sorbonne Université where she is supervised by Jean-Baptiste Minnaert. She studies retail market halls in major European cities from the late nineteenth up to the end of the twentieth century and more generally is interested in public urban planning and political history of European metropolises. She has worked at the Cité nationale de la Céramique, at the Pavillon de l'Arsenal and at the Département de l'histoire de l'architecture et d'archéologie de la Ville de Paris (DHAAP). She is also a Teaching Assistant at Gustave Eiffel University and at Sorbonne University.

Henriette Steiner is Associate Professor at the Section for Landscape Architecture and Planning at the University of Copenhagen. She holds a PhD in Architecture from the University of Cambridge, UK. She is joint project leader (with Svava Riesto) on Women in Danish Architecture 1925–1975, a three-year research project that aims to provide a more just and complete understanding of architecture history by highlighting women's contributions to the architectural disciplines in Denmark (www.womenindanisharchitecture.dk). Henriette's most recent book is *Tower to Tower: Gigantism in Architectural and Digital Culture* (Cambridge, MA: MIT Press 2020). Her next book will be on the spatial and affective consequences of the COVID-19 pandemic: *Touch in the Time of Corona: Reflections of Love, Care and Vulnerability in the Pandemic* (Berlin: De Gruyter, 2021). Both books are co-written with Kristin Veel.

Min Kyung Lee is Associate Professor in the Department of Growth and Structure of Cities at Bryn Mawr College. Her research centers on the relations between mapping, architecture, and modern cities, with a forthcoming book titled, *The Tyranny of the Straight Line: Mapping Modern Paris* (Yale University Press). She was the inaugural recipient of The Banister Fletcher Global Fellowship at the University of London Institute in Paris, The Bartlett School of Architecture and Queen Mary University in London for a project on the quantification of urban space.

Andrea Borghini is Associate Professor in Philosophy at the University of Milan and director of *Culinary Mind*, an international center promoting philosophical thinking on food. His research develops theoretical tools to rethink how we speak, structure, sense, and feel about food, eating, and culinary cultures. Recent publications include: *A Philosophy of Recipes: Making, Experiencing, and Valuing* (Bloomsbury, 2022, co-curated with Patrik Engisch); 'Cooking and Dining as Forms of Public Art' (*Food, Culture, and Society*, 2021, with Andrea Baldini); 'Eating Local: A Philosophical Toolbox' (*Philosophical Quarterly*, 2021, with Nicola Piras and Beatrice Serini). Personal page: https://sites.unimi.it/borghini/.

INDEX

abattoir 74, 106, 173
Acqua Marcia 233
Acqua Paola 233
activism 10–11, 15, 19–20, 33–35, 51–52, 178, 255, 261–263
Adamson Associates Architects 175–176
Aitken, Russell 63–64, 71–72, 74–75, 77, 80, 86
American Southwest 43
Andersen, Hans Christian 288, 292
Anishnabeg (people) 157
arcades 80, 145, 259, 261
architect 10, 32, 40–46, 48–49, 63–64, 70–72, 100, 106, 111, 133, 136, 229, 232, 234–235, 247–248, 250–256, 258–261, 263–267, 286, 290, 294, 306
Armstrong, Mary 165
Arretche, Louis 258–259, 263
Art Deco 12, 41, 43, 52, 111, 129, 133, 137
Art Nouveau 233
Asia 191, 305
Association de défense du marché Saint-Germain-des-Prés, Paris 263–265
Association Sauvons le Carreau du Temple, Paris 263
Atelier parisien d'urbanisme (APUR) 267
Atlantic World 20, 22
Atlas Corporation 175
Australia 305
autarchy 235–236
authority, authorities 9–10, 12, 64, 66, 68, 72, 74, 87, 100–103, 111, 113, 115–117, 129, 175, 198, 207, 211, 245, 248–249, 255, 262–264, 266, 268, 308
bacteriology 10, 27, 207
Baltard, Victor 14, 104, 230–231, 245, 250, 267–268
Baltimore 38
Bardon, Renaud 259–260
Bas, Paul 265
Bashford, Alison 103
Batignolles Market, Paris 256–257, 261–264
bazaar 22, 87, 101, 195–196
Beauvau Market, Paris 267
Beckham, David 285
behavior 34, 47, 64, 74, 109, 115, 294
Beijing (Peking) 10, 13, 191–197, 200–213
Beijing Municipal Council 198, 205–206, 209
Belluomini, Alfredo 306
Bengalee, Sorabji Shahpurji 68
Berlin 205, 261
Bilbao 295
biopolitics 13, 227, 236, 297
Bjarke Ingels Group (BIG) 291
Black 22, 34, 44, 47, 50
black market 236
Blackburne, S.L. 133
Blondel, Jean-Baptiste 259, 261
Blum, Sam 39

body politics 293, 297
Bombay (Mumbai) 10, 12, 61–74, 75–81, 84, 86–88, 105
Bombay Cathedral 87
Bombay Mint 69
Bonnier, Louis 135
Bornholm 285
Boston 205
Branche, Pierre 264
Brandt, Karl 136
Breslau (Wrocław) 104, 134, 136
brick 24, 27, 32, 35–36, 100, 113, 136, 161, 196, 202, 209, 233–234, 267
Britain 64, 66, 83, 100–101, 111, 134–136, 148
British East India Company 65
British Empire 11–12, 100, 136, 138, 166
British Municipal Council 105, 136
British Treasury 111
Bureau of Markets, New Orleans 38
Burges, William 70, 77, 80–81, 83–84
butchers 20, 27, 34, 64, 67, 69, 74, 87, 103, 142, 157, 160–162, 164–166, 169–172, 305, 309
Buttcon Limited 175
Butte-aux-Cailles 134–135
bylaws 103, 106, 157, 178
Bywater 24
Cacoub, Clément-Olivier 267
Calcutta 71
Canada 157, 166, 169
Capital Police Board, Beijing 198, 200, 209
car 13, 72, 74, 174, 230, 236, 246, 249, 252–253, 255
car park (parking) 133, 174–175, 246, 249–250, 253, 255, 257–258, 265
Carreau du Temple Market, Paris 257–259, 263–265, 267
Carrolton Market, New Orleans 23, 35
Cattle Market, Glasgow 205
Cendon, Paul 27
Central and Western Market Offices, Hong Kong 110
central market(s) 26, 70, 231, 245, 306–309
Central Market, Hong Kong 12, 99–101, 105–107, 110–117
Centrale Montemartini, Rome 233
Centre Pompidou, Paris 265
Chadwick, Edwin 66–67
Chadwick, Osbert 101, 105
Chicago 38
China 13, 105, 111, 114, 193, 196–197, 200–202, 204, 213, 305
Chinese 13, 69, 101–102, 105, 110–112, 115–116, 191, 194–195, 198, 201, 204, 207, 213
Chipperfield, David 268
Chippewa (people) 157
Chirac, Jacques 248, 264–265, 267
cholera 11, 101, 161–162
Christian 69
citizens 10, 15, 33, 36–37, 39, 43, 51, 70, 87, 174–175, 191, 196, 207–208, 211–213, 228, 234, 236
City Beautiful Movement 30, 51
City Board of Health, New Orleans 27
city council 27, 35, 39, 175, 249, 257, 261, 265, 267
city government 22, 26, 30, 33–35, 37–41, 51, 212
civic order 9–10, 235
cleanliness 12, 19, 32, 36, 40, 63, 83, 102–104, 112, 116, 133, 140, 160–161, 169, 206–207, 261, 299
Cleveland 32
cloth market 69
Colboc, Pierre 258, 260–261, 263
colonial 9–12, 20–22, 24, 51, 62, 64–65, 71, 74, 81, 88, 100–101,

103–104, 110–113, 115–117, 129, 132–133, 136–138, 140, 144, 146–148, 207, 211
Comité des habitants du 3e arrondissement, Paris 263
Commerce Board of Dongan Market, Beijing 210
Commission des sites, France 267
committee 34–36, 140, 161, 166, 172
community 9–11, 14–15, 19–20, 32, 35, 38–39, 47, 52, 63–64, 69–70, 74, 110, 112, 145, 147, 164, 177, 255, 261–263, 267–268, 307, 309–310
competition 25, 70, 77, 113, 175–176, 237–238, 248, 258–260, 264–266, 268
contagion 19, 161, 168, 305, 308
control 30, 47, 64, 68, 70, 72, 74, 87–88, 102–103, 106, 109–110, 136, 140, 146–147, 160, 203–204, 207–208, 210–213, 227, 234, 236, 257, 261, 307
Conybeare, Henry 66–67
Cooper, James 158
Copenhagen 10, 14, 285–298
coronavirus (see also COVID-19) 14, 285, 297–298
Council of Paris 250, 255, 257
Covent Garden 230
COVID-19 (see also coronavirus) 9–11, 14–15, 175, 286, 297–299, 305–308, 310
Crane, Walter 61, 80, 86
Crawford, Arthur 61, 63–65, 68–77, 83–84, 86–87, 105
Crawford Market, Bombay (renamed the Mahatma Jyotiba Phule Market and Mumbai respectively) 11, 61–63, 65, 68, 72, 74, 76, 79–80, 82–86, 88
crowds 61–62, 87, 116, 162, 210
Daoist 194
Davies, Philip 61, 86
Davies, William 166–167, 172–173
Davis, Mike 146
Dayan, Georges 265
Dayton 35
Deffontaines, François-Noël 265–266
Delamore Market, New Orleans 23, 35
Délégation permanente et commission supérieure des monuments historiques, France 267
demonstrations 210–211, 263
Denmark 285–287, 290, 294–299
design 10–12, 24, 26, 32–33, 35–36, 39–41, 43–44, 47, 52, 64, 70–72, 74, 77, 80–84, 86, 88, 99–100, 103, 106, 109, 113–114, 116–117, 135–137, 140–142, 144–146, 148, 175, 198, 202, 228–233, 245, 248, 250, 252–253, 255, 257–261, 263–268, 294, 299, 306–307
Detroit 38
Directorate of Economic Affairs, Paris 248–249
dirt 41, 110, 169
disease 10, 14, 19–20, 22, 26–27, 32, 37, 40–41, 50–52, 66–67, 101, 140, 160–161, 166, 168–169, 177, 204, 207
disgust 72, 88
disorder 178, 213
Dollar Loan 112
Dominati, Jacques 268
Dongan Market (Dongan Shichang or Eastern Peace Market), Beijing 13, 191–192, 195–213
Dongan Market Administrative Office 200, 204, 207, 212
Dongsi Department Store 195
Dryades Market, New Orleans 20, 23, 28–34, 38, 40–42, 44–46

Dumont, Georges 246–247
Duncan, Jonathan 69
Duncan Market, Bombay 69-70
Duplay, Michel 265–266
Dynamique urbaine 264
East Africa 12, 136
Easton, Murray 135
École Spéciale d'Architecture (ESA), Paris 264
egg market 232
Eight-Nation Alliance 194, 200
Emerson, William 63–64, 70–71, 75–84, 87
Enfants-Rouges Market, Paris 267
England 68, 70, 74–75, 77–78, 83, 86, 105, 134, 166, 205
enslaved 22
epidemic 11, 100
epidemiology 11, 19, 30, 51
Era Club 34
Esders clothing factory 135
Esplanade, Bombay 66–67, 69–70, 75–76, 79–80, 87
Ethiopia 236
Europe Market, Paris 253, 255, 257–258, 262–263
Ewing Market, New Orleans 23, 41, 46–47
fascism 13, 227, 230, 234–237
Favette, Maurice-André 250–252, 257
Fermigier, André 263
filth 169, 206
finance 68, 205, 291, 293
fish 12, 20, 24, 36, 40, 61, 75, 102–103, 106–109, 162, 169, 205–206, 308
fish market 22, 162, 177, 232–233
flies 26–27, 36, 211
Florence 231
flower market 232, 290
Food Commission 228–229
food market 9, 11, 19, 22, 108, 140, 205–206, 234, 285, 290–291, 295, 305
Forbes, James A. 68
Fort Area, Bombay 69, 78
Fort markets, Bombay 70
Forum des Halles, Paris 261
Foucault, Michel 207
Foyer du Fonctionnaire et de la Famille (FFF), Paris 250
Framjee, Dosabhoy 86
France 24, 104, 134–135, 148, 248
Frankfurt 104
free people of color 22, 24
French Market, New Orleans 22–24, 26, 47, 50
French Quarter, New Orleans 24
Frere, Bartle 66, 70–71, 74, 81
Frere Town, Bombay 70–71
Friends of Old City Hall, Toronto 174
fruit market 22, 75
Gamble, Sidney 194–195, 209, 211
gastrosexual 285–286, 294
Gehl, Jan 294
General Electric Company of China 114
germ theory 72, 307
Germany 134, 136, 148
Gillet, Guillaume 259
Ginsberg, Jean 257
Giroud, Françoise 264
Giscard d'Estaing, Valéry 264
Giunta Nathan (organization) 228, 233–234
Glasgow 205
glass 100, 104–105, 141, 196, 205, 230–234, 252, 259, 261, 285, 292, 296, 299
Global South 12
Gloucester 83–84
Gothenburg 291

government 9–13, 19–20, 22, 24–26, 30, 33–35, 37–41, 51, 69–71, 74, 87, 100–105, 110–117, 136–137, 146, 191, 194, 196, 198, 200, 202–213, 227, 233–236, 286, 307–308
Gracey, T. 140
grain market 75, 162
Grossmarkthalle 104, 230
Grunewald, Theodore 38–40
guard 146, 207
Guillotte Market, New Orleans 23, 35
Gujarat 78
Guomindang government 200, 210
Guy, Michel 263
Hagens, Hans Peter 290–293
Halles de Paris (Les Halles) 14, 26, 104, 205, 230–231, 245, 248, 258–259, 261, 263, 268
Haudenosaunee (people) 157
Haussmann, Georges-Eugène 68, 255
health 12, 14–15, 19, 26–27, 51, 74, 100–102, 106, 115, 137, 140–141, 160, 162, 168, 211, 227, 259, 310
Health Campaign Assemblies 210
Helsinki 291
Hindu 64, 71–72, 74–75
Hodges, Alfred Walter 100, 106
Hong Kong 10, 12, 99–117
Hongkew Market, Shanghai 105, 114
Housewives' League Division 34–36
Houston 35
Huanan wet market, Wuhan 305
hygiene 10–14, 63–64, 99–102, 110, 140, 196, 206–207, 211, 228, 248–249, 252, 258, 268, 299, 306
illness 27, 33, 206
imperial 9, 71, 103, 137, 146, 148, 227
improvement 20, 30, 37, 64, 68–70, 74, 83–84, 115, 140, 191, 204, 206, 208–209, 211–213
India 61–62, 65–66, 71, 74, 82–84, 88, 113
Indian National Congress 68
Indigenous (peoples) 22, 157
Indigenous 10, 64, 101
industrial 41, 100, 116, 166, 168, 172, 191, 228, 232, 237, 296
infestation 11, 26, 33
informal 142, 144–145, 163, 206, 232
infrastructure 10–11, 13, 67, 100–101, 103, 105, 111, 113, 116, 142, 161, 166, 168, 173, 177, 228, 230, 236, 290–291
Ingels, Bjarke 291
Inner City, Beijing 192, 196–198, 200, 207, 209–210
inspection 10, 34, 72, 74, 77, 99, 102–103, 110, 114–116, 160, 169, 209–210
Intergovernmental Panel on Climate Change (IPCC) 141
Inuit (people) 157
iron 12, 32, 35, 40, 63, 68, 70, 72, 74, 77, 83, 86–87, 104–105, 107, 196, 202, 206, 230–233, 259
Israels Plads (Israel's Place), Copenhagen 287–292, 297–298
Italy 11, 13, 227, 233, 235–236, 305
Jamsetjee Jeejeebhoy School of Art, Bombay 70, 77, 80–81, 83
Jew 287
Kabraji, K.N. 70
Kandjian, Abro 246–247
Kennedy Town, Hong Kong 106
Kentucky 164
Kenya 130, 132, 136, 138, 140, 142, 144–145, 148
Kipling, John Lockwood 83–86
Kipling, Rudyard 83
Koolhaas, Rem 237
Korniloff, André 257–258

Küster, Heinrich 136
Kwong, Sun 114
La Chapelle Market, Paris 267–268
Lafay, Bernard 249
Lafaye, E. 35–36
Lake Ontario 158, 166
Lake Pontchartrain 37
Lamy, Philippe-Georges 259–260
Lawrence Hall, London 105, 134–136
Legation Quarter, Beijing 191–192
Leith, Andrew 67–69, 72, 79
Lemercier-Brochant 257
license markets 102
light 10, 32, 40–41, 72, 79, 105, 110, 116, 141–142, 196, 231–232, 234, 252, 257, 306–307
Linnés Torv (Linnaeus's Square), Copenhagen 287
livable city 293, 295, 297
London 66, 70–71, 101–102, 105, 134–135, 230
Louisiana 11, 21, 24, 33, 41
Louisiana State Board of Health 33
Lower Manhattan Market, New York 230
Mackenzie, William Lyon 161
Magazine Market, New Orleans 23–25, 41, 48
Mahallawi, Ramzi 265
Mahatma Jyotiba Phule Market, Bombay (see Crawford Market) 61
malaria 101
Maloo Market, Shanghai 105, 109
Marboeuf, Auguste 249
Market Commission, Toronto 169
Market Committee 34, 36, 161
Market House 24–25, 32, 40, 46–48, 50, 158–162, 177
Massé, Georges 256–257
mayor 160–161, 227, 237–238, 248, 264–265, 268
McCants, Helen 35
McClellan Charles, Millie 50
meat 20, 22, 24–27, 30, 34, 36, 40, 65–66, 71–72, 74–75, 77, 87, 102, 107, 109–110, 132, 142, 147, 160, 164–166, 169, 171, 192, 205–206, 229, 232, 236, 295, 308
meat market 22, 68–69, 75, 142, 233
merchant 69, 78, 83, 86–87, 129, 136, 196, 198, 203–204, 209–210, 212–213, 236, 249
Messine Automobile (company) 253
Metropolitan Police Board (Inner City and Outer City), Beijing 196–198, 209–210
Meyer, Claus 285
miasma 66–67, 72, 161
migrant 22, 24, 27
Ministry for Construction, France 262
Ministry of Civil Affairs, China 209
Ministry of Internal Affairs, Denmark 290
Mississaugas of the Credit (people) 157
mobilization 10, 14, 157, 177, 211, 248, 262
mobs 161
modernization 13-15, 41, 43, 88, 145, 169, 191, 196, 208, 212–213, 227, 245, 248, 253, 255, 257, 268
Moines-Batignolles (organization) 257
Molinos, Jules de 265
Mumbai 10, 61–62
Munich 104, 230
Municipal Corporation of Bombay 68
Municipal Council 105, 109, 136, 198, 205–206, 209
municipal market 51, 109, 113, 132, 204–207, 231
Municipal Markets Commission, New Orleans 39
Muslim 64, 69, 71–72, 80

Mussolini, Benito 13, 227
Nairobi 10, 12, 105, 129–130, 132–138, 140–142, 144–148
Nairobi City Market (formerly Nairobi Municipal Market) 12, 105, 129–148
Nathan, Ernesto 227–228, 233–235
Native Town, Bombay 66–67, 69–70, 78–80
New Orleans 10–12, 19–51, 205
New Orleans Live Stock Exchange 39
New York 33, 38, 205, 230, 296
Ninth Street Market, New Orleans 23, 33
Noma 285, 292
Norberg-Schulz, Christian 148
Nørreport 287
North America 169
North American Convention of Colored Freemen 168–169
Norton, John 70
Nyhavn 292
Odense 285
Office of Food and Markets, Rome 234–235
Office of Metropolitan Architects (OMA) 237
Office of Urban Policing, Rome 234–235
officer 10, 68–69, 101, 115–116, 168, 204, 207
officials 20, 24–25, 27, 30, 32–34, 37–41, 47, 51, 109, 136, 169, 177, 196, 204, 211, 245
Ohio 32, 35, 164
Ontario Food Terminal, Toronto 173
order 9-14, 61, 63, 65, 69, 71, 74, 78, 85–87, 100–101, 109, 132, 137, 207, 209, 235–236, 307
ordinance 30, 35–37, 102, 105
Ørestaden 291
Orleans Club 38
ornament 65, 81–82
Ornano, Michel d' 264
Ørsted, H.C. 288
Ørstedsparken 288–290, 292
Ostia 228–230
Ostiense 228–229, 233, 237–238
Oudin, Alain 264
Overy, Rand 133
Ovipol Market, Rome 232–233
pandemic 11, 14–15, 176, 285–286, 298–299, 305–307, 310
Paris 10, 14, 26, 104, 135, 205, 230–231, 245–264, 266–268
Paris-Majorité 249
Passy Market, Paris 246, 250, 257
patrol 207
pavilion 24, 230–237
pavilion market 22, 32, 41
Pavillon Baltard, Paris 267
Peking (Beijing) 10, 13, 191–197, 200–213
Peking University 210–211
Perret brothers 135
Philadelphia 24, 38
Philippon, Jean-Paul 259–261
Piazzone market, Viareggio 306
Pisa 229–230
plague 88
Plan d'Urbanisme Directeur (PUD) 248
planning 9–12, 14, 37, 101, 136–138, 144, 211, 230, 248, 261–263, 267, 286, 294, 296
Plateforme des associations de participation à l'urbanisme 263
Poland 134, 136, 148
police 65, 68, 74, 102, 162, 204, 207, 228, 238
Police Board 196–198, 200, 209–210
politics 9–11, 13–15, 19, 33, 38, 100, 103, 117, 132, 136–137, 146, 158–159, 161–162, 168, 177–178,

191, 194, 196, 200, 207, 210, 212–213, 227, 235, 248, 263–264, 290–291, 293, 297, 305, 310
pollution 15, 22, 64, 72, 168, 249, 296
Poplar Baths, London 134, 136
Port Market, New Orleans 23–24
Porta Palazzo Market, Turin 231
postcolonial 12, 88, 129, 132, 137–138, 147–148
poultry 12, 24, 102–103, 107–109, 158, 160, 169, 231–232
poultry market 162, 232
Poydras Market, New Orleans 22–24, 33
Pratt, Miles A. 39
Préfecture Morland Building, Paris 268
private market 25, 27, 30, 33–37, 39, 69, 87
protest 19, 74, 87, 210, 248, 261, 263, 267–268
Prouté, Michèle 262, 264
Prytania Market, New Orleans 23, 33
Public Chamber of Commerce of Dongan Market, Beijing 198, 210
public health 10–12, 14–15, 19–20, 22, 27, 32–35, 37, 39, 41, 50–51, 99–101, 103, 105, 115, 117, 138, 140–141, 148, 157, 160–161, 163, 168–169, 176–178, 196, 206, 234, 238, 245, 248, 308
Public Health Department (PHD) 100, 140
Public Health Ordinance, Hong Kong 101–103, 116
public market 14, 19–20, 22–27, 30, 33–41, 50–51, 68–69, 86, 101, 105–106, 113, 115, 157, 191, 206
public market renewal 39
public market system 19, 24, 26, 33, 38
public space 10, 43, 160, 207, 238, 245, 286, 291, 305, 309
public works 103, 111, 116, 196–197, 200
Public Works Department, Hong Kong 100, 103, 111, 113, 116
Pugin, A.W.N. 80
Qingyun Pavilion, Beijing 195
quality 27, 37, 50, 117, 140, 147, 160, 168, 209–210, 255, 287, 290, 295, 297, 309
Quincy Market, Boston 205
Rabaud, Olivier 253
Rabourdin, Patrick 266
Raggi, Virginia 238
railroad 229–230, 232, 291
Railways Committee, Hong Kong 140
Rasmussen, Poul Nyrup 291
Readymoney, Cowasji Jehangir 83
reform 10–13, 20, 34, 36, 63–65, 68–72, 78, 80, 83, 86, 88, 103, 105, 198, 204, 207, 211–213, 248, 264
refrigeration 32, 34–35, 37, 40–41, 50, 232–233, 252
regeneration 14–15, 176, 286, 295
Registrar General, Hong Kong 102–103, 114
regulation 10, 13, 34, 40, 64, 100–101, 103, 110, 115, 138, 140, 145, 148, 160–162, 177, 198–200, 204–210, 213, 228, 262, 307–308
Ren, Qingtai 196–198
riot 162, 212
Riquet Market, Paris 250–253, 255–256, 258
Robertson, Howard 135, 158, 161–162, 172
Rogers Stirk Harbour + Partners 175–176
Rome 10, 13, 227–238
Rouslett, Louis 78
Roy, Fernand 256–257
Royal Horticultural Halls 135

Royal Institute of British Architects (RIBA) 71
rule 13, 36, 62, 64–66, 71, 83, 100–101, 113, 116, 140, 146, 173, 197, 213
safety 51, 79, 101, 116–117, 198, 204–205, 207, 212, 294, 306
Saffi, Emilio 229–235
Saint-Didier Market, Paris 267
Saint-Germain Market, Paris 257–265, 267–268
Saint-Honoré Market, Paris 246-247, 250, 252-253, 257
Saint-Martin Market, Paris 268
Saint-Quentin Market, Paris 257–258, 261, 265–266, 268
salmonella 19, 26–27
salubrity 246, 255
San Lorenzo Market, Florence 231
Sanchez, Rosio 292
Sanitary Board, Hong Kong 101–102
Sanitary Department, Hong Kong 102–103, 109, 112
sanitation 10–15, 30, 32–34, 36–37, 61, 63–68, 70, 72, 74–75, 79–80, 82–88, 100–105, 110–111, 114–117, 138, 140, 157, 161, 168–170, 173, 177, 196, 204–206, 208, 211, 213, 227–228, 231–233, 249, 255
Sargent, Gordon 34
Schlüter, Poul 290–291
Schmid, Christian 296
seafood 24–27, 30, 40, 229, 231–232
seafood market 230, 232-235
Secrétan Market, Paris 265, 267
Segonzac, Lionel de 264
segregation 12, 43–44, 47, 100, 115, 140, 146, 148
sewage 100, 233
sewers 36, 161, 168, 206
Shanghai 100, 105–106, 109, 114, 116
Simpson, J. 101
Singapore 104
Sivadjian, Jean-Louis 266
skylights 32, 169, 196, 234
slaughterhouse 67–74, 77, 102–103, 166, 228, 233
smells 61, 69, 110, 293
Smith, T. Roger 72, 74, 81
Social Work 200
Société pour la Protection des Paysages et de l'Esthétique de la France (SPPEF) 263
Soraparu Market, New Orleans 23, 35
Sorunpur, Bombay 69
SOS Paris 263
South, John S. 39
St. Bernard Market, New Orleans 23, 43, 49–50
St. John Market, New Orleans 23, 35
St. Lawrence Hall, Toronto 162–164, 168, 174, 177
St. Lawrence Market, Toronto (formerly the Old Market House, the New Market House and the St. Lawrence Arcade) 13, 157–166, 168–178
North Market, Toronto 169, 171, 174–175
North St. Lawrence Market Redevelopment 161, 175–177
South Market, Toronto 169, 171–172, 174–175, 177
St. Mary Market, New Orleans 22–24, 35
St. Roch Market, New Orleans 23, 41, 43–44
stall 10, 12, 24, 27, 40 41, 47, 61, 77, 87, 102–103, 105–107, 109, 113, 117, 132–133, 141–143, 146, 160, 162–166, 169, 171–173, 195, 198,

201, 203, 212, 231–234, 236, 257, 286, 290
State Board of Health, Louisiana 33–34, 37
stench 20, 66–68, 168
Stockholm 291
Stone, Sam (Jr) 41–46, 48–49
street market 13, 192, 195, 207
streetscape 133, 237
strike 74
Stuttgart 136
Suburban Market, New Orleans 23, 40–41
supermarket 11, 13, 37, 248, 262–263, 291, 294–295, 305–310
Supplementary inventory of historical monuments (ISMH), France 248, 267–268
surveillance 64–65, 77, 86–87, 100, 104, 116, 207–208
Surveyor General 102, 113
Sviluppo Centro Ostiense 237
Sweden 287, 291
Syndicat de Défense des riverains du marché de l'Europe, Paris 262
Tak Hing (construction firm) 114
technology 72, 83, 86–87, 104, 111, 116, 204
Telok Ayer Market, Singapore 104
temple market 192, 194–195, 210
Termini Station, Rome 233
Ternes Market, Paris 253–255, 257–258, 262–263
Testaccio 228, 233
The High Line, New York 295–296
Thwaites, C. 80
Tianjin (formerly Tientsin) 110, 198
Tiber (river) 228
Tientsin (see Tianjin) 105, 110, 136
Time and Place group, Toronto 174
Todd, Ronald Ruskin 106
Toronto 10, 13, 157–159, 161, 163, 166–168, 172–173, 175–178
Torvehallerne Market Halls 14, 285–299
transit 227–228, 236
Treeck, Martin Schulz van 252, 257
Treme Market, New Orleans 23–24, 33
trust 27, 51, 65, 308
tuberculosis 245
Turin 231
typhoid 168
typology 141, 147, 248, 307
Union féminine civique et sociale, Paris 262
United States 19–20, 24, 26, 41, 51, 230, 261
United States Department of Agriculture (USDA) 30
Upper and Lower Bazaars, Hong Kong 101
urban amenities 12, 99, 102, 105, 116
Urban Council, Hong Kong 101, 106, 116
Urban Renewal Authority, Hong Kong 117
urbanism 10, 13, 227, 138
Urry, John 294–295
Vasconi, Claude 261
vegetable market 22, 75, 77, 147, 206, 230, 232–233, 236, 287–288, 290
Veltroni, Walter 237
vendor 10–11, 19–20, 22, 27, 30, 34, 36–37, 40–41, 50–51, 63, 69, 116, 140, 142, 145, 157, 159, 162, 164, 166, 171–172, 178, 196, 290, 305–309
ventilation 10, 15, 22, 24, 32, 35–36, 40, 68, 72, 77, 110, 141–142, 160, 169, 206, 245–246, 257, 307
Viareggio 10–11, 305–307, 309–310
Vibro Piling Company 114

Vivre à Paris 262
Voirin-Marinoni Factory, Montataire 135
Wacha, Dinshaw E. 68–69
Wanchai Market, Hong Kong 114–115
Washington Market, New Orleans 22–24
water 12, 40, 66, 83–84, 100, 107, 109, 140, 160–162, 168–169, 205–206, 233–236, 252, 261, 267
Wellington, R. 101
Wendat (people) 157
West Side Market, Cleveland 32–33
Western Market, Philadelphia 24
wholesale market 75, 112, 170, 172, 227, 230
Wholesale Market, Rome 13, 227–238
Works Progress Administration (WPA) 39-40, 43-44, 51
Wrocław (Breslau) 104, 134, 136
Wrocław Market Hall 134
Wuhan 305
Xisi Department Store, Beijing 195
Zengel Market, New Orleans 23, 41
Zhu, Qiqian 205
Züblin, E. 136